The Social Origins of

Health and Well-being

The past decade has seen an exponential growth in research into the social determinants of health. This new research challenges the assumptions that investments in the health system and lifestyle behaviours are largely responsible for health gains. By focusing on persistent inequalities in health, the research has shed light on a wide range of factors that influence health and well-being. This book covers the differential health impacts of socio-economic status, family and early development, changes in work and work conditions, health systems, the physical environment of cities, indigenous peoples, social capital, culture, and global economic and environmental changes. It also discusses how inequality gets 'under the skin', through describing the physiological changes that follow from stress and behaviours. Particularly important is the 'natural experiment' represented by the different political and economic paths taken by Australia and New Zealand over the past two decades and the opportunity this provides to assess their effect on health. *The Social Origins of Health and Well-being* will be of great value to scholars and professionals internationally and to students in Australia and New Zealand.

Richard Eckersley, **Jane Dixon** and **Bob Douglas** are Fellows at the National Centre for Epidemiology and Population Health, Australian National University.

D1427687

The Social Origins of
Health and
Well-being

Edited by
Richard Eckersley, Jane Dixon and Bob Douglas
Australian National University

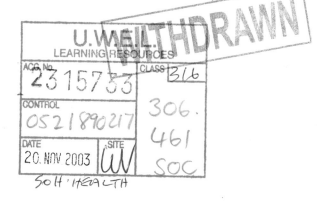
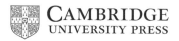

CAMBRIDGE
UNIVERSITY PRESS

PUBLISHED BY THE PRESS SYNDICATE OF THE UNIVERSITY OF CAMBRIDGE
The Pitt Building, Trumpington Street, Cambridge, United Kingdom

CAMBRIDGE UNIVERSITY PRESS
The Edinburgh Building, Cambridge CB2 2RU, UK
40 West 20th Street, New York, NY 10011–4211, USA
477 Williamstown Road, Port Melbourne, VIC 3207, Australia
Ruiz de Alarcón 13, 28014 Madrid, Spain
Dock House, The Waterfront, Cape Town 8001, South Africa

http://www.cambridge.org

First published 2001

Printed in Australia by Hyde Park Press

Typeface Goudy (*Adobe*) 10.5/13 pt.   *System* QuarkXPress® [M]

A catalogue record for this book is available from the British Library

National Library of Australia Cataloguing in Publication data
The social origins of health and well-being.
Bibliography.
Includes index.
ISBN 0 521 89021 7.
1. Health – Social aspects. 2. Health – History. I. Dixon,
Jane Meredith– . II. Douglas, Robert Matheson
III. Eckersley, Richard. IV. Title.

ISBN 0 521 89021 7 paperback

Contents

Figures and tables

Tables

Preface

Why publish yet another book about the social determinants of health? This was the initial reaction of a reader to whom Cambridge University Press sent our book proposal. The response is unsurprising. The past decade has seen the publication of some 15 books, major reports or special journal issues dealing with the social determinants of health. The number of individual journal articles has soared.

Can there really be a need for another overview of the subject? Cambridge's reader went on to say the initial scepticism was immediately dispelled by the originality of the material and the arguments put forward by the individual contributors: 'I am persuaded that this book will make a substantial, and novel, contribution to the literature, both in Australasia as well as internationally.'

We are also confident of the value of this book—for two main reasons. First, the existing literature has focused on the North American and European situations; we want to put the Antipodes on the social epidemiological map. Secondly, the recent literature has concentrated on socio-economic inequality as a prime determinant of health; we believe this book adds important historical, global and cultural dimensions to the social sources of health and well-being.

The book has its origins in the establishment of the Health Inequalities Research Collaboration by the Australian Commonwealth Department of Health and Aged Care to promote a better understanding of why some groups in the community are healthier than others. One of the early tasks of the Collaboration was to organise a major conference, held in Canberra in July 2000. Its aim was to build scientific, public and policy recognition of the importance of the social determinants of health. New Zealand participants and perspectives were included because research and policy development in this area are more advanced there than in Australia.

From the conference came the book. It brings together leading scholars from both countries to establish a baseline of what we know and what we need to do. There are, inevitably, omissions. Between conference and book, a few contributions fell by the wayside. But other perspectives were added, particularly on the implications for policy, intervention and research. We began the project with the view that economic and political institutions and social and cultural processes exert powerful influences over the opportunities and actions available to individuals and, ultimately, over their health and well-being: these factors 'produce health', and in ways that are unevenly distributed across populations.

Part A of the book lays out what many sociologists would consider to be the 'structural' determinants of health. These particular determinants are intergenerational mediators of social group behaviours, attitudes and experiences. The stage and nature of economic development is a particularly significant structural determinant that affects the character of national and global institutions, migration and settlement patterns, the financing and distribution of health and education systems and the use and abuse of the natural environment. The role of economic development is the dominant theme of the four chapters, which build a persuasive case against assuming a linear relationship between economic development and health gain.

John Powles argues that health improvement and health inequalities result from institutional and sub-population adaptations to economic development and that adaptive behaviours are not straightforward. Socio-economic inequalities in health can be explained, in part, by the idea that health status improves most for groups who can capture the benefits of economic development and minimise the attendant risks. Powles suggests that as the process of decision-making becomes more deliberative, subject to an array of choices and is grounded less upon custom, then inequalities based on social advantage will increase.

While for Powles, adaptation to new knowledge is fundamental, for David Legge, the ideologies which are woven around this present phase of global economic development have stopped the majority of the world's population from participating in a dialogue about inequalities. The capacity to 'make and assert truth'—ie, to contribute to the way in which development is defined and pursued—is a potent shaper of the contours of economic inequality and of health inequalities.

Colin D. Butler, Bob Douglas, and A.J. McMichael argue a key factor is the role that economic development plays in depleting natural environmental resources. We have long known that inadequate man-made environments encourage a range of diseases, especially amongst the world's poor, but what has not been so readily acknowledged is the contribution that the natural environment has to increasing health inequalities, both within and between countries. While we do not have consensus about the extent to which ecosystem health and population health are interrelated, there is sufficient evidence to include environmental degradation as a major determinant of health.

Without using the term, 'cultural determinants', all three chapters put substantial emphasis on what would be considered cultural factors: available knowledge, truth-making and judgements about progress and sustainability. Richard Eckersley, however, provides a detailed treatment of what we consider to be a major omission in the social determinants of health literature: culture. While epidemiologists have made sporadic use of cultural factors to explain differential and changing health status, culture has now been relegated to mere context. Eckersley challenges us to consider cultural factors to be as risk-laden for health and well-being as is socio-economic status.

The major output of social epidemiology has been on the relationship between socio-economic status and population health, which is the subject of **Part B**. Jake Najman sets the scene by proposing a general model of the social origins of health and well-being. In discussing many of the issues addressed in more detail in later chapters, Najman highlights the persistence and significance of health inequalities. If we are to understand these, he says, we must identify the causal pathways that link social contexts with the biological basis of disease. This includes addressing the confusion created by using different labels for the same phenomena or by emphasising different points along the pathways, and distinguishing major causes from minor.

The next two chapters in this section provide an overview of the dominant explanations that are competing to provide insights into how health inequalities are caused: the neo-materialist, psychosocial, social cohesion, behavioural and constitutional pathways are described. Gavin Turrell settles on the neo-materialist pathway as offering greatest explanatory potential for the relationship between income inequality and health status, while Richard Taylor opts for behavioural risk factors in concert with socio-economic status.

The chapter by Alistair Woodward, Colin Mathers and Martin Tobias illustrates the merits of being able to make national comparisons. By revealing a 'mortality cross-over' between Australia and New Zealand in the 1980s, and then analysing the different demographic, settlement, lifestyle and policy contexts of the two countries, the authors are able to put forward a rich range of propositions about why inequalities in health can change quite dramatically in a short period of time. Using data from New Zealand, Philippa Howden-Chapman and Des O'Dea argue that both low income and greater inequality are associated with poorer health. Like Woodward and his colleagues, they suggest that ethnicity is a separate, but interrelated, determinant of health.

The question of the degree to which health systems and health care contribute to health inequalities is also raised in these chapters and is the exclusive focus of Stephen Duckett's chapter. While Australia has an internationally recognised health system based on universal access to medical care, Duckett describes the barriers that hinder the equal uptake and effectiveness of that care. His argument adds to the growing evidence that the differential use of health services, due to the incentives and disincentives built into the overall system of care, can exacerbate health inequalities.

Part C contains chapters that examine how the ways in which societies organise themselves are fundamental to health and well-being. Cities, workplaces and communities are critical settings for shaping the distribution of income and other resources and for influencing lifestyle risk factors. They help to facilitate and inhibit relationships with other human beings and mediate interpersonal and intergroup trust, civic engagement and reciprocity: the ingredients of social capital. Not only do these forms of social organisation have a direct and indirect impact on social relationships, their physical manifestations can impact on rates of illness and sense of well-being.

Peter Newman casts a planner's eye over the healthy cities movement and outlines the many social and health problems created by the effects on the environment of automobile dependence. The chapter by Anne Marie Feyer and Dorothy Broom provides a detailed explication of how government-sanctioned changes to working life in Australia and New Zealand have the potential to have detrimental effects on population health.

It would be wrong, however, to cast cities, workplaces and communities as simply a backdrop or context in which individuals conduct their affairs. Those researching the relationship between social capital, health and well-being have shown how the nature of civic engagement, social networks and reciprocity produce different types of settings and how, in turn, these different settings structure opportunities to build different forms of capital that are advantageous for health and happiness.

Robert Bush and Fran Baum explore the potential for social capital to provide a framework for improving the health and life opportunities of poorer communities. Drawing on the Adelaide Health Development and Social Capital Study, they say that informal social participation predicts health status, and collective civic participation predicts sense of control. Both forms of participation were higher among the better off and better educated. The evidence warrants public policies that encourage trusting networks, support community-based organisations and foster environments which are conducive to social interaction.

From the coverage of upstream factors in parts A, B and C, **Part D** develops an argument that health inequalities are the result of a lifelong patterning of social, cultural, behavioural and biological factors. Within the population health field, one of the most exciting areas of investigation concerns the developmental perspective on health and well-being. This perspective is the result of the assembly of multi-disciplinary insights; being open to multiple causation and cumulative effects across the life course; and an emphasis on the interrelationship between brain development, human development and the social environment. If the grandmother's social status and social environment are determinants of the infant's health status, then public health has to deal with time and space in a way analogous to the perspective taken by those concerned with the sustainability of the eco-system.

Graham Vimpani's chapter provides an overview of the component parts of the developmental perspective and acts as an introduction to the fleshing out of three of these parts in the chapters that follow. Judy Cashmore explains in greater detail how what happens in the early years of life is instrumental to health and well-being in adolescence and adulthood. She addresses the question about how and why some individuals do well despite adversity and why others do poorly, using a mix of psychological and sociological concepts: risk, vulnerability, resilience and protective mechanisms.

Terry Dwyer, Ruth Morley and Leigh Blizzard go back even further, to before birth and to what has become known as the Barker hypothesis: that cardiovascular disease and diabetes have their origins in-utero, being more common in adults who were small at birth. Low birth weight is associated with low socio-economic status, raising the possibility that the well-known link between socio-economic status and these diseases is due to foetal exposures. However, their own study of twins suggests that individual factors are also involved.

The chapter by Kerin O'Dea and Mark Daniel focuses on one aspect of the brain–behaviour–emotion interrelationships: the neuroendocrine system, which affects hormonal and emotional functioning. If the neuroendocrine system develops in conditions of sustained stress, then it becomes wired to respond to social and physical environments in particular ways that are detrimental to health. Psychosocial factors, including depression, hostility and perceived stress, are associated with a range of health behaviours and are implicated in mediating the effects of broad social processes on physiologic responses relating to chronic and infectious disease.

Part E is devoted to the policy, research and political implications of the foregoing chapters, although many of these have sections devoted to the practical implications of the research. Ian Anderson says the conceptualisation of race and Aboriginality within social epidemiology and social policy requires attention. He criticises the prevailing models of the social determinants of health for generalising the impact of particular social institutions or responses across populations, ignoring the potential for differential impacts as a result of a variety of sub-population histories, contexts and starting points. One outcome of a different way of thinking about race and Aboriginality would be a demand for greater methodological sophistication in the way that evidence is both collected and interpreted.

Liz Harris, Don Nutbeam and Peter Sainsbury advance a similar web of causation for the health of poor Australians. They argue that poverty, like racism, has a multidimensional, multifactoral role in disease causation, and operates along complex pathways. On the basis of a study in western Sydney, the authors tease out what poverty means and they provide valuable insights into the experience of poverty beyond inadequate income. They, also, demand that public health researchers improve their research approaches and methods, and question the responsibility of the health sector for health outcomes that might have their origins in other sectors, such as finance and housing.

Ross Homel, Gordon Elias and Ian Hay address this very question by reporting on the early stages of a community intervention designed to tackle disadvantage in its many guises. By viewing a multiplicity of social problems, such as illicit drug abuse, child behaviour problems, poor health and low literacy, as the result of the same factors—material and social disadvantage and poor opportunities for optimal human development—it is possible to develop multi-pronged interventions that involve numerous portfolios. The authors detail what a developmental prevention approach looks like and how it might be evaluated.

In the final chapter, Bev Sibthorpe and Jane Dixon examine the reasons for a general lack of government attention to health inequalities, and focus on the 'lack of appropriate evidence'. They contend the evidence for the effectiveness of broad-based interventions is being sought using the wrong methods. They propose that, by rethinking the current divide between monitoring and research and orienting them to policy evaluation we will be able to gather the evidence needed for broad-based agendas for change.

This book offers a very broad perspective on the social determinants of health, ranging from the planetary to the molecular and from the theoretical to the practical. It includes social, economic, cultural, ecological and biological dimensions. While not as comprehensive in each area as some other publications, the scope of the book is unusual, perhaps unique, in the social epidemiological literature. It places this literature, clearly and influentially, within the context of wider debates about the nature of human development and social progress that seem set to dominate the politics of this century.

Richard Eckersley, Jane Dixon, Bob Douglas

Acknowledgements

We explain in the Preface that this book is the culmination of a process that included a national conference, *The Social Origins of Health and Well-being: From the Planetary to the Molecular*, held in July 2000. The Australian Department of Health and Aged Care provided funding and support for the conference and for the development and establishment of the Australian Health Inequalities Research Collaboration, the body which hosted the conference. We are grateful for this contribution. Liz Furler deserves special recognition for championing the Collaboration.

A number of colleagues overseas have contributed to the Australian initiative on health inequalities. Among those who have been particularly inspirational are, in no particular order, Leonard Syme, Fraser Mustard, Michael Marmot, Barbara Starfield, Michael Wolfson, Ichiro Kawachi, Johan Mackenbach, John Lynch, Hilary Graham and Alvin Tarlov. Other national and international colleagues provided chapter reviews. The book would not have come to fruition without the talents and commitment of Susan Lindsay, the diligent copy-editing of Valina Rainer, or the enthusiasm of Peter Debus and Paul Watt at CUP. Our thanks to all of them.

Contributors

Ian Anderson is Director of the Vichealth Koori Health Research and Community Development Unit at the Centre for the Study of Health and Society, University of Melbourne, 207–211 Grattan Street, Parkville, Vic 3052, Australia.
Email: i.anderson@cshs.unimelb.edu.au

Fran Baum is at the South Australian Community Health Research Unit, (SACHRU), Department of Public Health, Flinders University, GPO Box 2100, Adelaide, SA 5001, Australia.
Email: fran.baum@flinders.edu.au

Leigh Blizzard is a Research Fellow at the Menzies Centre for Population Health Research, University of Tasmania, GPO Box 252-23, Hobart, TAS 7001, Australia.
Email: leigh.blizzard@utas.edu.au

Dorothy Broom is a Senior Fellow at the National Centre for Epidemiology and Population Health, Australian National University, Canberra, ACT 0200, Australia.
Email: dorothy.broom@anu.edu.au

Robert Bush is at the Centre for Primary Health Care, Department of Social and Preventive Medicine, The University of Queensland, Princess Alexandra Hospital, Ipswich Road, Woolloongabba, Qld 4102, Australia.
Email: r.bush@sph.uq.edu.au

Colin Butler is a PhD student with the National Centre for Epidemiology and Population Health, Australian National University, Canberra, ACT 0200, Australia.
Email: colin.butler@anu.edu.au

Judy Cashmore is an Honorary Research Associate at the Social Policy Research Centre, University of New South Wales, Kensington, NSW 2052, Australia.
Email: judycash@nsw.bigpond.net.au

Mark Daniel is Assistant Professor of Health Behavior/Education and of Epidemiology, School of Public Health, CB #7400, Rosenau 306, The University of North Carolina 27599-7400, USA.
Email: danielm@email.unc.edu

Jane Dixon is a Fellow at the National Centre for Epidemiology and Population Health, Australian National University, Canberra, ACT 0200, Australia.
Email: jane.dixon@anu.edu.au

Bob Douglas is a Visiting Fellow at the National Centre for Epidemiology and Population Health, Australian National University, Canberra, ACT 0200, Australia.
Email: bob.douglas@anu.edu.au

Stephen Duckett is Professor of Health Policy and Dean of the Faculty of Health Sciences, La Trobe University, Vic 3086, Australia.
Email: s.duckett@latrobe.edu.au

Terry Dwyer is the Director of the Menzies Centre for Population Health Research, University of Tasmania, GPO Box 252-23, Hobart, TAS 7001, Australia.
Email: t.dwyer@utas.edu.au

Richard Eckersley is a Fellow at the National Centre for Epidemiology and Population Health, Australian National University, Canberra, ACT 0200, Australia.
Email: richard.eckersley@anu.edu.au

Gordon Elias is Senior Lecturer at the School of Cognition, Language and Special Education, Mt Gravatt Campus, Griffith University, Qld 4111, Australia.
Email: g.elias@mailbox.gu.edu.au

Anne-Marie Feyer is Director of the New Zealand Environmental and Occupational Health Research Centre and a Professorial Research Fellow in the Department of Preventive and Social Medicine, University of Otago, PO Box 913, Dunedin, New Zealand.
Email: afeyer@gandalf.otago.ac.nz

Elizabeth Harris is Director of the Centre for Health Equity Training, Research and Evaluation, and Lecturer at the School of Community Medicine, University of New South Wales, Liverpool Hospital, PO Box 103, Liverpool, NSW 2170, Australia.
Email: e.harris@unsw.edu.au

Ian Hay is Senior Lecturer at the School of Cognition, Language and Special Education, Mt Gravatt Campus, Griffith University, Qld. 4111, Australia.
Email: i.hay@mailbox.gu.edu.au

Ross Homel is Professor of Criminology and Criminal Justice, and Deputy Director, Key Centre for Ethics, Law, Justice and Governance, Mt Gravatt Campus, Griffith University, Qld 4111, Australia.
Email: r.homel@mailbox.gu.edu.au

Philippa Howden-Chapman is Director of the Housing and Health Research Program at the Department of Public Health, Wellington School of Medicine and Health Sciences, University of Otago, PO Box 7343, Wellington South, New Zealand.
Email: howdenc@wnmeds.ac.nz

David Legge is at the School of Public Health, La Trobe University, Vic 3086, Australia.
Email: d.legge@latrobe.edu.au

Colin Mathers is Principal Research Fellow in the Health Division of the Australian Institute of Health and Welfare, GPO Box 570, Canberra, ACT 2601, Australia.
Email: colin.mathers@aihw.gov.au

A.J. McMichael is Director of the National Centre for Epidemiology and Population Health, Australian National University, Canberra, ACT 0200, Australia.
Email: tony.mcmichael@anu.edu.au

Ruth Morley is Senior Research Fellow in the Department of Paediatrics, University of Melbourne, and the Murdoch Childrens Research Institute, Royal Children's Hospital, Parkville, Vic 3052, Australia.
Email: morleyr@cryptic.rch.unimelb.edu.au

Jake Najman is Professor of Sociology, School of Social Science and Director of the Queensland Alcohol and Drug Research and Education Centre, School of Population Health, University of Queensland, Qld 4072, Australia.
Email: j.najman@mailbox.uq.edu.au

Peter Newman is Professor of City Policy, Murdoch University, Perth, WA 6150, Australia, and Director of Sustainability Unit, Premier and Cabinet, Western Australian Government.
Email: newman@central.murdoch.edu.au

Don Nutbeam is a Visiting Professor in the Department of Public Health and Policy at the London School of Hygiene and Tropical Medicine, Keppel Street, London WC1 7HT, UK.
Email: don.nutbeam@doh.gsi.gov.uk

Des O'Dea is at the Department of Public Health, Wellington School of Medicine and Health Sciences, University of Otago, PO Box 7343, Wellington South, New Zealand.
Email: dodea@wnmeds.ac.nz

Kerin O'Dea is Director of the Menzies School of Health Research, PO Box 41096, Casuarina, NT 0811, Australia.
Email: kerin@menzies.du.au

John Powles is University Lecturer in Public Health Medicine, Institute of Public Health, Cambridge University, Robinson Way, Cambridge, CB2 2SR, UK.
Email: jwp11@cam.ac.uk

Peter Sainsbury is Director of the Division of Population Health, Central Sydney Area Health Service, and Associate Professor, Department of Public Health and Community Medicine, University of Sydney, NSW 2006, Australia.
Email: sainsburyp@email.cs.nsw.gov.au

Beverly Sibthorpe is a Fellow at the National Centre for Epidemiology and Population Health, Australian National University, Canberra, ACT 0200 Australia.
Email: beverly.sibthorpe@anu.edu.au

Richard Taylor is at the Department of Public Health and Community Medicine, Faculty of Medicine, University of Sydney, NSW 2006, Australia.
Email: richard t@pub.health.usyd.edu.au

Martin Tobias is Public Health Physician, Ministry of Health, PO Box 5013, Wellington, New Zealand.
Email: martin_tobias@moh.govt.nz

Gavin Turrell is a National Health and Medical Research Council Post-Doctoral Research Fellow at the School of Public Health, Queensland University of Technology, Victoria Park Road, Kelvin Grove, Qld 4059, Australia.
Email: g.turrell@qut.edu.au

Graham Vimpani is Head of Discipline of Paediatrics and Child Health, University of Newcastle, Locked Bag 1014, Wallsend, NSW 2287, Australia.
Email: gvimpani@mail.newcastle.edu.au

Alistair Woodward is Head of the Department of Public Health, Wellington School of Medicine and Health Sciences, University of Otago, PO Box 7343, Wellington South, New Zealand.
Email: woodward@wnmeds.ac.nz

Part A
Historical, global and cultural perspectives

Healthier progress:
historical perspectives on the social and economic determinants of health

John Powles

Introduction

The World Bank's seminal report 'Investing in health', published in 1993, has already established itself as one of the most influential public health documents of the late 20th century. In seeking to draw lessons from the past, it noted that 'three factors have been important in the dramatic and unprecedented mortality declines of the past hundred years . . . These factors are income growth, improvements in medical technology, and public health programs combined with the spread of knowledge about health' (World Bank 1993, p 34). When, as here, the past is used as a guide to the present, much rests on the truth of the interpretation offered. The purpose of this chapter is to examine underlying determinants of mortality change in adults in high income countries such as Australia, and, in the light of this, firstly, to suggest a re-formulation of the explanatory factors used in the 1993 World Development Report and finally to reflect briefly on some implications of this discussion for the social origins of health inequalities.

The chapter starts with an exploration of the complexities of the relationship between economic development and health improvement, noting both the health-favouring and health-damaging potentials of increased incomes. The underlying theme is that gains in health have often depended on complex institutional adaptations to the effects of economic development – with the measures found necessary to overcome the increased transmissibility of infection associated with rapid urbanisation in the 19th century providing the classic example. At the beginning of the 21st century, important adverse health effects of economic development remain to be solved.

Consideration then moves to the upward shift through the 20th century in the life expectancy attainable at given levels of real income. This points to the fundamental importance of increases in practical knowledge, which have enhanced capacities for health protection and improvement. The paths by which increases in knowledge may act to improve health are shown to be diverse and complex. Medicine therefore needs to be understood as an institution in which the whole of society participates and not merely as a vehicle for the professional deployment of 'medical technology'.

The argument pushes towards a rather abstract model in which health improvement is seen to depend on the interacting effects of increases in knowledge and economic and institutional development. The institutions influencing health are divided into three groups: institutions primarily concerned to protect and restore health (medicine and public health); institutions with major, but incidental, health effects (for example, dietary and drinking customs) and state and civil institutions that facilitate health protection and improvement. The major influences of these latter two categories help explain why mortality levels are so weakly related to levels of spending on professional medicine.

This broadly 'institutionalist' account of the sources of health improvement is in some accord with recent World Bank interpretations of the interrelated nature of economic and social development. As societies move towards 'late modernity', deliberation replaces custom in the regulation of social life. Health protection now depends on many adaptations that are complex and intrinsically difficult. This makes the secular increase in health inequalities by social rank unsurprising. It is concluded that solutions will need to be institutional.

Income

Increase in income may be thought of as an increase in command over commodities. Its most important health-favouring effect has been the increased command over food and the consequent increase in body size.

Fogel has described this transformation in body size as 'technophysio evolution' (Fogel and Costa 1997). He draws on the empirical work of Waaler who reported the relation between height and weight and subsequent mortality risks during the 1960s and 70s among more than 300,000 Norwegian males (Waaler 1984). From these data, Fogel and Kim constructed 'Waaler surfaces' illustrating relative mortality risks at different combinations of height and weight (figure 1.1). Estimates of the mean height and weight of French and English men in the 18th century were then plotted. Over calendar time, as average heights and weights increased, hypothetical paths could be traced down across the 'iso-mortality' contours and so down the valley – not, in this case, of death but of survival (1997, p 55).

Fogel estimates that, in 18th-century France, the agricultural population was producing only a small food surplus. Those in the bottom deciles of the income distribution commanded barely enough food for survival, and certainly not enough to support full-time labour. With mean body weights around 50 kg and heights just above 160 cm, their meagre diets left them vulnerable to early death. Fogel and Costa (1997, p 54) took their calculations to show that '. . . while factors associated with height and weight jointly explain about 90% of the estimated decline in French mortality rates over the period between about 1785 and 1870, they explain only about 50% of the decline in mortality rates during the last century.'

Their rather enthusiastic causal interpretation is not without problems. Findings on the relationship between body size and mortality have not been consistent, and relations appear to vary with the risks faced: taller is usually better for vascular risk but certainly not for breast

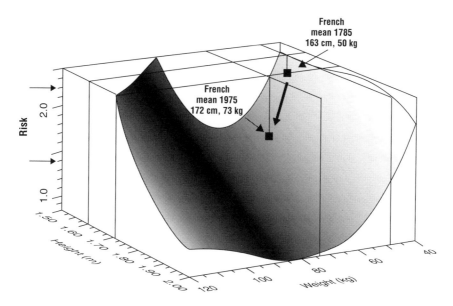

Figure 1.1 'Waaler surface' relating body size in adult males to mortality risk*, with illustrative estimates of mean body size change in French men and potential effect on mortality

* Based on data from 309,000 Norwegian males aged 40–59 and followed between 1963 and 1979. Reading from the vertical scale for (relative) risk implies that the increase in body size could account for a 36% decline in mortality (from 2.2 to 1.4).

Source: Reproduced from Fogel, 1993, p 35, with the illustrative data for French men added by the author. Reproduced with permission from RW Fogel; copyright 1993 by RW Fogel.

cancer (Cold 1998); fatter is better when your leading risk is TB (but being tall isn't) (Edwards et al. 1971); but, fatter is not better when your main risk is heart attack (Calle et al. 1999). Furthermore, increased body size can hardly be a pre-requisite for mortality decline, as many populations have attained low mortality before attaining high stature (eg, Greek, Italian and Spanish women over 50; Sri Lankans). Leaving these cavils aside, it is striking that these authors' enthusiasm for the health benefits of economic development is undimmed by evidence showing *deteriorations* in both height and longevity during the second and third quarters of the 19th century – a period of rapid economic development. Their own figure of trends in native-born white American males through the 19th century illustrates this deterioration dramatically (figure 1.2).

Fogel and Costa note, in relation to this deterioration, that one factor 'stands out more than any other: rapid urbanisation'. In the 'United States around 1830, cities with 50,000 or more persons had more than twice the death rates of rural areas; similar patterns have been observed for Europe'. The rapidity of the increase in urban populations 'exceeded the capacity of the cities to supply clean water, to remove waste, and to contain the spread of infection'. What these authors fail to note is that major institutional changes were found necessary in order 'to supply clean water, to remove waste, and to contain the spread of infection'; and their

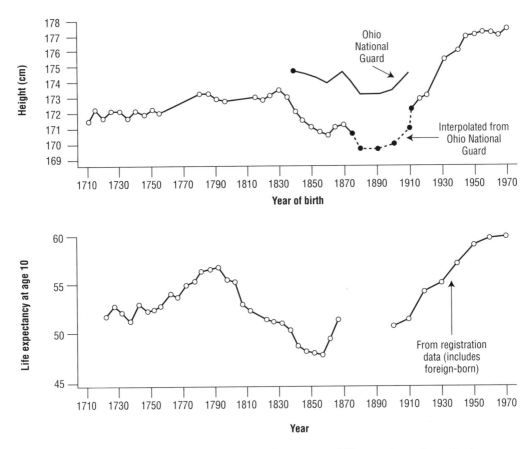

Figure 1.2 Time trends since the early 18th century in stature and life expectancy for native-born, white, United States males

Source: Fogel and Costa 1997, p 61. Reproduced with permission from Demography; copyright 1997 by Population Association of America.

silence on this serves to place them in the camp of those who regard unregulated economic development as consistently beneficial to health.

Szreter (1988, 1999) has shown, for the case of Great Britain, how fanciful it is to assume that the urban mortality penalty was removed by unregulated economic expansion. In the half-century from the 1820s to the 1870s, there was no overall improvement in life expectancy in the increasing number of British provincial cities with populations over 100,000. In these cities, rapid improvement had to await the breaking of the dominance of small businessmen over local government (by the extension of the franchise around 1870) and the invention of 'municipal socialism' by new civic leaders such as Birmingham businessman Joseph Chamberlain. For the United States, Leavitt (1982) documents a broadly analogous institutional history for Milwaukee, which, after an insalubrious beginning, attained a national 'healthiest city' award in 1929. Once discovered, institutional solutions that effectively countered the extra transmissibility of infection in cities rapidly became incorporated into the material and cultural infrastructure of modernity. Later modernising countries were able to cut short their suffering of the 'urban penalty' by borrowing solutions developed by the pioneers. In today's low-income countries, mortality even tends to be lower in urban areas. The securing of net gains to health from economic development thus depended on the institutional adaptations necessary to counter the increased transmissibility of infection in the enlarging settlements that economic development was itself creating.

Enthusiastic interpretations of the health benefits of rising incomes also tend to overlook the fact that the increasing command over commodities has not been limited to those that favour health. A global pandemic of nicotine addiction has followed in the wake of rising incomes with around 30% of adult deaths under 70 in developed countries now attributable to smoking (Peto et al. 1994). Not surprisingly, such societies have been developing increasingly strong counter-measures in an attempt to suppress this, their commonest avoidable cause of pre-mature death. Such measures include luxury taxes (accounting for two-thirds or more of retail prices in high-income countries), advertising bans and restrictions on smoking in public places (Chaloupka et al. 2000, p 238).

Economic development is also having other effects with substantial current or potential capacity to harm health. As development proceeds, mechanical slaves replace muscular exertion – both in production and in moving around. Physical Activity Levels, defined as energy expenditure divided by requirement for basal metabolism (Shetty et al. 1996), have declined substantially, especially since the mid-20th century (Prentice and Jebb 1995a). Data for trends in energy consumption, which provide the best available measure of energy expenditure, are given for England in figure 1.3.

Declining Physical Activity Levels harm health directly (Wareham et al. 2000) and are associated, probably causally, with the rising prevalence of obesity (Prentice and Jebb 1995a).

Economic development is also depleting natural capital and disrupting natural systems. Such disruptions could bring substantial future harm. Ambient temperatures are now rising around 30 times faster than at the end of the last glaciation, apparently because of the production of 'greenhouse gases' associated with global industrialisation (McMichael 1993). This could produce serious adverse effects on food production: for example, a consequential 1.0 m rise in sea levels could deprive Bangladesh of half its productive cropland (World Bank 1999a, pp 99–100). More frequent extreme weather events could also produce casualties of many kinds.

It is improbable that industrialism, as we now know it, can be both generalised to the whole human population and sustained indefinitely. Levelling up current average world incomes to rich country levels would require, other things being equal, an approximately four-fold increase in the global material economy. When multiplied by the expected approximate 50% increase in world population, we have an approximately six-fold increase in the global material economy – if nothing else changes. So to reduce current rates of aggregate ecological disruption, which have passed thresholds of sustainability (Loh et al. 1998), something like a 10-fold reduction in ecological disruption per unit of economic product would be required. Some optimists believe a 'factor 10' increase in 'ecological efficiency' to be feasible (OECD 1998), but this would clearly have us living within material economies that were qualitatively very different from 'industrialism as we have known it'.

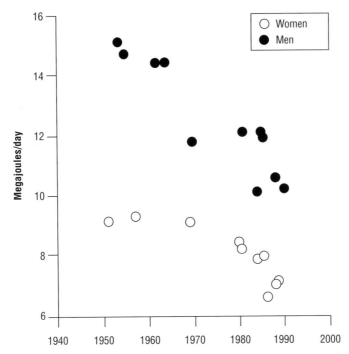

Figure 1.3 Secular decline in mean energy consumption per day in samples of the English population since 1950*

*These data are unadjusted for increasing body size; the decline in energy turnover per unit of lean body mass will have been greater.

Source: Prentice and Jebb, 1995b. Reproduced with permission from British Medical Journal; copyright 1993 by BMJ Publishing Group.

The increasing awareness of losses of natural capital, and of need to think about legacies for future generations, directs attention to the importance of stocks as well as flows. Sustainability, in its weakest form, implies that each generation passes on to the next a non-depleted total stock of capital – created, human and natural. Although 'in economics and finance one does not deplete one's capital and consider it an income stream', the current practice in national income accounts does just this, because it ignores the depletion of natural capital (Serageldin 1996, p 3).

In principle, capital is valued by the flow of benefits it generates. But in health matters, it may often be easier to see connections between changes in capital stocks and health than between changes in income flows and health (Anand and Chen 1996). During economic development, roads, schools and communications networks are built and teachers are trained. Schooling augments human capital, and mothers who have been to school care for their children in ways that make them less likely to die. Falls in child mortality were almost universal in low-income countries between 1980 and 1995 (Zambia being the only exception), and the proportional falls were just as great in countries where incomes fell as in countries where incomes rose (World Bank 1999a, p 19). This remarkable phenomenon suggests either, that economic development has recently had no important effect on child mortality in low-income countries or, more plausibly, that concurrent 'income growth' does not capture all the important effects of economic development on health. For this reason, it seems appropriate to add a pathway from economic development to better health via the health benefits of increases in stocks.

To complete this brief overview of the more important connections between economic development and health, it needs to be noted that the flows are not all one-way. Better health enhances productivity and persons who expect to live longer are likely to save more and thereby enhance levels of investment.

A graphical model is given in figure 1.4.

In the light of this brief overview, the representation in the World Bank report of the connections between economic development and health is deficient in these respects:

1 It tendentiously abstracts health-favouring effects of increased incomes from other processes integral to economic development that have also had important influences on health – both favourable and unfavourable.

2 It fails to acknowledge that optimising health outcomes has typically depended on a dynamic interaction between economic and institutional developments and not on economic development alone.

3 It fails to acknowledge that there are important emergent (*energy expenditure/obesity*) and potential (*ecological disruption*) adverse health effects of economic development that remain to be solved.

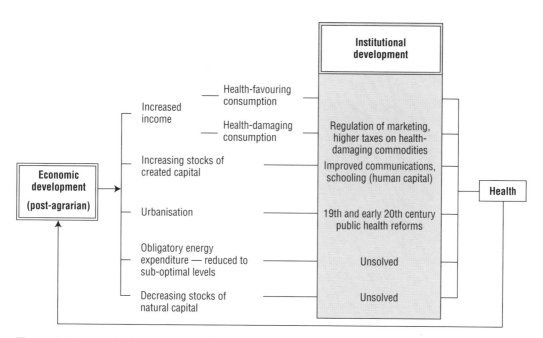

Figure 1.4 Economic development and health: main pathways and interactions with institutional development

Medicine and the increase of knowledge

The authors of the Bank report were well aware of the limited capacity of changes in income to explain changes in mortality levels and cited Preston et al.'s graph of the changing relation between these over calendar time (figure 1.5).

To account for other major influences on mortality trends, 'improvements in medical technology' and 'public health and the spread of knowledge' were invoked in the Bank report. The increase in knowledge was seen to underlie both.

Increased knowledge acts, in part, by enhancing the effectiveness of professional medicine, and evidence of significant health gains from this source has been accumulating. Bunker and colleagues have estimated that professional medicine has added several years to United States life expectancy since 1950 (Bunker 1995); Mackenbach and colleagues have produced more modest estimates for the Netherlands (Mackenbach 1996).

Factors contributing to changing heart disease mortality in 31 cohorts in 21 countries have recently been reported from the World Health Organisation Multinational Monitoring of Trends and Determinants in Cardiovascular Disease (MONICA) project. It was found that enhanced use of effective treatments accounted for far more of the variance than did

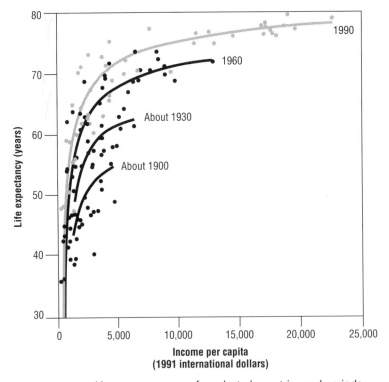

Figure 1.5 Life expectancy and income per person for selected countries and periods

Source: World Bank 1993, p 34, citing Preston et al. Reproduced with permission from Oxford University Press; copyright 1993 by Oxford University Press.

favourable changes in the three classic risk factors – blood pressure, blood cholesterol concentration and cigarette smoking (Tunstall-Pedoe et al. 2000, p 698). However, low treatment levels were strongly confounded with location in a former socialist country. For coronary mortality rates, variance explained fell from 64% to 18% when the nine cohorts in the former socialist economies, plus China, were excluded. The 'treatment effects' also lacked specificity – for example, use of thrombolysis during heart attacks was more strongly associated, paradoxically, with event rates than with case fatality. The authors commented that 'economically successful populations, which rapidly implement new treatments, may be adaptive and successful in controlling disease in other ways, including lifestyle behaviours such as diet'. This idea – that favourable health trends in highly 'medicalised' societies may owe more to their capacity to adapt to new knowledge about the causes and management of disease than to the specific effects of professional medicine or formal public health programs – finds support elsewhere. Three examples of public health 'success without interventions' can be cited briefly.

First, smoking cessation in the USA during the 1950s and 60s: Pierce and Gilpin have shown that cessation rates by calendar year closely mirrored coverage of the health effects of tobacco in the most widely read print media (Pierce and Gilpin 2001). A sequence occurred whereby advances in medical knowledge were marshalled by professional groups and state institutions, most notably by the Royal College of Physicians in 1962 (Royal College of Physicians 1962) and the US Surgeon General in 1964 (US Surgeon General 1964), and then disseminated through the general news media (Pollock 1999). There were no specific 'interventions'.

Second is the case of HIV transmission in homosexual men in England in the early 1980s. The behaviours responsible for transmission apparently changed markedly between 1983 and 1985 (De Angelis et al. 1998), well ahead of the formal public health program (Acheson 1993) (figure 1.6).

Third, the decline in Sudden Infant Death Syndrome (SIDS) in England followed discussions in the letters pages of the Lancet during 1988 of the relationship between sleeping position and risk of SIDS (Beal 1988). This and other theories were widely discussed in magazines commonly read by mothers with young infants. Death rates from SIDS fell by more than a third in the following three years *before* the UK government's formal 'Back to sleep' began in December 1991 (Office of Population, Censuses and Statistics 1988 and 1995; Hiley and Morley 1994) – again suggesting that mass behaviour change had occurred in response to new information flowing through the general news media and, in an uncoordinated way, via health professionals. In this case however, the rate of decline did accelerate sharply after the formal program, halving in the following 12 months.

These three examples suffice to show that health benefits from new medical knowledge need not depend on the specific 'interventions' of physicians or public health professionals and officials. Such knowledge may also be directly conveyed to the public and, by changing popular medical understandings, lead to important health-favouring changes in behaviour. Medicine therefore needs to be understood broadly, not just as a domain of professional practice, nor as a bundle of commodities to be 'delivered' but rather as an institution in which the whole of society participates.

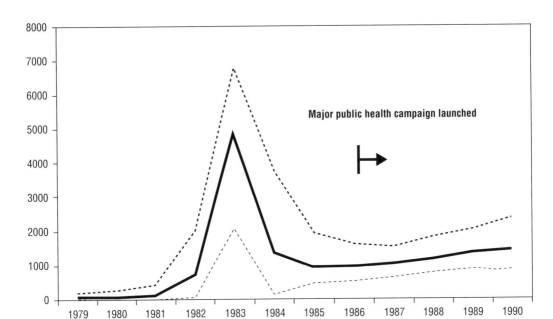

Figure 1.6 HIV incidence in homosexual and bisexual males, England and Wales, estimates by back-projection for 1979–90 (with 95% credible interval) and timing of main public health campaign

Source of data: De Angelis, personal communication.

Although the World Bank's report acknowledges the importance of knowledge flowing to the general public (under the head 'public health and the spread of knowledge'), this is separated from the influence of medicine, which is seen as flowing through 'medical technology'. It seems more appropriate to view medical knowledge as an evolving, interconnected whole, with clinical and public health applications flowing from the same sources. This points to the increase of knowledge as the underlying engine of change and to medicine, broadly conceived, as one of its channels of influence.

Advances in knowledge in many fields outside medicine also have a capacity to influence health – whether the advances are in scientific, technical or organisational understanding. The development of production systems for the counter-seasonal supply of fresh fruits and vegetables may be taken as an example (in part, because of its potential relevance to the east/west mortality difference in Europe, which is taken up further below).

It took from the 1920s to the 1970s to develop methods for producing lettuce year round in California (W Friedland, personal communication, March 1995). To convey this highly perishable product to distant markets special techniques had to be developed. The requirements are quite demanding:

> Not only must temperature be controlled but it must be controlled within a few degrees; there is little leeway available because a few degrees rise in temperature will drastically shorten the shelf life of the lettuce, whereas a few degrees of temperature drop will freeze it and turn it into slime. (Friedland et al. 1981, p 54).

These and other technical and organisational developments have provided western populations with year-round access to fresh fruit and vegetables. This achievement was unmatched by the former socialist economies of Europe. Over the couple of decades to 1990, the extent of counter-seasonal supplies of fresh fruits and vegetables constituted the most striking dietary divide between east and west. Even in the most affluent of the former socialist economies, concentrations of Vitamin C in the blood fell to low levels each spring in a significant fraction of the population (L Heinemann, personal communication, 1995; Thiel et al. 1994). By this time, in western countries, the transition to year round salads was substantially complete. Figure 1.7 shows the contrast in the seasonal swings of fresh food supplies in Hungary and Bulgaria (fruit and vegetable exporters within the former socialist block) and in Britain. (Because the comparability of the absolute values cannot be assured, the seasonal variation within each data series is given.)

It was not, of course, due to a lack of knowledge alone, that these systems were not developed in the former socialist economies. The nature of the command economy and its unresponsiveness to consumer demand was a critical determinant as well. This particular example thus illustrates how interactions of the advance of knowledge, economic development, and institutional factors, have plausibly contributed to the most dramatic differences in health attainments yet experienced in the developed world.

To summarise so far: Realising health benefits from economic development has depended

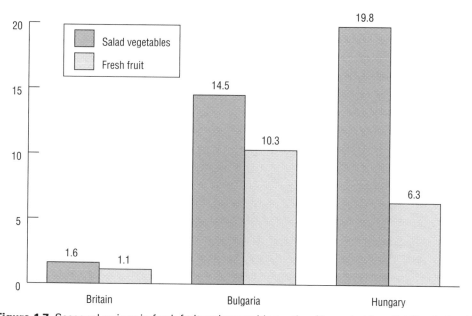

Figure 1.7 Seasonal swings in fresh fruit and vegetables: ratio of household availability during May to October to availability in November to April, Britain compared to Bulgaria and Hungary, 1989

Note: The reported absolute intakes are higher in summer in the two eastern countries but very much lower in winter. However, comparability of methods cannot be assured.

Sources: National Food Survey Committee, 1990; Bulgaria National Statistical Institute, 1989, p 42; P Szivos, personal communication, 1995.

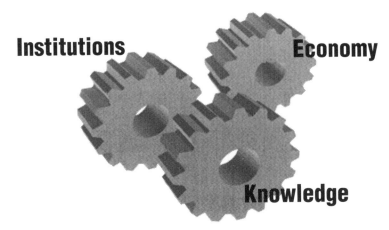

Figure 1.8 Underlying determinants of levels and trends of adult mortality in high-income countries

in large part on adaptive institutional changes. Further, new knowledge has contributed to health improvement by multiple pathways, not just via professional medicine, nor, as the commodifiers would have it, by the 'delivery' of 'medical technology' or 'health care'.

We have thus been pushed towards abstraction with a three-factor model that seems perhaps to say little more than that everything matters and everything is connected to everything else. Its defence is that models that are more specific and concrete have been shown to fail to capture important parts of reality. To be meaningful, models of this kind need to be illustrated by more examples, especially those illustrating interaction of the three domains.

Do organised efforts to protect health make much difference?

I shall now consider the role of institutions a little further and begin by asking whether organised and intensive efforts to protect health in high-income countries can be shown to produce visible effects on trends in mortality from major causes. I shall take as an example traffic injury control in the state of Victoria, Australia.

Changes in economy, knowledge and institutions have all played roles in the evolution of traffic injury rates and such injuries have recently ranked fourth as contributors to lost disability-adjusted life years (DALYS) in Europe and the Americas (World Health Organization 1999, p 110). Smeed (1972) showed that there was a very general tendency for deaths per unit vehicles to decrease as vehicle density increases in populations: deaths/vehicle = 0.0003(vehicles/population)$^{-0.66}$. As familiarity with motor vehicles and resources available for safety increase, so it seems, societies learn how to reduce the associated risks (see also van Beeck et al. 2000).

Trends in Victoria since 1920 are shown in figure 1.9. Over 80% of the reduction in fatalities per 10,000 vehicles that occurred between 1920 and 1995 had been achieved before the intensification of control measures began around 1970. During this 'pre-reform' period, Victoria was a poor performer with deaths per vehicle lying well above Smeed's prediction.

Then, from the 1960s, there was a growing political conviction that something more

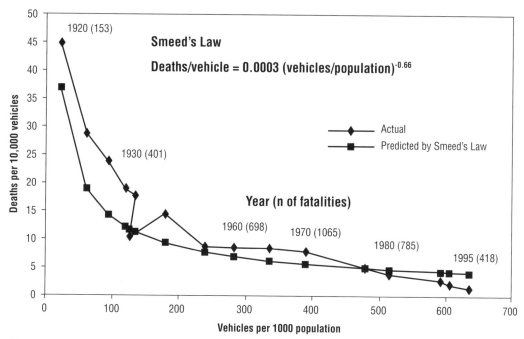

Figure 1.9 Decline in traffic fatalities per 10,000 vehicles, Victoria, Australia, 1920–95

Sources: Hawthorne 1991, chapter 5; Smeed 1972.

needed to be done to reduce deaths from road injuries. In December 1970, Victoria became the first jurisdiction in the world to make the wearing of seat belts compulsory. Other legislative measures followed, including random breath testing for drivers in 1977. The results were initially impressive, but improvement began to fade in the late 1980s (figure 1.10). At that time, compulsory third party injury insurance had been 'de-privatised', creating a single 'pot of gold' to fund the prevention of road injuries and the compensation of victims. Using these funds, a strong social marketing campaign backed by intensive policing was introduced (Powles and Gifford 1993). Death rates fell promptly and substantially. During the early 1990s, the Traffic Accident Commission (TAC) was spending substantial sums on injury control measures – several dollars per person over a few years. In 1994, 1.6 million random breath tests were performed, a number equal to about half the driving-age population. Programs of this intensity might appear costly, but car crashes are costly, and economic evaluations performed on behalf of the TAC concluded that the financial benefits to costs ratio was at least 3:1 (Cameron and Newstead 1996).

This story illustrates several points relevant to our theme. Economic progress brings adverse as well as favourable effects on health – in this case, high-speed collisions between the human body and hard objects. Societies learn, in multifarious ways, to cope with these new challenges. New knowledge is generated about the nature of the risks and the kinds of counter-strategies that might be tried. On top of these more or less universal institutional adjustments, some societies have mounted more specific and determined institutional responses. In

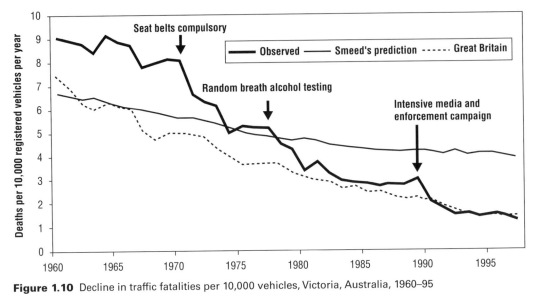

Figure 1.10 Decline in traffic fatalities per 10,000 vehicles, Victoria, Australia, 1960–95

Sources: VicRoads (multiple years); Smeed 1972; Department of the Environment, Transport and the Regions (1998).

the Victorian case, it seems that extra effort was well rewarded. The trend line for Britain (now with levels among the lowest in Europe) also makes a point. It shows that persistent but less dramatic institutional responses may also be effective.

Vascular disease and overall mortality levels

Cardiovascular diseases are the leading cause both of life-years and of DALYS lost in high-income countries. In many countries, the incidence of these diseases has been falling substantially and the relative importance of the factors contributing to these falls is clearly of great interest. The MONICA program results showing associations with the adoption of effective treatments have already been cited (along with their authors' assessment that more diffuse social responses to the challenge of premature vascular disease have probably also played a major role in their reduction).

Now if the favourable effects of economic development on adult mortality risks tended to outweigh the unfavourable effects and if there were additional benefits flowing from organised efforts to control disease and injury, then we might expect that these two variables could account for much of the variation in the attainment of low mortality. This, though, does not seem to be the case.

As a preliminary, the amount of recognisable 'noise' affecting especially adult male mortality levels needs to be noted. Levels and trends in adult mortality in high-income countries are substantially influenced by the timing and magnitude of their smoking epidemics. For example, amongst European males, those in England and Finland were early adopters of cigarette smoking and early abandoners – in contrast, say, to Spanish males. Past falls in smoking prevalence in the former countries are currently pulling down mortality from smoking-caused cancers and from vascular disease, whereas in Spanish men, the overall decline in mortality is being retarded by the continuing rise of mortality attributable to smoking.

Attempts to explain mortality levels and trends in high-income countries thus need either to account for the timing and magnitude of the smoking epidemic and incorporate this within the explanatory model, or to use methods such as those developed by Peto and colleagues (1992) to estimate smoking-attributable mortality and then to peel this away and see what remains to be explained. With sufficient time and resources, the latter might be preferable. For our purposes here, however, there is a shortcut that minimises noise from this source: namely concentrating on data for females. This also has the merit of minimising noise from the culturally variable determinants of male injury rates. From ages 35 to 69, smoking-attributable mortality and injuries account for about 46% of male mortality in developed countries, but only for about 18 % of female mortality (Peto et al. 1994). All-cause mortality rates in females may therefore be expected to be more sensitive to the effects of income levels and endeavours to control disease.

The relationship of mortality and income in females in high-income countries

Figure 1.11 provides a scatterplot of the relationship of adult female mortality to income levels in high-income countries.

It is apparent on visual inspection, that relationships with income levels are not impressive. (Fiddling with regression models and using the log of income and the log of income squared, it is possible to account for something approaching 20% of variance. But it is not clear that the assumptions of the method are being met, because variance is not constant across levels of income.) There is no association in these data between the gini index measure of inequality of income distribution and mortality level (*pace* Kawachi et al. 1999a). The poor performance of Denmark, where female smoking continues at high levels, and the favourable performance of Costa Rica (lower mortality than the USA) and Sri Lanka (lower mortality than Denmark) are striking.

The relationship of mortality and spending on professional medicine in high-income countries

Given the close association between income levels and both relative and absolute spending on medicine (mostly, of course, professional medicine) and the weak association of mortality and income, we would not expect to find – and do not in fact find – associations of any magnitude between medical spending and mortality levels (figure 1.12).

These essentially null findings are perhaps surprising. Estimates of increasing benefits from professional medicine in the USA and the Netherlands since the mid-20th century have

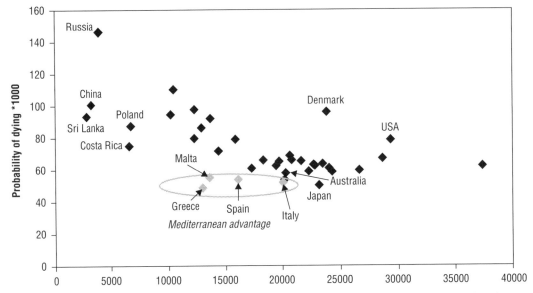

Figure 1.11 Scatterplot of probabilities of death between ages 15 and 60 (times 1000) for the female populations of high-income countries,* by income, 1998 (with corresponding points for selected other countries)

* Countries with populations over 250,000 and purchasing power parity adjusted incomes per person over 10,000 international dollars in 1998.

Sources of data: World Health Organization, 1999, Table 1; World Bank, 1999 pp 23–1.

already been noted. It would also seem inappropriate to assume that deliberate efforts to protect health by public health measures have been without appreciable effect, and such efforts probably increase in intensity with increasing national income. The reduction of road traffic injury in Victoria has been cited.

Why is it so difficult to account for mortality variation by income and spending on medicine?

There is a genuine puzzle here. The first possibility is that the effects of income and medicine are negatively confounded: that more income produces more disease while at the same time paying for the extra medicine to take care of it, leaving us back where we started. For women in the chosen age range, leading causes of death are ischaemic heart disease and breast cancer. Both of these show positive relationships with national income across at least the lower part of the income range being considered here. The negative confounding hypothesis has some plausibility and needs more rigorous testing.

Perhaps more persuasive is the idea that institutions other than those primarily concerned to protect health have substantial effects on health and that these are obscuring other relationships. A clue is provided by the countries (apart from Japan) with lowest female mor-

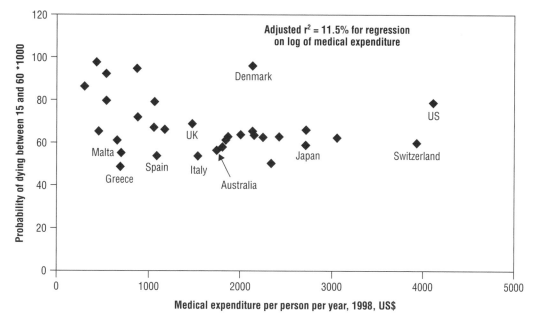

Figure 1.12 Scatterplot of probabilities of death between ages 15 and 60 (times 1000) for the female populations of high-income countries, by level of medical expenditures, 1998

Note: Adjusted r^2 = 11.5% for regression on log of medical expenditure.

Source of data: World Health Organization, 1999; World Bank, 1999a. Expenditure has been estimated by applying estimates for medical spending as a percentage of gross domestic product in 1995 from World Health Organisation with estimates of gross national product per capita in 1998 from the World Bank.

tality. These happen to be in the low–middle part of the income range: Greece, Malta, Spain and Italy. Australia almost makes it as an honorary member of the group. These countries exemplify the Mediterranean advantage, with especially low mortality levels for vascular causes, though this is now somewhat less true for Greece. France, often cited as a member of this group, lies closer to the centre of the mortality range in these data. Now if we suppose that the Mediterranean advantage is mainly attributable to diet (and not, for example, to genes), we have here a situation where the local food culture – itself a function of history, geography and economic development – is playing a major role in determining mortality levels. Clearly, any explanatory schema of the social determinants of health needs to leave a prominent place for influences such as dietary customs: that is, for institutions with major direct influences on health even though the protection of health is not their primary purpose.

An interesting feature of the Mediterranean advantage is that, far from disappearing with globalisation and apparent homogenisation of food cultures, it appears, at least in most of these populations, to be actually enhanced by affluence (figure 1.13). This effect is also observed amongst Greek and Italian migrants to Australia, despite their apparent loss of the favourable blood pressure levels and blood cholesterol concentrations typical of their homeland. Trends among Greeks remaining in Greece have been the exception in showing

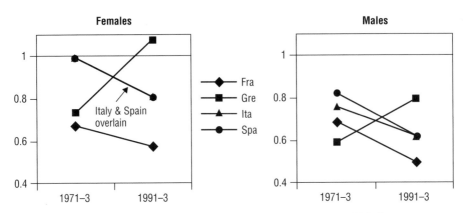

Figure 1.13 Estimated non-smoker mortality from vascular causes: ratios of Mediterranean countries to eleven other European countries, 1971–3 and 1991–3, ages 45–64

Source of estimates: Powles and Sanz 1999, p 37.

less favourable secular trends in vascular mortality – an anomaly that calls for further research. We see in this example a beneficial interaction between economic development and health-favouring customary institutions – in the absence of an explicit concern for health. Just why the Mediterranean advantage may be enhanced by affluence is a question a number of us are pursuing in studies of migrants to Melbourne.

The plight of Russia

No survey of mortality levels in the contemporary developed world can ignore the plight of Russia (although it does not meet criteria for being a high-income country). Even after the recent modest reductions in mortality from their peak in 1994, mortality levels remain extremely high. Russian females have, on current levels, a 14.6% chance of dying between 15 and 60, worse by a substantial margin than Denmark (on 9.6%), which is an outlier among high-income countries. For Russian males, the corresponding figure is an extraordinary 40%, within the range for sub-Saharan countries.

For all causes of death combined, the ratio of death rates in Russian women to the average for the European Union (EU) is not much less than the corresponding ratio for men, and for all vascular causes combined, the proportional difference is actually greater for females. Russia/EU ratios for 1990 for ages 35 to 69 (Peto et al. 1994) were:

	Males	Females
All causes	2.1	1.7
Vascular causes	2.6	2.8

These ratios suggest that the custom of binge drinking, which has been widely cited as a major contributor to the Russian excess (Leon et al. 1997), is only part of the explanation. Vascular disease contributes strongly to this excess mortality, and the proportional excess for vascular disease is not greater in males, among whom binge drinking is more prevalent. In relation to the extremely high rates of death from injury however (4.2 times higher than in the EU for men 35 to 69), binge drinking clearly plays a major role.

Thus, part of the explanation for Russia's sad state centres on an inheritance of particular drinking customs (shared also by Finland and other northern countries) and on the way alcohol use changed during a period of economic collapse and political and social upheaval (White 1996). The breakdown of state regulation and the more general malfunctioning of state institutions contributed to the extremely high levels of harm from alcohol use in the early 1990s. (In Poland, this period of deregulated alcohol sales has been referred to by Zatonski as 'schnappsgate' (personal communication, Zatonski, 1998). The Russian state has recently been ineffective not only in regulating alcohol production and sales but also in collecting taxes, paying salaries, maintaining law and order, regulating financial institutions, establishing property rights etc.

Richard Rose, following Max Weber, has described modern societies as those in which large-scale organisations function predictably. Russia is an 'anti-modern society' because large-scale organisations do not function predictably (Rose 2000). The cultural foundations for such functioning – in the form of modern bureaucratic culture – had not been laid during the Soviet era. Under the previous regime, society was simultaneously over-organised and under-bureaucratised, in the sense that decision-making was not rule-based and authority flowed from political position and not from formal offices. ('Bureau-cracy' understood sociologically refers to systems of authority based on 'office' – in both state and commercial organisations. This needs to be distinguished from its common pejorative usage.)

Just as the successful functioning of modern economies relies heavily on the effectiveness of state institutions (World Bank 1997a), so too do deliberate efforts to protect health. Societies that are not protected by custom (as the cited Mediterranean countries are), may be supposed to be especially vulnerable to the adverse effects of malfunctioning state institutions. Russians trust government and large organisations far less than people in western countries (Rose 2000). Without such trust, modern public health programs can hardly begin.

Trust exists not only between citizens and governments. The strength of informal social networks and of forms of local civic engagement (Lasch 1995) are now much discussed, often under the head of 'social capital', both for their favourable influence on economic performance and for their effects on the attainment of social well-being independent of income levels (Dasgupta and Serageldin 2000). One might thus posit a third class of health-influencing institutions: those that facilitate health protection.

In summary, this survey has identified three main types of institution exerting important influences on health, namely those that:
1 Have the protection of health as their primary objective. Medicine, professional and popular, and public health are examples.
2 Have major direct health effects even though the protection of health is not their primary objective. Dietary and drinking customs are examples.
3 Play an important facilitating role in health protection. The state, civil organisations and informal networks are examples.

Although advances in knowledge provide the most powerful and important underlying engine for health improvement, prediction of the future effects of such advances is notoriously difficult. It would be hazardous to speculate, for example, about the likely effects of the rapid expansion of genetic knowledge. In the long run, these are likely to be substantial.

Health and the 'new institutionalism'

Although the advance of knowledge will continue to expand the horizon of the possible, the extent to which this knowledge is put to work will continue to depend on institutions. In this respect, the preceding emphasis on their role is justified. This 'institutionalist' emphasis is in accord with a developing viewpoint within organisations such as the World Bank. In the 1997 World Development Report on 'the state in a changing world', the view of states as enemies of markets was clearly rejected: 'we now see that markets and governments are complementary' (p 4). The World Development Report for 1999/2000 (1999), which addressed 'the changing development landscape of the early 21st century' is explicitly agnostic about the adequacy of 'single, overarching policy prescriptions' – including, one must assume, neo-liberalism. 'The situations in which success and failure occur differ so much that it is sometimes not apparent which lessons should be extracted or whether they can be applied in other countries' (p 17). This new prescriptive caution recognises the complexity of human societies and the differing ways in which they order their affairs. It should follow that progress is not to be sought by the remote control of a few key national economic policies (understood to be universally important) but rather by much more encompassing proposals that include, for example, the encouragement of civil engagement at all levels of society.

It was noted above that the female populations with the lowest mortality were those apparently protected by a fortuitous interaction of dietary customs and increasing affluence. In countries such as Spain and Italy, the prevention of ischaemic heart disease by deliberate efforts to change diet therefore assumes lesser importance as a priority for formal public health programs. Such countries have different challenges to face: high rates of traffic injury in Spain and Greece (van Beeck et al. 2000) and of HIV infection among intravenous drug users, for example.

However, it is in the nature of late modernity that deliberation is replacing custom. With time, action to protect health becomes ever more explicit and deliberate.

Implications for inequality

A broad interpretation can now be advanced relating these thoughts to health inequalities: as health becomes less determined by conditions given by custom and circumstance and depends more on complex and deliberate adaptations, so will differences between individuals in their personal capacities and in their access to social resources assume a greater importance in determining health levels. Inequalities might therefore be expected to increase with time.

Some observations consistent with this hypothesis:

1 The British aristocracy. Life expectancy among British aristocrats was lower than in the general population until mortality began to improve in the later 18th century. Then,

whatever it was that served to reduce mortality, worked better for the aristocrats and their life expectancy began to exceed that of the rest of the population (Wrigley et al. 1997, p 206).

2 Child mortality in the USA. Preston has shown that, around 1900, rates were relatively equal by paternal occupational group, with rates among the children of farmers lower than those for the 'professional, managerial and clerical' group. Given the relative lack of knowledge about what might be done to reduce child death, advantages in income and even schooling counted for less (though this was just beginning to change). In today's low income countries there are, surprisingly, more possibilities for protecting the health of one's children. So whether you have the schooling and the resources that enable you to do so counts for more (Preston 1985). Hence, inequalities are greater.

3 Smoking. In the early stages of the smoking epidemic, uptake may be higher among the rich. Recently, in England although '. . . poor people are somewhat more likely to become smokers, the strongest association is with persisting smoking. What we need to explain above all is not so much why poor people start smoking, but why they do not give it up' (Jarvis 1999, p 247). Disadvantaged groups are no less likely to want to quit, but the task itself is formidably difficult: 'the chances of succeeding for at least a year in a serious unaided quit attempt are no better than about 1 in 100' (*ibid.*, p 251). In countries with mature smoking epidemics, smoking prevalences decline first among more advantaged groups, increasing the social gradient in smoking and therefore in smoking-attributable mortality. Such mortality now accounts for more than half of the social gradient in male mortality in such populations (Bobák et al. 2000b).

4 With declining energy expenditure during obligatory daily activities, those who are genetically susceptible to obesity find it more and more difficult to avoid. In the 18th century, obesity was mainly confined to the wealthy. Now, in females at least, it is most common in the lowest socio-economic strata.

5 Male mortality gradients in western Europe. Ratios of mortality rates in manual workers to those in non-manual workers, tend, if anything to be smaller in the south (Spain, Italy) than in the north (Sweden, Norway) despite the strongly egalitarian social and economic policies of the latter (Kunst et al. 1998). This may partly reflect the earlier stage of the smoking epidemic in the south (during which stage, uptake may even be higher in upper socio-economic groups) but could also be largely due to the protective effects of dietary customs. Everyone benefits from these in the south. Because an affluent version of a traditional northern diet increases risk of vascular disease, lowering risk requires conscious efforts to change dietary practices for health reasons. Such change would be expected to show a social gradient with more advantaged groups having more 'cultural access' to lower risk diets eg, from holidays in the south.

To the extent that the adaptations that serve to protect health depend on deliberation and on choices that are difficult to make and even more difficult to implement, it is not surprising that success is increasingly dependent on social advantage. Working to reverse this tendency will require more than emphasising the responsibilities of disadvantaged individuals. It will require health-favouring institutional changes at all levels. Revisiting past successes, especially those that have depended least on the unequal capacities of individuals, will remain a useful guide to what is needed today.

Further Reading

Preston, S H & Haines, M 1991, Fatal Years: Child mortality in late nineteenth-century America, Princeton University Press, Princeton.
  – *Provides a detailed and robust account of child mortality differences by location and social rank, and shows how increases in knowledge and more effective social organisation rather than increases in income must account for the marked improvements since the beginning of the 20th century.*
Szreter, S 1988, The importance of social intervention in Britain's mortality decline c 1850–1914: a re-interpretation of the role of public health, Journal of the Society for the Social History of Medicine 1: 1–37.
  – *Emphasises the contribution of institutional reform to mortality decline in late nineteenth century Britain. It provides a critique of interpretations that emphasise either increases in income and nutrition or technical advances within medicine and public health.*
World Bank. 1993, Investing in Health: World development report 1993. Oxford University Press for the World Bank, Oxford.
  – *Signalled the World Bank's increasing interest in public health policy, especially in low and middle income countries and illustrates attempts to systematically quantify health gained for money spent.*

Health inequalilties in the New World Order

David Legge

The international health gap is widening

Life expectancy is increasing, yet the health gap between the rich world and the poor world is widening. From the 1950s to the 1990s, the mortality gap between the developing world and the richer world (aggregating the formerly socialist economies and established market economies together) more than doubled for the under-fives age group and almost doubled for the 5–14 years group (see table 2.1).

In 1980, the probability of dying before the age of five was 16/1000 in the high-income countries and 135 in the middle and lower-income countries (table 3.2). The rate in the middle and lower income countries combined was 8.4 times that of the rich countries. By 1998, the probability of dying before the age of five in middle and lower income countries had improved (from 135/1000 to 79/1000), but the improvement in the rich countries had been proportionately greater (from 16/1000 to 6/1000). As a consequence, the rate for the middle and lower income countries had gone from 8.4 times that of the rich countries to 13.2 times, an increase of 57%.

Table 2.1 The widening global health gap, 1950–90

Age group	1950	1980	1990
< 5	3.4	6 4	8.8
5–14	3.8	6.5	7.0
15–59	2.2	1.8	1.7
60+	1.3	1.4	1.4

Note: Age-specific death rates expressed as the rate ratio {DDC}/{FSE+EME}; the ratio of the age-specific death rates in the demographically developing countries {DDC} to the combined rates of the formerly socialist economies {FSE} and the established market economies {EME}.

Source: Calculated from World Bank 1993, p 203, table A.5.

Table 2.2 Probability of dying before the age of five years (per 1000)

Country group	1980	1998
High-income countries	15	6
Middle and lower-income countries	135	79
Rate ratio: {low + mid}/{high}	8.4	13.2

Source: From World Bank 2000a, p 276, table 2.

The immediate reasons for the lagging health status of the developing world are well known. They may be categorised as: lack of access to health care, barriers to healthier ways of living, and hazardous living environments. These are the proximal causes of poor health. They reflect and mediate influences that need to be understood in more macro terms: lack of resources and barriers to economic and social development. Lack of access to care is associated with family and national poverty and user pays health care systems, increasingly privatisatised and without insurance. Barriers to healthier ways of living include poverty, powerlessness, alienation and violence. Hazardous living environments are associated with family, regional and national poverty, war, lagging infrastructure development and environmental degradation.

Welcome to the New World Order, the global village, buzzing with exciting new technologies and escalating productivity. But the New World Order (NWO) has some downsides too including widening economic polarisation and the rising challenges to democratic sovereignty.

The NWO presents both promises and opportunities for health as well as threats and hazards. The opportunities include: powerful sick care technologies, improved knowledge about the pre-conditions for better health and the resources to create healthy, safe and supportive environments. However, for many millions of people, the threats to health associated with the New World Order are far more immediate: poverty, alienation and violence, collapse of social infrastructure, unemployment and underemployment and environmental degradation. (Some useful recent references: United Nations Research Institute for Social Development 1995, Werner and Sanders 1997, Sabha 2000, Kim et al. 2000 and Raghuram 2000.)

Widening health inequalities correspond closely to widening economic inequalities, both within and between countries. From 1960 to 1995, the relative wealth of the richest 20 countries and the poorest 20 countries, measured in terms of per capita gross domestic product, has widened from a 14-fold gap to a 29-fold gap (World Bank 2000a, p 51, box 3.3). Income inequality between individuals has also increased globally over the last two decades (ibid.). This widening gap reflects the structured unfairness of the global economy. It is a steeply sloping playing field.

Industry and trade are the sectors of social life where wealth is produced and where the distribution of wealth is determined. To narrow the income gap and the health gap, conditions for productive industry and mutually beneficial trade must be created. However, the structures and rules currently determining the production and distribution of wealth are strongly biased in favour of the rich strata of the rich countries. This can be demonstrated in relation to agriculture, commodities, manufacturing, technology, capital and labour. Examination of each of these sectors of production and trade demonstrates how widening inequality is structured into the New World Order.

The regulation of global agriculture has involved one-way trade liberalisation. Developing countries have been forced to stop supporting subsistence farming and to move to export production including the encouragement of agribusiness. However, the industrialised countries continue to subsidise and protect their own farming, and in some cases, dump subsidised products in Third World markets. Global trade in commodities is largely a buyers' market. There are many sellers and a small number of powerful buyers. There is generally tight price competition and with changing technologies many of the markets are quite static. Where producer countries have tried to get together as producer cartels, they have faced strong opposition and threats of retaliation.

Manufacturing globally is dominated by the big corporates and there is fierce competition between them in many of their markets. However, in these markets brand competition and technological innovation play a major role and the producers have some discretion with respect to price. This contributes to 'sticky pricing' where increases in input costs are passed on in prices but productivity savings flow to profit. Where poor countries, selling agricultural produce and other commodities, trade with rich countries, selling manufactures, technology and services, there tends to be a progressive deterioration in the terms of trade. Prices for agricultural products and commodities fall relative to the prices for manufactures. Farmers have to produce more to buy the same basket of imported goods.

Trade in technology is likewise a one-way street. Poor countries have to pay for patented know-how from the large corporates whose property rights are protected by the World Trade Organisation. Poor countries are further disadvantaged by the barriers they face in producing new technologies; building a technologically trained workforce and building institutional capacity for research and development.

Like technology, access to capital is controlled in the heartlands of capitalism, by the transnational corporations (TNCs), banks and the money markets. Capital flows to poor countries are generally conditional upon free market reform and social stability and even then they carry a high premium for risk. The barriers to poor countries developing their own indigenous manufacturing are huge; not just the price of capital and technology but the exposure to cheaper imports consequent upon the forced dismantling of import protection.

Labour markets are where free trade stops (except for the trade in 'symbolic analysts'). Reich has coined the terms 'routine production workers', 'personal service workers' and the 'symbolic analysts' to describe the new structures of stratification and polarisation emerging across global labour markets (Reich 1992). Immigration barriers to the movement of labour within the routine production and personal service sectors mean that while the distribution of work is determined by the owners of capital and technology, the movement of labour is tightly contained by national boundaries. Where capital chooses not to go, there will be no work. The structured unfairness of this regime has two dimensions: the capacity of TNCs to take mass production to very-low-wage sites; and the protection of living standards in the rich countries. The symbolic analysts are of course the exception. They compete in a labour market that is increasingly integrated globally, face growing demand for their skills and command proportionately higher salaries. The ways in which the rich countries encourage the brain drain by selectively admitting symbolic analysts provides a metaphor for the continuing flow of value from South to North.

     This is a very brief overview of a very complex field. For an introduction to what is a very large literature, see Hettne (1995), Coote (1992) or Nader et al. (1993).

Structured unfairness

The structured unfairness of the New World Order is not an accident. It is a direct consequence of the economic policies of the last two decades that have restructured the world economy in ways that favour the interests of the rich capitalist metropolis. These policies have been packaged separately for the poor world and the rich world. In the poor world, they are called 'structural adjustment' (see Gibbon 1995 and Jeebhay et al. 1997) and in the rich world, they are labelled more generally as 'neoliberalism' (Boyer and Drache 1996) or 'economic rationalism' in Australia (Pusey 1991). However, despite the different packaging, these two policy regimes are very similar.

     Structural adjustment packages, which are commonly forced on developing countries as a condition of debt relief, generally include:

- re-orienting the economy to export markets (and withdrawing support for subsistence agriculture);
- reducing import barriers;
- making the economy more attractive for foreign investment;
- creating more 'competitive' labour markets (and weakening unions); and
- moving to small government, with low taxes, privatisation and reduced public sector provision.

     A very similar package of policies has been implemented in many industrialised countries (especially the Anglophone countries) under the flag of neoliberalism. The main difference in the industrialised countries is the somewhat greater focus on eliminating barriers to international capital flows rather than on being more receptive to foreign investment. The emphasis on reducing import barriers is also modulated somewhat according to the strengths of local producers.

     At the heart of neoliberalism is a suspicion of government and of democratic process; an argument for limiting the role of government to certain core functions, such as law and order, while allowing the free market to achieve its efficiencies unconstrained by public sector competition or regulation. Such policies are very much about adapting the economies of both poor and rich countries to take their assigned places in the emerging New World Order.

The success of neoliberalism

So why are these policies so persuasive? Have they been imposed through the power of those whom they benefit? And if so, how and by whom? Or have people been persuaded by their particular rationality? In which case, what is the story and what is the evidence? Perhaps it is a bit of both: power and rationality. Understanding how this situation has developed is critical for public health advocates who wish to argue for a different set of policies to create a fairer (and more sustainable) world order and reduce global health inequalities.

There are very powerful forces driving the implementation of neoliberal policies. In the developing world the pre-eminent disciplinarian is the International Monetary Fund backed up by the World Bank. In the case of structural adjustment lending, or the 'bailouts' of Mexico (1995) and Indonesia and Thailand (1997), the sanctions behind the adoption of shock therapy policies are crude and public. (Although more extreme discipline may sometimes be called upon, as with the economic boycotts of Cuba, Vietnam and Iraq and the bombing of Iraq and Yugoslavia.)

The adoption of corresponding policies in the industrialised countries is also the focus of powerful forces although not so blatant. The two major institutions through which this pressure is expressed are the mass media and the financial markets. The forums of representative democracy are both the focus of this attack and one of the key places where the argument will be determined. The corporate interest is well represented in government through the involvement of big money and powerful media groups in electoral politics and helps to explain the rise of Tweedledum politics in government. With instantaneous global news, the financial markets are very aware of the policy directions that governments all over the world are considering, and business sentiment in relation to such decision-making can be communicated equally rapidly through currency sell-offs and exchange rates fall-offs.

Clearly, there are forces associated with the elites of metropolitan capitalism who are able to exercise powerful influence on policy debate and the reshaping of the New World Order.

However, there is a rationality to neoliberalism also: a rationality that can be articulated in terms of the 'wealth through growth' proposition. This story argues that global well-being depends on new wealth creation (reflected in economic growth). Wealth creation is driven by new technologies (enhanced productivity); new frontiers of industrialisation (where people with energy and needs gain new access to technology and capital); creation of new domestic markets (commodifying functions previously performed outside the market); and by the exploitation of natural resources. These developments are all best managed by market forces (hence the need for deregulation and small government). This story is told very persuasively in successive annual reports of the World Bank and the World Trade Organisation.

'Wealth through growth' is a plausible story and is consistent with some histories. It is also consistent also with the material interests and perspectives of the elites of the rich world. It provides the rationale for structural adjustment and neoliberalism.

Global crisis deferred

There are alternative stories. The story of 'wealth through growth' can be relativised by considering the story of 'global crisis deferred'. This story is not disseminated through the mass media but it circulates widely in oppositional movements and in developing countries. It was certainly present at Seattle in November 1999 and at the People's Health Assembly at Gonoshathaya Kendra in Bangladesh in 2000 (see http://www.phamovement.org/). Two recent accounts that develop this story are presented by Shutt (1998) and by Went (2000a).

According to this story, the global economy faces a looming crisis which is continually deferred through adaptive policies, many of which make the structural crisis worse. The threat of crisis stems from the imbalance of accelerating productivity over constrained demand. Increasingly efficient production for increasingly global markets tends to a decline in aggregate employment and therefore a decline in demand. Corporations see sluggish demand growth as a threat to profits and respond by strategies aimed at cost cutting (especially labour costs) and expanding market share (reflected in the rapid increase in mergers and acquisitions). Both strategies contribute to reducing the buying power of the workforce: cost cutting by replacing labour with technology and replacing high wage labour with low wage labour and the market share strategy through concentration of production (and reduced aggregate employment). The declining buying power of the labour force further threatens profits and reinforces the need for strategies of cost cutting and market share. Nevertheless, the crisis (due to declining demand associated with lower wages and slower jobs growth) is continually deferred, because consumption levels are maintained (although not high growth rates) through other channels including:

- increasing household debt in the North (as corporate profit is diverted from new investment, parked in the financial sector and available for consumer credit);
- bubble consumption among small shareholders (due to overly optimistic income expectations associated with inflated asset values);
- consumption by the new global middle class, including wealthy minorities in low and middle income countries (relatively small proportionately but large in absolute numbers in the case of China, India, Indonesia, Brazil, Pakistan, Bangladesh, Mexico, etc.);
- the continuing flow of funds from the economies of the South to the banks of the North through national debt repayment;
- the continuing flow of value from the South to the North through unequal and unfair trading relationships; and
- the conversion of environmental assets into current income flows.

Making sense of widening global health inequalities

To review the argument. Global inequalities in health are widening. They are clearly related to widening economic inequalities. Widening economic inequalities are related to the structured unfairness of the New World Order. The structured unfairness of the New World Order has been actively created through a raft of policies implemented through the muscle of structural adjustment and the logic of economic rationalism.

We have compared two stories which claim to make sense of what is happening in the global economy and which therefore might provide some guidance with respect to inequalities in health. These I have labelled: 'wealth through growth' and 'global crisis deferred'.

In terms of health futures, 'wealth through growth' counsels the poor to 'suffer now for better health later'. The apologists for 'wealth through growth' recognise that this is a bitter pill but they argue:

- that the glass is actually half full – that in almost all countries life expectancy is actually increasing (and focusing on inequality merely reflects the politics of envy);
- that the widening of income inequality in the late 20th century was not as bad as during the 19th century;
- that widening health inequalities are not actually due to economic reform;
- that although health inequalities may be partly due to economic reform, these costs are offset by the benefits;
- that the health consequences of economic reform can be ameliorated by better policy and governance; and
- that they have now learned from their earlier mistakes and their revised policy package can now be trusted (see, in particular, World Bank 1993 and 2000a).

'Global crisis deferred' suggests on the other hand that the burden of disease associated with economic inequality globally reflects the costs of maintaining the well-being of the North (at the cost of the health of the South), maintaining the new global middle class (at the cost of the health of the poor) and of maintaining the health of the symbolic analysts (at the cost of the health of the routine production and personal service workers). Further, the 'crisis deferred' analysis points to a number of practical policy directions which might help to recreate the conditions for Health for All. These include reregulating the financial sector, cancelling Third World debt, decentering the export-led growth paradigm, moving to sustainable production, controlling the labour process, redistributing work, redistributing income, and applying democracy and planning in economic and social development (Went 2000).

However, moving from broad principles to the practical implementation of new institutions and regulatory frameworks will involve a great deal of policy discussion and movement-building. The social movements that will drive the implementation of such policies will involve new forms of solidarity and new ways of organising. The 2000 People's Health Assembly (http://www.phamovement.org/) brought together public health activists and grass roots community organisations from 93 countries; working together to build the links, the ideas and the confidence that will be necessary.

Scissors, stone, paper: my truth overrides yours

Which story is really true? The global economy is impossibly complex and we are all inside it. Different problems and opportunities confront different stakeholders in different places and times and suggest different explanations and strategies. 'Wealth through growth' has some explanatory and strategic power and some merit as a basis for policy. However, the story of 'crisis deferred' throws a different light on some of the longer term and system dynamics which are ignored by 'wealth through growth' and also on the distributional consequences. However, 'crisis deferred', like 'wealth through growth', reflects a particular set of concerns expressed at a particular time in history. There are many more stories which can be told, which are being told; the truth of each story is bound up with the context, interests and perspectives of the story teller.

One of the most potent and subtle projections of power is the privileged access to truth which is claimed by the spokes-institutions for global capitalism, led by the World Bank. The theories and models which underly the earnest concern of the Bank and the blustering of the World Trade Organisation are based on a (claim of) privileged access to truth. Their truth overrides the misapprehensions and illusions of people who see things differently. There are two ways of responding to this arrogance. One way is to make counter claims for different truths. Another way is to recognise the aspiration to singular truth as a fantasy in the face of impossible complexity and our own embeddedness in the system we are trying to understand.

'Wealth through growth' and 'crisis deferred' reflect two different perspectives on the contemporary global economy. However, they serve different purposes, take different time frames, assign different values, and have different implications for different stakeholders.

Many of the protagonists on different sides of economic debate are united by this paradox: that somewhere, there is a singular truth; likewise, the proposition that it can be revealed, through whatever methodology. I am suggesting, to the contrary, that economic policy debate needs to go beyond the logic and facts of abstract argument. It needs to include a sharing of the worldviews and life experiences and hopes and fears that set the frameworks and orientation of the different stories and perspectives. Debate in this sense involves a deep listening to the life worlds that animate the different stories, listening to the farmers of the Third World as well as the capitalists of the metropolis.

Implications for practice

I draw four conclusions from the argument I have presented:
- The political economy tradition provides theoretical models and descriptive frameworks that can help us to understand the wider context that frames inequality in health.
- Debates about economic policy and structural reform are key determinants of the fairness of the New World Order. Public health people must be able to speak in the language of political economy if they are to take part in these debates.
- The fairness of the New World Order will not be determined by debate alone. Public health people who would reduce inequalities through fairer structures may also need to participate in the organisational politics through which the new rules and new institutions are being shaped.
- Activists who wish to advance the interests of poor countries in debates about economic policy and the fairness of global structures need to do so in collaboration with people in those countries, giving voice to their experience and aspirations as well as their argument.

If public health activists are to engage in debates over the fairness and the politics of the New World Order, it is important that we are reflexive about the particularities of our own positions.

Further Reading

Hettne, B 1995, Development theory and the three worlds, Longman Scientific and Technical, Harlow.
  – *One of the most accessible yet broadly based accounts of development theory in the context of the ascendancy of fin de siècle transnational capitalism, providing a broadly based analysis from a pro-Third World perspective.*
United Nations Research Institute for Social Development 1995, States of disarray: the social effects of globalisation, UNRISD, London.
  – *A survey of the social effects of globalisation. It is publications like this that make the US Congress refuse to pay their dues to the UN system.*
Went, R 2000, Globalisation: neoliberal challenge, radical responses, Pluto Press with International Institute for Research and Education, London.
  – *A challenging analysis of the current crisis of global capitalism.*

3
Globalisation and environmental change:
implications for health and health inequalities

Colin D. Butler, Bob Douglas and A.J. McMichael

Introduction

Contemporary globalisation has three key elements. Two – long-distance trade and the diffusion of ideas and technology – have existed, albeit in less intense forms, for millennia (Landes 1999). Its third element, increasingly free of social constraint, is capitalism, still in many ways intellectually wedded to a time when human impact on the earth was puny. This triad, with increasing technological capacity, now threatens the ecological and social fabric of civilisation.

Two writers were especially influential in the development of capitalism. Adam Smith, though mindful of the risk of monopolies (Schlefer 1998), enumerated numerous advantages to material production made possible by specialisation, self-interest, and the rule of law. David Ricardo's theory of 'comparative advantage' demonstrated how, under certain assumptions, free trade could result in mutual gains. Taken at the most extreme, these theories lead to the view that an 'invisible hand' can act automatically to maximise economic efficiency, and, implicitly, public welfare. The laissez-faire capitalism that marked early and mid-19th century Britain accompanied, though it did not necessarily cause, spectacular increases in productivity. But soon, this extreme form of capitalism proved socially unsustainable (Gray 1999).

During the early industrial revolution, life expectancy in the provincial British towns and cities probably deteriorated (Szreter 1997), and few of the health gains which eventually emerged should be uncritically attributed to the market economy. Much credit belongs to policies initiated by reformers, often wealthy, reacting to the excesses of 'blind' capitalism, detailed, for example, by the novelist Charles Dickens. Other reforms included improved occupational safety standards, a widened franchise, an upgrading of state-provided education (Gray 1999, p 14) and a resurgence of smallpox vaccination (Szreter 1997). Internationally, agitation helped to end the slave trade. None of these reforms were 'economically rational'. Smith's invisible hand clearly needed guidance.

The resurgence of marketism

The 25 years following World War II, a time of comparatively restrained marketism, witnessed the highest growth rates in history. Primary health care, decolonisation, war-fostered technological and organisational improvements, and greater intellectual and public support from the more advanced economies helped to spread the wealth and create the hope needed to make significant improvements in the living standards of the newly described 'developing countries' also seem plausible.

The inaugural speeches of presidents Truman and Kennedy each pledged to reduce Third World poverty (Butler 2000a). The desire to help the South escape poverty was expressed by many institutions, especially the World Health Organisation, and by commissions such as the Pearson Report (Pearson 1969). But the 1960s, starting as the 'decade of development', also saw the failure of U.S. President Johnson's Great Society and increasing US entanglement in Vietnam. Third World development, formerly seen as a bulwark against Marxist ideology, was replaced by a strategy of supporting Third World strongmen who proclaimed anti-Communism (Hopkinson 1999).

In the 1970s, Keynesianism suffered its own crisis when its policies were unable to solve the oil price rise, 'stagflation' and rising unemployment. Public support faltered, and a shift to the right occurred, especially in English-speaking economies. A new economic dogma arose with a central commitment to marketism – a swing back to the more laissez-faire economic theories of the 19th century, once thought totally discredited.

Marketism remains an integral component of contemporary globalisation. However, though increased international interdependence has been accelerated by trade deregulation, the next stage of globalisation may operate under far more restrained market principles. Gray also warns of 'wild' globalisation, in which the effort to deregulate trade globally is replaced by bilateral agreements and a resurgence of protectionism (Gray 2000).

Initially, supporters of marketism sought public support, from populations that retained a comparatively strong belief in social justice, by asserting that real wages for the poor, in both North and South, would increase through a process of 'trickle down'. It was argued that cutting government services, including to social security and education, would liberate efficiency and entrepreneurial zest. Claims were made that free trade and 'level playing fields' would benefit everyone through the 'inviolable' economic law of comparative advantage (Toohey 1994, Navarro 1998).

Problems of marketism

But other commentators pointed out that level playing fields are illusory. There is an inherent contradiction between principles of marketism which promote and reward self-interest and the possibility of mutual benefit through comparative advantage. Mehmet describes this paradox as the 'Eurocentrism' of economic theories. He argues that Western economists selectively promote economic principles that result in the maintenance or increase, rather than reversal, of existing international inequality (Mehmet 1995). For example, impartial 'market forces' are used to justify the divergence of domestic wage rates between the skilled and unskilled, and of per capita national incomes between the North and South.

In exchange for continued credit lines, many countries of the Third World were obliged to take strong doses of marketism's medicine, in the form of 'structural adjustment programs' (Bello et al. 1994, Chossudovsky 1997). These involved the reduction of already slender government services, including for health care and education. They contributed to health losses in many extremely poor countries, and have been identified as contributing to the tuberculosis (Grange and Zumia 1999) and HIV epidemics in sub-Saharan Africa (Anonymous 1994a) and also to the Rwandan genocide (Chossudovsky 1997, pp 111–22). Partly as a result, serious communicable diseases, once hoped to be largely controlled by the year 2000, remain common among the poor, following 'fault lines' of poverty between countries (Farmer 1996).

Supporters of globalisation point to substantial improvements of many indicators of well-being, including global life expectancy (Castles 2000) and literacy rates as evidence of its success. But these indicators have many social and technological causes, many of which operated either before the demise of Keynesianism or independently of marketism.

Average global life expectancy has increased, and it is difficult to disentangle the relative causal contributions. However, it would be premature to attribute sole, or even major, credit to 'globalisation' for this improvement. Improved access to both health care and education in many poor countries, particularly in the early post-World War II decades, occurred because of deliberate intervention by both the state and non-government sectors. An example is primary health care, whether that envisaged by the drafters of the Alma Ata declaration (Werner and Sanders 1987), or more targeted approaches such as the expanded program of immunisation and oral rehydration therapy (Wisner 1988, Taylor and Jolly 1988). It is possible that the lagged effect of such interventions in the post-World War II era has been of more benefit than the policies of accelerated globalisation. Also of concern is that, in both sub-Saharan Africa and parts of Eastern Europe, life expectancy has fallen (United Nations Population Division 1999, Leon et al. 1997). In Russia, the decline appears to have started several decades earlier in rural areas, perhaps because of the sacrifice of social needs to military purposes during the Cold War (Demine 2000).

Is there a relationship between capitalism and moral values?

Hirschmann (1982) reviews a centuries-long debate about the effect of trade and capitalism upon the moral values of society. He argues that the relationship is cyclic, subject, at least partially, to self-correction by reformers whose influence increases whenever the harshness of unrestrained capitalism becomes too visible. Many early capitalist theorisers predicted that commerce would improve civil society, by linking consumers together in mutual self-interest. A century later, reverse views were dominant, with fears expressed that capitalist society was undermining the moral foundations upon which society rested. Reduced 'offshoring' of capitalism's excesses may have contributed to this perceptual change. In the 17th century, many of capitalism's unpleasant aspects, including the slavery and forced labour which were transforming the Old World and its offshoots (Landes 1999), were hidden from its main beneficiaries in Europe. The inhumanity and excesses of the industrial revolution, however, occurred at home.

Morality is subjective, and the examples of slave-labour camps in Stalinist Russia and the barbarity of the Chinese Cultural Revolution (Salisbury 1992, pp 248–50) illustrate that capitalism has no monopoly on immoral behaviour. However, in our time, in wealthy liberal democracies, concerns are increasingly expressed that the influence of marketism is negatively permeating social value systems, illustrated, for example, by the popularity of expressions such as 'greed is good' (Beatty 1999, Totaro and Brown 2000 pp 1, 8). Aid budgets to developing countries have fallen well below previously adopted targets. Marked differentials in income and access to resources are not only tolerated, but positively encouraged as evidence of societal success.

Increasing domestic and international inequality

Inequality within many developed and developing countries, including China, has risen in recent decades (Barrett et al. 2000, OECD 1995, Deininger and Squires 2000, Xu and Zou 2000). Real wages for the low-skilled have been static or declining, while, at the same time, wages of executives and the highly skilled have increased (Frank and Cook 1995). Publicly provided services have declined; for the poor and middle classes, promises of 'trickle down' and 'increased capacity' are wearing thin. Many anti-World Trade Organisation protestors claim to lobby for a better deal for the South, although this motivation is probably conflated, by many, with the fear of further low-skilled job transfers from the North.

Global income inequality, measured using exchange-adjusted currency, has increased enormously in recent decades (Butler and Smith 1999, United Nations Development Program 1999). Figure 3.1 shows a Lorenz curve, which plots the global distribution of exchange-adjusted income in US dollars, allowing calculation of the Gini coefficient for 1997. In 1997, after adjustment for income inequality within nations, the global Gini coefficient was 79.3% (Butler and Smith 1999). Figure 3.2 shows the trend in global income inequality between 1964 and 1999.

The purchasing power parity debate

Some workers contend that the trend of global income inequality measured by income adjusted for purchasing power parity (PPP) is far less clear (Berry et al. 1983, Summers and Heston 1991, Firebaugh 2000, Melchior et al. 2000). PPP incomes attempt to measure the 'real' value of goods and services consumed in any economy (Summers and Heston 1991). 'Real' in this case means purchasing power adjusted, not for inflation, but for the lower cost of many goods and services in many relatively poor economies, especially those that are not internationally traded. Proponents of this measure argue that PPP incomes more accurately reflect the consumption of goods and services, and thus of genuine living standards. We argue that, while neither method is perfect, the use of PPP adjusted incomes is a particularly flawed measure of comparative international bargaining power. Lack of space, unfortunately, restricts further discussion of this here (Butler and Smith, in preparation).

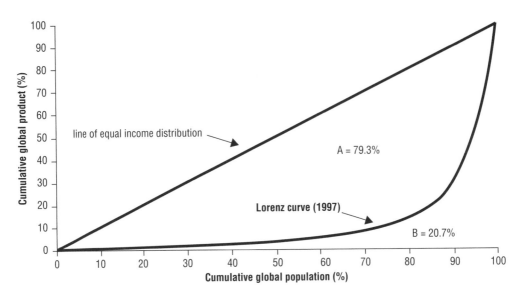

Figure 3.1 Global distribution of exchange-adjusted income in United States dollars, 1997

Note: The Lorenz curve plots the cumulative income received by the cumulative population. If income is distributed equally, the curve will follow the diagonal line. The Gini coefficient is derived by calculating the ratio of the area between the straight line and the Lorenz curve to the area under the straight line [a/(a+b)]. It can vary between 0% (perfectly equal distribution) and 100% (all income received by a single person). The above distribution has a Gini coefficient of 79.3%. In comparison, the Gini coefficient for Australia, in 1993, was 30.2%.

Does inequality matter?

Some economists argue that inequality is irrelevant, provided absolute incomes are rising for the poorest. However, inequality fails to maximise the health and living standard gains of increasing average incomes and has many adverse social effects (Wilkinson 1996a, Berkman and Kawachi 2000). While no population, even pre-agricultural, is truly egalitarian (Price and Feinman 1995), excessive inequality impairs social cohesion and shifts average expenditure towards private consumption and away from public goods (Magnani 2000).

Both the scale and trend of global exchange-adjusted income demonstrate that globali-sation is not meeting its stated goal of wealth for all. International power, rather than becoming more evenly shared over time, has increasingly been concentrated. Brazil, recog-nised as a country of substantial income and power inequality (Martin and Schumann 1997), has a lower Gini coefficient (60.1% in 1995, World Bank 1999b) than the world now has, measured in either exchange or PPP-adjusted terms. This supports claims that the wealthy countries of the North practise economic slavery, economic racism (Abbasi 1999, Korten 1995, pp 230–2) and environmental neocolonialism (Aggarwal and Narain 1991).

The recent slight fall in global inequality is encouraging and intriguing. It appears to be

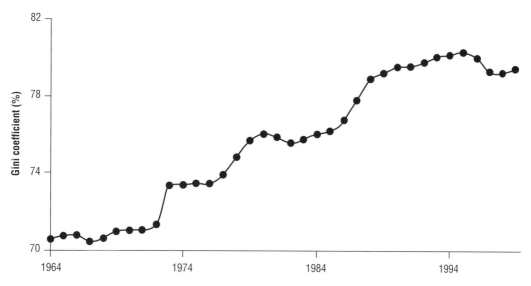

Figure 3.2 Global income distribution (adjusted for national income distribution), 1964–99

Note: This shows a time series of Gini coefficients for 1964–99, measuring the distribution of global income in US$. The coefficient increased from 70.5% in 1964 to greater than 80% in 1995, before falling slightly to 79.4% in 1999. In comparison, the Gini coefficient for Brazil, which has the most unequal income distribution for any nation, is less than 65%. The data are adjusted for national income distributions and make the assumption that these remained constant at their most recently known levels. This is conservative because there is evidence that national income has become more unequally distributed in recent years (Deininger and Squires, 1996; Butler and Smith, in preparation). Therefore, global income distribution in the earlier part of the time series is likely to have been more equal than shown.

Source: Original national data (foreign exchange-adjusted income, income distribution and population, all at national levels) from World Bank

caused mainly by unusually large increases in the per capita incomes of several populous poor nations, including China, India, Indonesia and Bangladesh. These economies all grew faster than the global average in 1997. However, the decline in global inequality was partially reversed in 1999, reflecting a decline in the Indonesian economy. Adjusting for the recent increase in Chinese domestic inequality (Xu and Zhou 2000) is likely to further erode this improvement.

Courting global environmental failure

Globalisation's unprecedented power and scale jeopardise civilisation (Union of Concerned Scientists 1992) in another fundamental way: by changing the environment at an unprecedented scale and rate. For example, it is estimated that 33–50% of the world's land surface has been transformed by human action (Vitousek et al. 1997). More atmospheric nitrogen is fixed by industrial processes than from all combined natural terrestrial sources; more than 50% of all accessible surface fresh water is now used by humanity (Postel et al. 1996, Vitousek et al. 1997). Well over a decade ago, when global population was only 75% of its current level, Vitousek et al. (1986) estimated that 40% of the products of terrestrial photosynthesis were appropriated by humans.

To optimists, these figures demonstrate increasing human mastery over the environment (Simon and Kahn 1984). But there is a growing global consensus that these developments are of critical concern. This is reflected, for example, by the efforts to limit stratospheric ozone depletion, the work of the Intergovernmental Panel on Climate Change and the proposal for a similar international body, the Millennium Assessment, designed to assess the extent to which ecosystems can support ongoing human needs (Masood 2000).

Declining biodiversity and ecosystem health

The decline in global biodiversity has been characterised as the sixth major extinction in Earth's history, the first to be caused by a single species (Chapin et al. 2000). Biodiversity decline also leads to profound alterations in ecosystem functioning, particularly by the removal of top predators (Diamond 1991, pp 322–323, Purvis and Hector 2000, Williams 1998). The resulting 'eco-impoverisation' (Butler 1997) is likely to have adverse, human health effects, through several possible mechanisms.

Possibly the best recognised of these is the loss of genetic material for research into pharmaceutical or alternative food crops (Cassis 1998, Lister and Schrire 1999, Tanne 1998). However, declining biodiversity is also likely to have substantial impacts by impairing eco-system services, which currently provide large economic benefits to humanity (Costanza et al. 1997). The value of these (usually uncosted) benefits may exceed the total value of the global human economy, which ecological economists argue is a subset of the wider natural economy (Daly 1996). Examples of ecosystem services to humanity include pollination, reduction of water runoff and erosion during storms and heavy rain, resulting in reduced flooding and drought, and water purification through natural filters (Chichlinisky and Head 1998). Mangrove ecosystems foster fish breeding and provide protection from seasurges, which are likely to be of greater significance in association with the rising sea levels predicted as a con-sequence of climatic warming. Declining biodiversity reduces the resilience of ecosystems, and may leave them more vulnerable to future natural and anthropogenic perturbations.

Falling biodiversity may interact with climate change, leading to a reduced terrestrial carbon sink, which, in turn causes more warming and more eco-impoverisation. This might occur through intensification and prolongation of the El Niño phase (Guilderson and Schrag 1998), in association with increased logging, burning and, possibly changes to the flowering and fruiting patterns, which reduce the effectiveness of forest reproduction (Curran et al. 1999, Gascon et al. 2000, Hartshorn and Bynum 1999). The progressive decline in ecosystem productivity and stability would be expected ultimately to affect human health and well-being, particularly by adverse flow-on effects to infrastructure and aspects of the measured economy.

Climate change

Irrespective of further decline in global emissions, the atmospheric concentration of the major greenhouse gas, carbon dioxide, will increase for at least another century, because of its long atmospheric life (Houghton et al. 1996, pp 15–6). There is increasing recognition that significant climate change is occurring (Schiermeier 2001), although the precise cause or causes (Ackerman et al. 2000, Lockwood et al. 1999, Keeling and Whorf 2000) and extent (Allen et al. 2000) remain uncertain. Human health effects are predicted to include changes in the distribution of vector-borne diseases, increased heatwaves and increased allergies (McMichael et al. 1996). Climate change is also likely to have many adverse economic effects likely to harm human health, including from sea level rise (Mitrovica et al. 2001). Changes in agricultural and fisheries productivity (O'Brien et al. 2000) may also reduce regional food security (Parry et al. 1999). Increased extreme weather events (Easterling et al. 2000, Knutson et al. 1998) not only from storms but also from droughts and floods are a climatic wild card, which could substantially impair food security, the reinsurance industry, tourism and morale.

There are many interactions which involve climate change. Recently, an interaction between climate change and ozone depletion has been hypothesised to partially explain the persistence of significant global stratospheric ozone depletion (Shindell et al. 1998). Global warming, in turn, may be aggravated by a number of feedback mechanisms, including not only deforestation (Myers 1997) but also changes in the ocean leading to decreased uptake of carbon dioxide (Joos et al. 1999) and warming of tundra, which may liberate additional quantities of both carbon dioxide and the second most important anthropogenic greenhouse gas, methane (Cicerone 1988).

The deteriorating global environment

Figure 3.3 shows a time series index using three categories of global environmental data: biodiversity, the atmosphere and stratospheric ozone. Each category has shown a progressive decline. It is conceivable that some of components of this index may be shown by subsequent research to be of less importance than currently believed. For example, the significance of carbon dioxide as the most important greenhouse gas has recently been questioned (Hansen et al. 2000, Smaglik 2000, Veizer et al. 2000). However, there are likely to be other changes, not measured with the same accuracy over time, that are at least as important.

Critics may respond that the decline in the different environmental indices shown is a small price to pay for the much larger increase – almost 400% – which has occurred in the human population over the past century. However, previous increases in human population resulted in far less disturbance to these global environmental indicators. A threshold has been passed, beyond which human activities have altered multiple environmental sectors on a global scale. The indices are continuing to decline. If, as seems inevitable, these trends continue, a point may be reached where irreversible adverse consequences, possibly to our entire civilisation, become unstoppable (Butler 2000a, Butler 2000b, Butler 2001).

The rate of decline in the index depends on the scale. Zero for each element represents

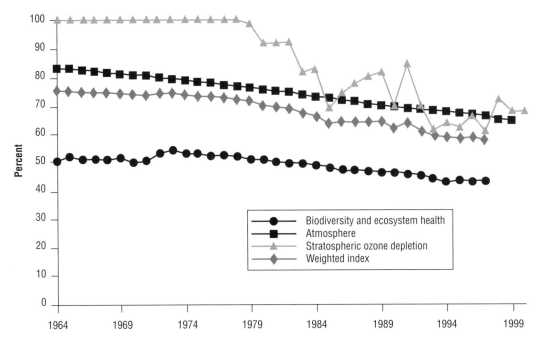

Figure 3.3 Indices of global environmental change, 1964–99

Note: This shows time series indices for three categories of the global environment of concern: biodiversity and ecosystem health; greenhouse gas accumulation; and stratospheric ozone depletion (SOD). Each category incorporates several elements. The maximum (100%) reflects the level in nature prior to human-associated changes. Monitoring of SOD commenced in 1978, and we made the conservative assumption that no decline had occurred before then. The SOD index is weighted for surface area (of the earth beneath the thinning ozone layer), but not cloud cover. For most of these indicators, the trend in nature (eg, tropical forest cover or the average trophic level of the marine fish harvest) has declined. In contrast, the concentration of the two major human-generated greenhouse gases, carbon dioxide and methane, has increased. Sensitivity analysis demonstrates a similar trend for the combined index, irrespective of the weightings given to the components of the various sub-indices. Each index has shown a gradual decline, and the combined index has fallen from 75% in 1964 to 57.5% in 1997.

a clearly undesirable level, such as a doubling in concentration of the main greenhouse gas, carbon dioxide, or a decline in moist tropical forest cover to 20% of its original area. Scientific uncertainty regarding a 'safe' level of decline is substantial, and we caution that the level we have selected as zero may be too optimistic. Because of inertial factors, further decline in the index appears inevitable during this century. However, concerted human effort may reduce the rate of decline, and, eventually, change the direction of the trend.

'Gray economics'

Classical economics, born in the 18th century when human impact on the natural world was modest, made little allowance for ecological limits, despite Malthus's concerns. Even today, many economists, untempered by an appreciation of ecological limits, continue to assert that supply and demand, together with substitution and science, can safely steer humanity through the shoals of the future (Simon and Kahn 1984, Singer 1989, Anonymous 1994b, Daly 1996, Anonymous 1997).

Past successes from this approach have fuelled the illusion of future indefinite success (Hamilton 1994). But the short-term priorities of capitalism, the inertia of a still-growing global population trying to catch up with Northern levels of consumption (Butler 1997), and the failure of leadership by the advanced nations now risks runaway climate change and unprecedented ecoimpoverisation, with uncertain and probably harmful impacts upon future generations (Costanza et al. 2000). Numerous books (Daly 1996, Daly and Cobb 1989, Hamilton 1994, Henderson 1981), articles (Butler 1994), and an increasingly influential subset of the economics discipline (Dasgupta 1996) argue that the prevalent method of measuring national and global wealth is seriously misleading, particularly because of its failure to account for the depletion of natural capital (Cobb et al. 1995, Costanza et al. 1997).

Linking inequality, globalisation and environmental brinkmanship

Accelerated globalisation has exacerbated inequality at both domestic and global levels. By increasing social tensions, inequality can cause significant social disruption. Accelerated globalisation has created an unprecedented efficiency of production, particularly by the conversion of natural capital to goods and services which humans demand. Both expectations and the means to fulfil them for many people, at least in the short-term, have been raised, though millions in countries in the South, for example in South Africa, remain disappointed.

The global income inequality of recent decades (in either foreign exchange or purchasing power parity adjusted terms) quantifies an enormous division in the daily lives of billions of humans. In the world's more privileged quarters, conflict may involve the choice of TV channel to watch or the brand of pizza to choose for delivery. The information and entertainment choices generally available to and selected by such populations focus mainly on the lives of similarly endowed or wealthier people. Travel to a developing country by this population, if it occurs at all, is generally to a resort or game park, where there will be little contact with ordinary people. Much of the media coverage provided in the North about the 80% of the global population who, in 1997, shared less than 13% of the total global foreign exchange-adjusted income, is paid for by aid organisations, frequently requesting funds for child sponsorship, or concerns periodic catastrophes, wars and epidemics. Economic forecasts are generally confined to predicting the future only for the comparatively wealthy fraction of the global population. The extent of this division is also demonstrated by the frequently exhibited desperation of asylum seekers.

Thus, despite the rhetoric of globalisation and exaggerated claims that the internet will forge global understanding, our world is cleft broadly into two divisions, which know comparatively little of each other (Butler 2000a). Given the restricted education, media exposure, family links, and life-experience of the wealthier population, it is not surprising that the concerns of the poorer world are of little concern to them.

Kaplan (1994) has suggested that some of the chaos, disease, and environmental degradation found in developing countries, especially in Africa, will spread to more privileged parts of the world. Though some politicians in wealthy countries, reportedly including former US president Bill Clinton (Anonymous 1994b), have taken this seriously, few of his constituents seem likely to.

Growing divisions in wealthy countries, illustrated for example by the homeless in Britain and the incarcerated in the US, also seem to be tolerated increasingly (and, often, justified) by the comparatively wealthy.

We suggest that the magnitude of global inequality partially accounts for the continued refusal by national governments to properly account for changes in natural and social capital, despite some tentative steps in this direction by the World Bank (Munasinghe and Shearer 1995, Daly 1996, World Bank 1997b). Instead, existing national accounting measures, though not intended for such a purpose (Cobb et al. 1995, Daly 1996), provide the standard guideposts to measure progress.

Despite the many limitations of these measures (Eckersley 1998a), governments, stock markets and shareholders are reassured by 'growth' in such indicators. But it is increasingly likely that a continuation of 'business as usual' approach to economic growth is unsustainable. Regional declines in such growth seem more likely because of adverse social and environmental change.

The impact of globalisation upon health in Australia

Globalisation has resulted in a focus on economic efficiency, loss of tariff protection and the withdrawal of agricultural subsidies. This has, for example, resulted in many small rural farm holdings becoming unprofitable in Australia. The rationalisation of the dairy industry is symptomatic of the changes that are taking place. High-density, hand-fed dairy herds farmed in new peri-urban areas that can take advantage of economies of scale, with easy access to factories and markets, are expected to render more distant grazing properties, based on small family holdings, increasingly unprofitable. As governments remove trade barriers, subsidies and commodity floor price support, a number of primary farm industries including those connected to grain, wool and meat production are being forced to adapt to the new economic imperatives. Small family farms either close or become burdened by further debt. Consequently, segments of the rural hinterland become marginalised, rural towns lose services, and critical mass and rural infrastructure decline (Douglas 2000).

From the health perspective, male youth suicide, depression and the psychological stress of unemployment are impacting on the social fabric of rural areas across Australia (Dudley et al. 1997). In the cities, globalisation is producing other mental health effects. The drive for competitiveness with cheap labour overseas has resulted in substantial restructuring of manufacturing industries and in the public service. Industrial awards are giving way to enterprise bargaining. For those in employment, job security is diminishing. Many in employment work long, unpaid hours, and the economic 'imperative' for two incomes in a family adds to the mental stresses upon families

Food production and distribution is increasingly globalised. A modern mouthful of

Australian food can contain components from across the planet. The bovine spongiform encephalitis/Creutzfeldt-Jakob disease (BSE/CJD) saga in Europe demonstrates several downsides of this, including from deregulation and the unqualified pursuit of 'efficiency' (Butler 1998). In many parts of the world, microbial food poisoning is increasing. There is a suspicion, but not yet convincing evidence, that the same is happening in Australia (Australian and New Zealand Food Authority 1999, p 17). As globalisation affects the food chain, the need for sophisticated surveillance to guarantee the fitness of food for human consumption will increase.

The impact of global environmental change upon Australian health

Insect vectors responsible for the transmission of malaria, dengue fever, Japanese encephalitis and Ross River virus disease all occur in Australia, and these can be expected to change their habitats and seasonality with climatic change. There have been increases in Australian cases of dengue fever and Ross River virus disease. Japanese encephalitis has appeared in the Torres Strait Islands. Transmission of malaria could re-occur in North Australia (Bryan et al. 1996).

Increasing climatic instability also exposes Australian populations to increased risks of flooding, droughts and bushfires with their various public health consequences. The recent significant flooding – for the third year in succession – along the Darling River basin illustrates a local example of the interaction between climate change and health. Lives may not be lost, but crops, income and morale are all harmed. Another example is the predicted extensive coral bleaching of the Great Barrier Reef, forecast as a consequence of global warming (Pockley 1999). If this occurs, it will inevitably harm the economic viability of parts of North Queensland.

Ozone depletion has allowed more ultra-violet radiation to reach the earth's surface, increasing the potential for DNA damage, skin cancers, cataracts and immunological disturbances. Human-made ozone depletion is almost certainly contributing at the margin to our high skin cancer rate. It could also be playing a subtle role in a number of auto-immune diseases which show variations in latitudinal incidence.

Demonstrating the causal relationship between environmental change and disease patterns in affluent countries like Australia is not simple, and precise health impacts are difficult to quantify. The United Nations Environment Programme (1998) estimates that Europe and (white) US populations will experience 5–10% increases in skin cancer incidence during the middle decades of this century. Australia is at the forefront of the skin cancer epidemic, a consequence both of our geographic location and our behavioural patterns of sun exposure.

Young people in Australia face chronic uncertainty about the effects of both globalisation and environmental change. They bear the brunt of unemployment and the changing nature of work (Eckersley 1997). Many are alienated and feel increasingly impotent to control their future. We speculate that the current epidemic in drug taking and escapist behaviour is particularly attributable to urbanisation, homogenisation, globalisation – particularly its element of marketism – and environmental deterioration. Several decades ago, René Dubos predicted the loss of sensory stimulation from contact with nature would be compensated by increased artificial stimulation, including by drugs (Moberg and Cohn 1991). In parts of Australia, the drug culture is becoming a way of life (Hall et al. 2000).

There is thus much uncertainty about the magnitude of the current impact of globalisation and environmental change on the health of Australians. But there is little doubt that the association is real and that the cost of these phenomena to the health of Australians is growing.

Figure 3.4 presents an overview of possible causal pathways connecting economic globalisation, global environmental change, poverty and inequity and poor health. Simple linear explanations for these linkages do not do justice to the complexities of the likely interactions, but the health of human communities can be considered an index of their economic and environmental sustainability. Affluent countries like Australia are still experiencing rising life expectancy. Australia also is currently on the winning side of the global market economy. Falling life expectancy is occurring in a number of Eastern Block countries which have less successfully adapted to global economic and environmental change (Notzon et al. 1998).

Inertial forces and long turn-around times cause dilemmas for cautious scientists and for policy makers. To delay action until they convince every sceptic of these arguments is to ignore the precautionary principle. In all but best-case scenarios, future policy makers are likely to have more pressure to act, yet less ability to influence outcomes positively. These issues entail unavoidable complexities and uncertainties; the likely changes are large-scale, unprecedented, and partially irreversible. Where possible, at the minimum, 'no regrets' policies should be adopted.

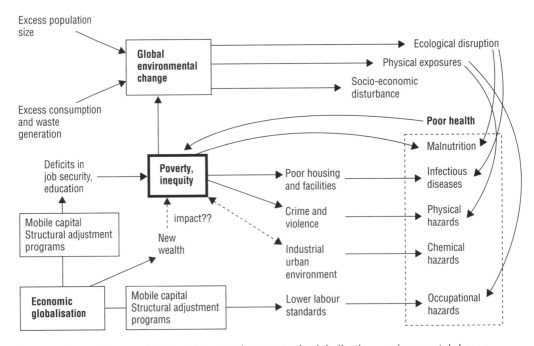

Figure 3.4 Possible causal pathways connecting economic globalisation, environmental change, inequity and poor health

Distorted goals

The negative consequences of globalisation are attributable in part to a world-view that consumption and economic transactions of almost any kind will contribute to the net well-being of humanity. This model of 'progress' fails to properly value and preserve the global commons, ignores the vital place of social capital and fails to address expanding inequality. Globalisation has given a pre-eminence to wealth creation and to the consumption of material goods, even if undermining environmental and social sustainability. The daily movement of capital, the hourly change in the Dow-Jones index, the monthly change in the national deficit and the annual change in the rate of economic growth have become the central game, ignoring the physical and social well-being of many of the world's human inhabitants. The multi-billion dollar globalised illicit drug industry, which is ravaging the health of young people worldwide, nevertheless contributes to the growth in the gross domestic product (GDP) when its black money is laundered. At the same time, the progressive destruction of environmental heritage fails to register a 'bleep' on our economic indicators, where the central objective continues to be economic growth.

What should be done?

There are evolving social and political moods that suggest that the dominance of marketism can be reversed (Saul 1997). The undoubted creativity and energy of capitalism should be harnessed for the public good. Persistent, unadjusted adherence to marketism, interacting with global environmental change, plausibly threatens the viability of civilisation as we know it (Butler 2000a; 2000b; 2001). The challenge of the coming decades may prove to be crucial for the global sustainability of *Homo sapiens*.

The health of humankind will depend increasingly on how we manage inequality and both social and ecological sustainability. Social stability and, ultimately, economic productivity demand that we discover ways of arresting expanding inequality. Sustainability must move to the centre of social policy. We urgently need to redefine what we mean by social progress and to adopt new ways of measuring it.

Simply relying upon technological progress to rescue the world for our descendants is extraordinarily risky; rather, technological progress is likely to be facilitated by full-cost accounting, including to natural and social capital. Delaying the transition to sustainability (McMichael et al. 2000) risks harming population health. Addressing global threats to the sustainability of human health will require changed commitments by many national and international agencies.

Indicators of progress

While economists agree that the GDP per capita is an imperfect index of progress (Gregory 1998), it has nevertheless become the international benchmark which influences social policy

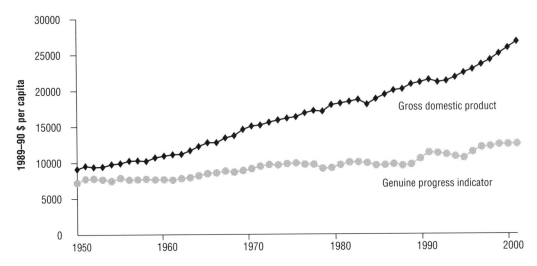

Figure 3.5 Per capita gross domestic product and genuine progress indicator, 1950–2000 (constant 1990 prices)

Note: The trajectories of these two indicators continue to diverge.

Source: The Australia Institute.

everywhere. The goal of economic growth measured by a rise in the GDP per capita dominates our social and political policy without proper regard to social and environmental consequences.

GDP per capita fails to recognise the way resources are distributed within societies and ignores the way markets affect the environment. It treats economic transactions as equal, regardless of their social or environmental consequences. Its pre-eminence as the world's social barometer contributes substantially to the distortion of our social goals.

The 'genuine progress indicator' (GPI) has been developed in Australia by researchers at The Australia Institute (Hamilton and Denniss 2000; Hamilton 1999) to help to put the GDP into perspective. Like its American counterpart, and the European 'index of sustainable economic welfare', the Australian GPI adjusts the conventional measure of personal consumption by a range of factors including changes in the distribution of national income, the value of housework, the costs of unemployment and overwork, the costs of atmospheric and water pollution, the costs of car accidents and congestion, and the depletion of non-renewable natural resources. When the GDP is adjusted in this way, the Australian GPI trajectory presents a very different picture to the unadjusted GDP.

Social sustainability

We suggest that the dominance of the market ethos increasingly threatens social sustainability. Australia is a society characterised by growing litigation and attempts to assign blame and seek compensation. We observe increasing social preoccupation with individual wealth, greed and self-fulfilment and a diminishing societal capacity and willingness to provide support for those in need. Undiluted marketism risks distilling life's purposes to mere winning, losing, consuming and getting rich; it ignores spiritual values, purpose and the wonder of human existence. The market end-product of spiralling consumption, in our view, is a social and environmental dead-end. An unrestricted market ethos forces competition when often collaboration is what is required. Contrary to believers in 'Homo economicus', unrestrained competition may counteract evolutionarily programmed human cooperative behaviour (Roberts and Sherratt 1998, Wedekind and Milinski 2000).

We are not arguing that we can, or should, arrest the market in its tracks or revert to state control, but that there is an urgent need to devise countervailing mechanisms to enable human society to reassert human values, and to place human health and genuine well-being at the centre of the social engine.

Conclusion

The autonomous nation state is becoming an anachronism. Australians are not yet facing the harsh realities of the near future. Retreating into a 'fortress Australia' mentality, trying to ignore climate change and global poverty is likely to increase justifiable resentment by the rest of the world. Australians must and can find new ways to redistribute resources and incomes and modify marketism so that it can deliver its benefits, while minimising its costs.

In summary, globalisation and environmental change are harming the social fabric and the health of the Australian and indeed of the global population. We must learn to manage this challenge, substantially through social organisation; technology alone will be insufficient. We must recognise global interdependence and re-order individual, national and global priorities.

National governments in wealthy countries like Australia need to lead in promoting sustainability. We need new frameworks for ecological, economic, social and cultural sustainability. We may measure our success or failure in terms of global health expectancy, equity and social well-being. We need a new approach to internationalism that recognises the delicate nature of our interdependence.

We would like to see Australia commit to the global community by way of supporting debt alleviation, education, preventive health care and international governance. As a nation, we need to place social and environmental sustainability and population health ahead of economic growth as a national goal, and develop social policies that can enhance equity, social stability and trust.

Globalisation and environmental destruction pose new threats to the health and well-being, not only of Australians but of the entire human species. Our response must extend beyond conventional frameworks for social and economic policy. A response that entrusts the future to technological solutions without a strong focus on strengthening the social determinants of human well-being and health and a commitment to achieving ecological sustainability is entirely inadequate.

Acknowledgement

Special thanks to G Bodeker, E Dlugokencky, D Pauly and E Houlahan for provision of data used to compute the Index of Global Environmental Change.

Further Reading

Bales, K 1999, Disposable People: New slavery in the global economy, University of California Press, Berkeley.
- *A carefully documented and very readable book that describes some of the human suffering behind the dry figures of global income inequality.*
Daily, GC (Ed.) 1997, Nature's Services: Societal dependence on natural ecosystems, Island Press, Washington DC.
- *Provides a wealth of detail about the dependency of the human economy, and ultimately human health, on nature.*
Butler, CD 2000, Inequality, global change and the sustainability of civilisation, Global Change and Human Health 1: 156–72. <www.baltzer.nl/kaphtml.htm/GLOBI>
- *Argues that global inequality is so pervasive and extensive that it warrants a new word – 'claste' (a hybrid of 'class' and 'caste') – and that the most powerful clastes practise 'environmental brinkmanship', which at the worst case threatens civilisation.*
McMichael, AJ 2001, Human Frontiers, Environments and Disease: Past patterns, uncertain futures, Cambridge University Press, Cambridge.
- *Explores the long history of social and environmental changes as the fundamental determinants of human survival and patterns of disease. This ecological perspective is critically important in addressing the new, unfamiliar challenges to human population well-being and health posed by global environmental changes.*

4
Culture, health and well-being

Richard Eckersley

Introduction

In the 1970s, I spent two years travelling overseas – through Africa, Western and Eastern Europe, the Soviet Union and Asia. The most difficult cultural adjustment I had to make was on my return to Australia. My initial celebration of the material abundance and comfort of the Western way of life soon gave way to a growing apprehension about its emotional harshness and spiritual desiccation. In a way I hadn't anticipated, the experience allowed me to view my native culture from the outside, and in ways I hadn't appreciated before, I realised ours was a tough culture.

In his book, *Biology and the Riddle of Life*, the biologist Charles Birch says science inevitably leads to mechanical analyses. Is there nothing more to be said, he asks:

> I think there is. It is to propose that there are two points of view – *the inside and the outside, the subjective and the objective, from within and from without* . . . There is an enormous gap between what science describes and what we experience . . . (T)he solution to the riddle of life is only possible through the proper connection of the outer with the inner experience (1999, p 58, italics in original).

This chapter is concerned with this connection as it relates to the social determinants of health, and as it is expressed in the relationships between cultural and socio-economic factors. 'Culture' is a difficult concept because it is defined and used differently between different disciplines, and even within the same discipline. Culture can be taken to include all aspects of society, to describe an entire way of life of a people. However, it is often distinguished from social structure, with a key research goal being a better understanding of how the two interact (Swidler 1986). Larazus (1991, pp 349–83), in his study of emotion and adaptation, distinguishes between 'culture' and 'social structure' in this way: 'culture' provides a set of internalised meanings that we carry into our interactions with the social and physical environment; 'social structure' refers to the detailed patterns of social relationships and transactions among people with different roles and status within a social system.

However, Hays (1994) challenges the separation of culture and social structure. Culture, she argues, is a social structure, both internal and external, subjective and objective, ideal and material. The notion that culture is arbitrary and objectively inaccessible would make many (sensible) social scientists hesitate to analyse culture at all, she says. It raises the image of a 'rational scientist' studying 'material reality', while a 'star-struck' interpretative sociologist studies 'subjective meanings'. Hays favours regarding social structure as consisting of two central, interconnected elements: systems of social relations (patterns of roles, relationships and domination that define categories of class, gender, race, education etc.) and systems of meaning (which is what is often called 'culture').

The literature on the social determinants of health, to the extent that it discusses culture at all, treats it as separate from the social structures on which research focuses (so tending to confirm the conceptual danger against which Hays warns). Given this separation already exists in the literature, and given her definitions of systems of social relations and meanings are similar to Lazarus's of culture and social structure, I will, for the sake of clarity, retain the distinction between culture and social structure in this chapter. However, my arguments could equally be framed in Hays' terms.

My key points are that: research into the social determinants of health has unduly neglected culture, in favour of socio-economic factors, notably inequality; cultural determinants can influence health and well-being by amplifying or moderating the impact of socio-economic factors, and also in other ways; they do this through the same psychosocial pathways by which socio-economic factors are thought to influence health; and recognition of the role of culture has important implications for our understanding of the social determinants of health and well-being and for what we should do about it. In essence, I argue that while socio-economic inequality is important, it is far from being the only important social determinant of population health and may not be the most important.

The chapter discusses, in turn: the research on social determinants of health and its treatment of culture; key trends in modern Western culture and their social significance; the psychology of well-being and its links to culture; and young people's psychosocial well-being. An important aspect of the chapter's perspective is that it goes beyond the usual 'mortality/ morbidity' framework of health and draws on a different body of research than is usual in the mainly epidemiological literature on the social determinants of health.

Social determinants of health

In the remarkable resurgence over the past decade or so in scientific interest in the social determinants of health, culture has been largely excluded from consideration. In the social models, the role of culture is seen as distal and diffuse, exerting a pervasive but unspecified influence on health (see figure 4.1 and Turrell, this volume, p 98). Of the many books and reports on the subject published in this period, few give cultural determinants more than a passing mention (Evans et al. 1994; Daedalus 1994; Amick et al. 1995; Blane et al. 1996; Wilkinson 1996a; Bartley et al. 1998; Strickland and Shetty 1998; Adler et al. 1999; Keating and Hertzman 1999; Marmot and Wilkinson 1999; Turrell et al. 1999; Berkman and Kawachi

2000). None offers a comprehensive account of the health implications of the cultural characteristics of modern Western societies such as individualism and consumerism.

The overwhelming emphasis of this research is on socio-economic inequalities in
health – the inequalities associated with income, education, occupation, residential area and
class. Even social capital, with its basis in the qualities of trust, participation, cooperation and
reciprocity, is discussed largely in terms of inequality (Kawachi et al. 1997a; Kawachi 1999;
Wilkinson 1998a, 1999a). This focus is perhaps not surprising. Against a historical background
of improving health, especially as measured by mortality rates and life expectancies, and the
clear evidence of persistent and even increasing socio-economic gradients in health, it is logical
to concentrate on reducing inequality as a means of further improving population health.

However, the very pathways by which inequality is believed to 'get under the skin' to
affect health are also those by which culture could affect health. These pathways present a
critical issue in opening the way for cultural influences. To date, they remain unclear and contested. A central issue of debate is whether health inequalities derive primarily from material

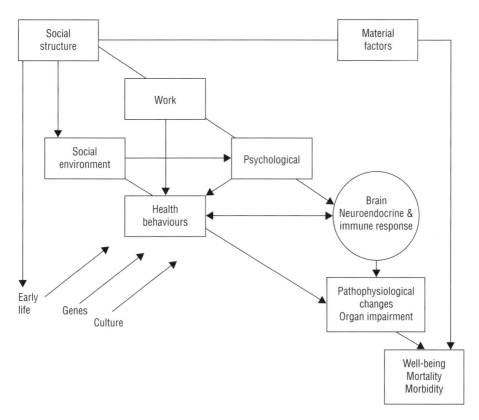

Figure 4.1 Model of the social determinants of health, linking social structure to health and disease via
material, psychosocial and behavioural pathways. Genetic, early life and cultural factors are further
important influences.

Source: Brunner and Marmot 1999. Reproduced with permission from Oxford University Press;
copyright 1999 by Oxford University Press.

deprivation and disadvantage – from differential access to the material resources necessary for optimal health – or whether they result mainly from the psychosocial consequences of inequality (Marmot 1999; Lynch et al. 2000a; Lynch 2000). Put another way, are health inequalities a matter of (degrees of) absolute deprivation or relative deprivation? These different perspectives are labelled 'materialist' (or 'neo-materialist') and 'psychosocial', respectively.

Materialists emphasise factors such as the poorer quality housing, food, working conditions, neighbourhoods and access to services such as health care, transport and leisure that are associated with low socio-economic position. While affecting the poorest most, these absolute differences in material conditions can also affect health across the socio-economic spectrum. Advocates of the psychosocial perspective argue that the relatively uniform gradient in health, even among people who are not poor, indicates material deprivation is not the most important factor. They emphasise the significance of people's relative position in the social hierarchy.

How people's relative social position is translated into health outcomes remains uncertain. At the social level, inequality reduces social capital, weakening social cohesion and increasing social fragmentation. At the personal level, it may decrease social support and increase isolation. Socio-economic differences in the prevalence of behavioural risk factors such as smoking, drinking, diet and exercise explain at least some of inequalities in health. However, inequality also affects qualities such as personal control or mastery, optimism, hostility, coping style, and parenting, all of which may be important to health (Marmot 1999; Taylor and Seeman 1999).

While the stress associated with inequality can impact on health via direct adverse physiological effects, another important pathway may be through affective states or emotions (Gallo and Matthews 1999; Kubzansky and Kawachi 2000). Depression, hopelessness, anxiety and anger have been associated with higher risks of death and disease (the evidence is strongest for coronary heart disease, weaker for cancer). Conversely, happiness appears to be associated with good health (Argyle 1997). All these affective states tend to show a social gradient, making them a plausible pathway. However, the causal links remain to be clearly established.

The debate between the materialist and psychosocial perspectives is one of relative emphasis or importance, not mutual exclusivity, with the recent contributions focusing on issues of causality and intervention. Thus Lynch (2000), while acknowledging psychosocial factors are involved, argues that 'there are real-world living conditions that should be the basis for understanding and analysing inequality'. It is hard to see, he says, how a psychosocial theory of health inequalities 'can form the basis for an effective policy agenda to improve overall levels of population health and reduce health inequalities'. However, the need for a perspective that takes in more than material inequalities has been reinforced by recent findings that challenge the belief that there is a straightforward relationship between socio-economic inequality and health inequality.

A study of occupational class mortality in European nations found that while inequalities in health occur in all countries, these do not correlate with income inequality; in other words, the most equal nations do not necessarily have the most equal health (Mackenbach 1998; Mackenbach et al. 2000). A study of well-being (measured by life expectancy, self-reported health and happiness) and state welfare (social security expenditure) in 40 nations revealed no connection between the size of state welfare and either the overall level of well-being or the equality of well-being (Veenhoven 2000).

If psychosocial factors are important in explaining health inequalities, then culture must be an important part of the equation of social determination. Once we allow a role in health for perceptions, expectations and emotions, then cultural factors have to be taken into consideration, not only with respect to inequality but also in other ways. As Lazarus (1991, p 361) states: 'The most obvious way in which cultural meaning can influence the experience and expression of emotion is through how a person *perceives*, *understands*, and *appraises* what is happening socially . . .' (italics in original).

The most complete accounts of cultural factors in the recent social determinants literature are those by Corin (1994, 1995). She warns that socio-economic status far from encompasses all the ways in which the social environment may influence health, and that an exclusive emphasis on it could have 'the perverse effect of enforcing a purely objective and deterministic conception of environmental influences on the health of individuals and groups' (Corin 1994). Corin (1994) attributes epidemiology's neglect of culture to its origins in the conceptual framework of medicine. Its 'categorical' approach to sociocultural factors, which fits comfortably within prevailing scientific paradigms, strips human realities of much of their social context and disregards and dismisses other approaches to social and cultural realities, she says. Whereas epidemiological research defines culture through variables such as ethnicity, place of birth or language, anthropology considers it as a web or matrix of collective influences that shape people's lives.

> . . . culture is above all a system of meanings and symbols. This system shapes every area of life, defines a world view that gives meaning to personal and collective experience, and frames the way people locate themselves within the world, perceive the world, and behave in it. *Every aspect of reality is seen embedded within webs of meaning that define a certain world view and that cannot be studied or understood apart from this collective frame* (Corin 1995, p 273, italics added).

Corin (1995) argues that cultural factors shape the experience of stress and psychosocial factors such as social support and coping strategies. Humans do not live in a purely objective world in which objects and events possess an inherent and objective significance; instead, these things are imbued with meanings that vary with individuals, times and societies, and which emerge from a network of associations. There is a complex interaction between the objective and subjective worlds, and between reality, expectations and values, she says. Within these interactions, values play an important role, mediating the effects of an experience by regulating its meaning and its importance.

Corin (1994) notes that cultural influences are always easier to identify in unfamiliar societies. Thus most studies of culture and health have not involved Western societies, but have examined other societies or specific sub-populations such as migrants and ethnic minorities. However, their conclusions, which indicate a potential role of culture in health and disease, also apply to Western societies:

> Cross-cultural studies reveal the larger influence of culture and social structure that shapes the daily lives of individuals and collectivities . . . As long as one remains within one's own cultural boundaries, the ways of thinking, living, and behaving peculiar to that culture are transparent or invisible; they appear to constitute a natural order that is not itself an object of study. But this impression is an unsupported ethnocentric illusion (Corin 1994, p 119).

DiGiacomo (1999) also says that while epidemiology and anthropology may be natural allies in the study of population health, bioscientific uses of the concept of culture have led to 'the medicalisation of culture understood as "difference", which often stands in for social class'. Coming from a different perspective, Coburn (2000) has criticised the 'startling lack of attention' in the recent literature to the social, political and economic context of the relationships between health and inequalities in socio-economic status or income. He urges more examination of the causes of these inequalities, especially neoliberal (market-dominated) political doctrines and their impact on both inequality and social cohesion. Thus his focus is more limited than mine here, although it does bear on the cultural trends discussed in the next section.

To argue that the 'social determinants of health' literature downplays culture is not to claim that epidemiology has totally ignored its study. Indeed, one of the more curious aspects of the current situation is that the neglect occurs despite the existing evidence of its importance. Examples of influential research into the health effects of culture, including Western culture, are: the work of Marmot and his colleagues on the negative effect of exposure to Western influence on coronary heart disease in Japanese (Corin 1994, 1995); Wolf and Bruhn's long study of the role of social cohesion and egalitarianism in explaining unusually low mortality rates, especially from heart disease, in the small town of Roseto in Pennsylvania (Amick et al. 1995, pp 6–7; Wilkinson 1996a, pp 116–18); and the Stirling County Study, a classic study in psychiatric epidemiology by Leighton and his colleagues, which showed that social disintegration, as measured by the degree of consensus about values, meaning and shared sentiments, was directly related to the prevalence of psychiatric disorders (Corin, 1994, 1995; Amick et al. 1995, p 6).

So evidence of cultural influences on health exists, but much of this research dates back to the 1950s, 1960s and 1970s, and is overshadowed by the emphasis in contemporary research on socio-economic inequalities. Nowhere in the recent literature on the social determinants of health, to my knowledge, is there a detailed discussion of the characteristics of modern Western culture and their implications for health and well-being. These will be considered in the following sections.

Cultural trends

There are many patterns and trends in Western culture that we might expect to be significant to health. Cultural factors interact closely with structural social and economic factors, both as causes and effects. At one level, inequality and whether it increases or decreases could be said to be a consequence of culture, specifically the values reflected in public policy. However, cultural qualities may also act on health in other ways.

A vast literature exists on the nature of modern Western society and its culture, ranging from the works of the great 19th century social philosophers and sociologists such as de Tocqueville, Weber, Marx and Durkheim, to contemporary social theorists such as Habermas, Bourdieu, Beck and Giddens. I am not going to attempt to discuss Western culture within the context of this literature. While drawing partly on this work (and making some specific references to it), I am basing what follows largely on my own analysis and observations, and on the more popular debate about modern life.

Several cultural qualities are widely considered to characterise Western culture (although they are not necessarily confined to it, and are, in fact, becoming increasingly global in their influence). I am not suggesting these qualities exert a uniform effect on everyone, regardless of gender, class and ethnicity; or that individuals are cultural sponges, passively absorbing cultural influences, rather than interacting actively with these factors; or that there is not a variety of subcultures marked by sometimes very different values, meanings and beliefs. Nevertheless, I believe the trends in these qualities are historically important and their effects pervasive, including on the health and well-being of populations. Here are a few 'isms' of modern Western culture:

Consumerism: Consumerism (often equated with materialism) refers to a lifestyle characterised by the acquisition and consumption of goods and services produced in the market economy. The trend in consumerism is broadly reflected in growth in per capita gross domestic product or GDP (about 60% of which is derived from private consumption). By this measure, consumerism has increased about five-fold in Australia and many other Western nations in the past 100 years.

Individualism: Individualism is a defining characteristic of Western nations, often contrasted with the collectivism of Eastern societies. Individualism places the individual, rather than the community or group, at the centre of a framework of values, norms and beliefs. It is exemplified by the former British Prime Minister, Margaret Thatcher's famous comment: 'There is no such thing as Society. There are individual men and women, and there are families.' (The reference to families is often omitted when this remark is quoted.)

Economism: Many might equate economism with capitalism, economic rationalism or neoliberalism. However, I use the term to embrace more than an ideological faith in free markets. It refers to a tendency to view the world through the prism of economics: to regard human society as an economic system, and to believe that choice is, or should be, based primarily on economic considerations. Again, GDP growth probably provides some sort of proxy measure of the trend in economism. A good example of economism is the Australian Prime Minister John Howard's statement in a speech to a 1998 World Economic Forum dinner that: 'The overriding aim of our agenda is to deliver Australia an annual (economic) growth rate of over four percent on average during the decade to 2010'.

Postmodernism: This includes a suite of related cultural qualities that characterise contemporary society. Postmodernity, or late modernity, is marked by the loss of grand narratives, universal truths and unifying creeds. Its characteristics include relativism, pluralism, ambiguity, ambivalence, transience, fragmentation and contingency. Postmodern life is episodic, uncertain, flexible and reflexive. Meaning in life is no longer a social given, but is individually chosen, or constructed, from a proliferation of options.

All these cultural qualities are interrelated, and interact: economism with consumerism, consumerism with individualism, individualism with postmodernism, for example. In a review of Zygmunt Bauman's *Life in fragments: essays in postmodern morality* (1995), Elliott, also a scholar of postmodernity, says that while postmodernism is identified with the political Left, it is much less obvious that it is itself a radical concern:

What has happened in so-called postmodern society is the collapse of core community values and ethical foundations, and the reorganisation of everyday cultural life within the ideological structures of the globalised capitalist economy itself. From this angle, the advent of postmodernism – with its deconstruction of metaphysical foundations, its dazzling globalisation of social institutions, its reifying of high-tech, and its cult of hedonism – fits hand in glove with the imperatives of a market logic in which everything goes but nothing much counts (1995).

There are other cultural factors and trends besides these: for example, *secularism* – not so much the decline of religious belief, but its exclusion from large parts of private and public life; and *pessimism* – the foreboding many people feel about humanity's future, even while they remain optimistic about their own lives. Yet other cultural trends might be described as countervailing: *feminism* – not just the movement for gender equality, but also the greater recognition and expression of the 'feminine' in human nature; *environmentalism* – the shift from an ethic of ignorance and exploitation of the natural environment to one of awareness and conservation; and *universalism* – the growing consciousness of other peoples, our affects on each other, and our obligations to each other. So there is profound conflict as well as powerful synergy between contemporary cultural forces in Western societies.

All these cultural trends have benefits to health and well-being: consumerism has contributed to making our lives safer and more comfortable; individualism has enhanced human rights, self-determination and political participation; economism has increased economic efficiency and productivity; postmodernism is associated with greater tolerance and diversity; secularism has helped to loosen the chains of bigotry and dogma; feminism has enhanced the status of women and given them more control over their lives; even pessimism, if it does not destroy hope, can be an incentive to change. Both environmentalism and universalism are prerequisites for a sustainable and harmonious planetary existence.

In a commentary on the paper by Coburn (2000) on the role of neoliberalism in health inequalities, Hertzman (2000) lists several factors that he suggests might explain why health is continuing to improve despite the growing influence of neoliberal economics. These include growing social tolerance, diversity, pluralism and flexibility: 'an end to the social respectability of religious, gender, ethnic, and racial discrimination . . . a general loosening of social norms and behavioural expectations and an increase in the range of lifestyles which are considered socially acceptable'. These changes, he says, may increase the level of 'psychosocial equality' in society (so, again, the focus remains on inequality).

Yet taken too far, too fast, and together, the cultural forces I have discussed also present risks to health and well-being. This is especially true of consumerism, individualism, economism and postmodernism, as we shall see, but problems arise even where the essential cultural direction is positive. For example, feminism, in the transitional stages, creates a conflict of roles and goals for both women and men, and can be influenced by other cultural forces such as economism and individualism (that is, these affect how the equality feminism seeks is defined). Environmental consciousness, pitted against the cultural power of consumerism, can produce a sense of despondency and futility.

The conflicts and contradictions include a tension between cultural ideal and social reality. While modern Western societies can be characterised as offering excessive choice and freedom, it is also the case that these can be illusory. Social constraints remain, and in some cases are increasing, whether these concern having sex or driving cars (both powerful symbols of freedom which are highly prescribed by rules and realities), or class and privilege (which still substantially define opportunity). Furthermore, the postmodern ideal is really a Trojan horse for the social promotion of *particular* choices and values. Western societies present a façade of virtually unlimited freedom that disguises a powerful preference shaped by cultural forces such as consumerism and economism. The media are a potent source of this tension. For all the cultural celebration of autonomy and self-realisation, never before have people lived so little within their own lives; never before have our images of social realities been so filtered and distorted. While cultures are rarely, if ever, completely internally consistent, modern Western culture is deeply incoherent.

One critical consequence of the cultural trends of consumerism, individualism, economism, postmodernism (and secularism) has been their effect on moral values. Values provide the framework for deciding what is important, true, right and good, and so have a central role in defining relationships and meanings. Most societies have tended to reinforce values that emphasise social obligations and self-restraint and discourage those that promote self-indulgence and anti-social behaviour (Campbell 1975; Funkhouser 1989; Ridley 1996). 'We define virtue almost exclusively as pro-social behaviour, and vice as anti-social behaviour', Ridley (1996, p 6) observes in his analysis of human nature and society, *The origins of virtue*. This is not to argue that other societies have always been paragons of virtue, or that they did not often deal brutally with 'out' groups, or that 'pro-social' values such as conformity and deference to authority do not have costs when they, too, are taken too far and become blind obedience. There is also an important distinction to be made between abstract values and the often highly prescribed and proscribed behaviours into which they are socially translated.

Social virtues serve to maintain a balance – always dynamic, always shifting – between individual needs and freedom, and social stability and order. The 13th-century theologian, St Thomas Aquinas, listed the seven deadly sins as pride (self-centredness), envy, avarice (greed), wrath (anger, violence), gluttony, sloth (laziness, apathy) and lust; the seven cardinal virtues as faith, hope, charity (compassion), prudence (good sense), temperance (moderation), fortitude (courage, perseverance) and religion (spirituality). Other values widely regarded as virtues include patience, honesty, fidelity and forgiveness. Virtues, then, are concerned with building and maintaining strong, harmonious personal relationships and social attachments, and the strength to endure adversity. Vices, on the other hand, are about the unrestrained satisfaction of individual wants and desires, or the capitulation to human weaknesses.

Modern Western culture undermines, even reverses, traditional (or universal) values. Thus most consumption today (beyond meeting basic needs) is located within the vices, little within the virtues. We cannot quarantine other aspects of life from the moral consequences of ever-increasing consumption. The results of this cultural shift include not so much a collapse of personal morality, but its blurring into ambivalence and conflict. Individuals are encouraged to make themselves the centre of their moral universe, to assess everything – from personal relationships to paying taxes – in terms of 'what's in it for me?'. This promotes a preoccupation with personal expectations that keep rising, and with wants that are never sated because new ones keep being created. As consumerism reaches increasingly beyond the acquisition of things to the enhancement of the person, the goal of marketing becomes not only to make people dissatisfied with what they have, but also with who they are.

Economism is important to values because economics is amoral – that is, it is not concerned with the morality of the choices consumers make to maximise their utility or satisfaction. The more economic choices govern people's lives, the more marginalised moral considerations become. Money itself becomes the dominant value. Social status is ever-more narrowly defined in terms of income and wealth, and the 'opportunity costs' of spending time on things other than making money grow (Csikszentmihalyi 1999). The risks of postmodernism include the trivialisation of conviction and commitment by an 'anything goes' morality: a belief that values are just a matter of personal opinion, and that one set of values is no better or worse than another. Values cease to require any external validation or to have any authority or reference beyond the individual and the moment.

Surveys suggest a deep tension between people's professed values and the lifestyle promoted by modern Western societies (Eckersley 1999, 2000a, 2000b). Traditional sources of moral guidance such as religion, although weakened, no doubt fuel this tension, as would other cultural trends such as environmentalism and universalism. Many people are concerned about the greed, excess and materialism they believe drive society today, underlie social ills, and threaten their children's future. They yearn for a better balance in their lives, believing that when it comes to things like freedom and material abundance, they don't seem 'to know where to stop' or now have 'too much of a good thing'. People perceive a widening gulf between private and public morality, between their own standards and those reflected by institutions such as the media, government and business, even religion. This produces a growing sense of alienation and disengagement, a rising cynicism about social institutions and their roles.

As Durkheim (1970, pp 361–92) observed in his seminal sociological study of suicide a century ago, a crucial function of social institutions such as the family and religion is to bind individuals to society, to keep 'a firmer grip' on them and to draw them out of their 'state of moral isolation'. 'Man cannot become attached to higher aims and submit to a rule if he sees nothing above him to which he belongs', Durkheim (1970, p 389) writes. 'To free him from all social pressure is to abandon him to himself and demoralise him.' While he focused on social structures, Durkheim saw clearly the distinction between material and moral causes of despair, noting (in the language of an earlier time):

> If more suicides occur today than formerly, this is not because, to maintain ourselves, we have to make more painful efforts, nor that our legitimate needs are less satisfied, but because we no longer know the limits of legitimate needs nor perceive the direction of our efforts . . . The maladjustment from which we suffer does not exist because the objective causes of suffering have increased in number or intensity; it bears witness not to greater economic poverty, but to an alarming poverty of morality (1970, pp 386–7).

The cultural qualities I have discussed, while pervasive, can show gender and socio-economic differences in their expression and impact. Thus while Western culture promotes a view of the self as individualistic, autonomous and independent of others and social influences, this may be truer of men than of women, for whom the self is more likely to be construed as interdependent, with others considered part of the self (Cross and Madson 1997). The gender differences in self-construal might, however, be narrowing under the influence of contemporary cultural trends.

In terms of socio-economic differences, consumerism and economism, for example, would cause most stress among low-income groups because of the emphasis they place on money and material well-being. Less obvious is the evidence of a social gradient in postmodern qualities, which also illustrates how culture can accentuate disadvantage. Elchardus (1991, 1994) has shown that the attitudes associated with the 'cultural flexibility' that characterises post-modernity – religious and philosophical indifference, a 'here-and-now' hedonism and an individualism that extends well beyond emancipation from traditional restrictions – are negatively correlated with education and occupation. Cultural flexibility is related to low educational levels, high risk of unemployment, low occupational status, and low degrees of autonomy on the job. Elchardus (1994) criticises the linking of cultural flexibility to a 'progressive vision of individualisation', saying it has resulted in 'a somewhat shameful legitimation of increases in uncertainty and unpredictability in the life of the poor and socially weak'.

> Cultural flexibility . . . seems to be a form of withdrawal of commitment and emotion from a social order in which one is losing out. Such a reaction cannot really be considered a form of resistance, let alone revolt, for its very form makes organised action unlikely. Cultural flexibility rather seems to be the meek acceptance of the flexibilisation of one's life for the purposes of economic efficiency and organisational control (Elchardus 1991, p 721).

In summary, modern Western culture, its strengths and benefits notwithstanding, displays several characteristics that have the potential to harm health and well-being. These include: its promotion of anti-social values; the moral ambivalence and confusion arising from its openness and its inherent contradictions; and the tension generated between cultural ideals and social realities. Cultural influences can interact with structural conditions to modify their social effects.

Well-being

The importance of culture to health and well-being emerges more clearly from the research into psychological well-being than it does from epidemiological studies on health. There is very little cross-referencing between this mainly psychological literature and social epidemiology. A significant body of research concerns subjective well-being. In several important respects, this research supports the psychosocial perspective on health inequalities. However, it also reveals some interesting differences between health and well-being. Subjective well-being is not a single construct, but comprises three distinct and to some extent independent dimensions: a cognitive aspect; life satisfaction; and pleasant and unpleasant affect (moods and emotions) (Myers and Diener 1995; Wearing and Headey 1998; Diener et al. 1999). It differs from the concept of 'health' in excluding physical health and in including positive emotions; it is thus less focused on illness and disease (both physical and mental).

Subjective well-being, which is often loosely equated with happiness, is, like health, positively correlated with control, optimism and social support (unless otherwise indicated, much of what follows on subjective well-being is taken from: Myers and Diener 1995; Wearing and Headey 1998; Diener et al. 1999; Diener 2000; Myers 2000). It is also positively correlated with extroversion, and negatively with neuroticism. It is associated with self-esteem, which, however, does not seem to be important to health (Taylor and Seeman 1999). The significance of self-esteem to well-being is culturally variable, which might help to explain this discrepancy.

Looking at other factors, being married and religious enhances well-being. So does the ability to adapt, to set goals and progress towards them, and viewing the world as understandable, controllable and meaningful. These qualities are interrelated. Meaning in life is strongly related to well-being (more so to its positive dimensions than its negative) and is, in turn, related to self-transcendent values, strong religious beliefs, membership of groups, dedication to a cause and clear life goals (Zika and Chamberlain 1992). Diener and Suh (1997) note that the central elements of well-being are based on people's most important values and goals: subjective well-being 'is most likely to be experienced when people work for and make progress towards personal goals that derive from their important values'. Goal conflict or ambivalence, on the other hand, is associated with diminished well-being (Diener et al. 1999).

The most interesting findings on subjective well-being, compared to health, concern its relationship to income. As with health, there are income gradients between and within populations: average well-being is higher in rich countries than in poor (although this may also be due to factors other than wealth, such as literacy, democracy and equality), and within countries, the rich have more of it than the poor. As with health, the biggest gains in well-being with rising income come at low-income levels, and taper off at higher levels. Increased income appears to matter when it helps people meet basic needs; beyond that, the relationship becomes more complex.

Neither in comparisons between nor within countries, however, is the gradient in well-being as pronounced as it is with health. In contrast to the wide disparities between rich and poor countries in life expectancy, Cummins (1998) has demonstrated the uniformity in population estimates of life satisfaction. When life satisfaction is measured as a percentage of the scale maximum, the population average for countries across all major geographic regions is about 70% with a standard deviation (SD) of 5% (for Western nations, the average is about 75%, SD 2.5%). Within countries, only in the poorest is income a good indicator of well-being; in most nations the correlation is small, and even the very rich are only slightly happier than the average person (figure 4.2).

Another striking difference between health and well-being is that while health, as measured by mortality and life expectancy, has improved steadily over past decades, well-being has not, at least not in developed nations. The proportion of people in developed societies who are happy or satisfied with their lives has remained stable over the past several decades (50 years in the US), even though they have become, on average, much richer. Indeed, one of the most striking findings of research into subjective well-being is the often small correlation with objective resources and conditions. One recent estimate is that external circumstances account for only about 15% of the variance in subjective well-being (Diener et al. 1999, Diener 2000).

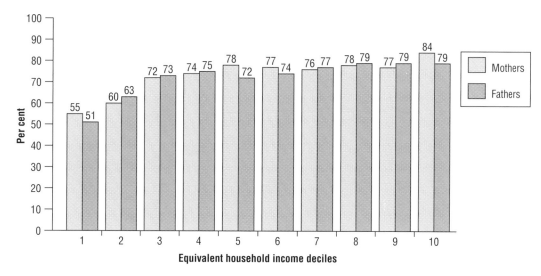

Figure 4.2 Australians' life satisfaction by income, 1991–2

Notes: Figures represent the proportion of parents in each income decile scoring 7–9 on a nine-point scale of life satisfaction. The survey involved parents with at least one child under 20 in nine urban and two rural areas (N = ~ 8,500). Equivalent household income refers to combined incomes of parents and children over 15, expressed as a percentage of the Henderson Poverty Line.

Source: Australian Living Standards Survey, 1991–92, Australian Institute of Family Studies, Melbourne; personal communication with Ruth Weston.

In a recent review of research on subjective well-being, Diener et al. (1999) conclude that there is no simple answer to what causes happiness. Instead, there is a complex interplay between genes and environment: between life events and circumstances, culture, personality, goals and various adaptation and coping strategies. The evidence suggests that people adjust goals and expectations and use illusions and rationalisations to maintain over time a relatively stable, and positive, rating of life satisfaction and happiness. This characteristic of subjective well-being might explain the key differences with health, despite the similarities in their social determinants. It might also explain why, despite the apparent links between health and emotions, the relationship between health and subjective well-being is not clear-cut: subjective well-being correlates strongly with self-reported health, but only weakly with objective health (Diener et al. 1999).

All in all, the literature on subjective well-being paints a pretty positive picture: most people are mostly happy and satisfied most of the time. However, there is a range of evidence that suggests a positive bias in the results of happiness and life satisfaction surveys (Eckersley 2000b, 2001). For example, while Australians' overall life satisfaction has remained relatively stable over the past two decades, their satisfaction with many of the life domains that are important to life satisfaction – friends, family, community, freedom – has declined (figure 4.3) (Jones 1999). And when people are asked about social conditions, rather than about their own lives, responses are more negative: in 1999, only a quarter of adult Australians believed overall

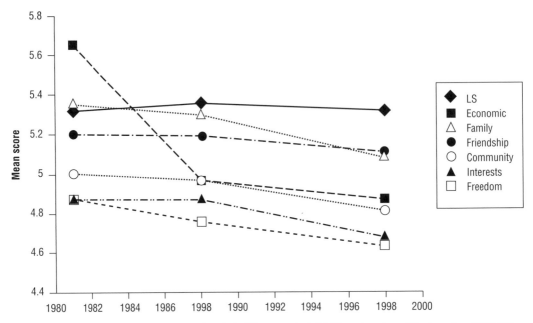

Figure 4.3 Australians' satisfaction with their 'life as a whole' (LS) and various life domains, 1981–98

Notes: Scores are based on a 7-point scale, terrible (1) to delighted (7). Domain scores are means of responses to a range of items in each of the domains of: economic circumstances and well-being (job, income, standard of living, housing); family (time, adult relationships, responsibilities); friendship and respect (love, acceptance, inclusion, honesty, kindness); community (as a place to live, safety, schools, health services); life's interests and diversity (enjoyment, sex, fun, challenge, spare time); and freedom (pressure, relaxation, sleep, independence, privacy). Data are based on a national sample of 1,000 Australians aged 18 and over.

Source: based on data from Jones 1999.

quality of life in Australia was improving and the same proportion that the 1990s were the decade of highest quality of life (Eckersley 1999, 2000a, 2000b).

If qualities such as meaning, goals and values are important to well-being, then so is culture. Drawing on cross-cultural studies of happiness, Diener et al. (1999) conclude: '. . . culture can have a profound effect on the causes of happiness by influencing the goals people pursue as well as the resources available to attain goals'.

People for whom 'extrinsic goals' such as fame, fortune and glamour are a priority in life experience more anxiety and depression and lower overall well-being than people oriented towards 'intrinsic goals' of close relationships, self-acceptance and contributing to the community (Kasser and Ryan 1993, 1996; Kasser 2000). People with extrinsic goals tend to have shorter relationships with friends and lovers, and relationships characterised more by jealousy and less by trust and caring. Materialistic values are positively correlated with social alienation (Khanna and Kasser, in preparation; personal communication with Tim Kasser, Knox College, Illinois), with depression, anxiety and anger, and negatively correlated with life satisfaction

(Saunders and Munro 2000). While these correlations do not prove that materialism and related values cause a deterioration in well-being, they do suggest their cultural promotion is not conducive to it. The cause–effect relationship is likely to be complex and two-way.

Despite the positive correlation between personal control and well-being, individualism, considered more broadly, has been associated with diminished well-being, especially when taken to the extreme (although in cross-country studies, individualism correlates positively with happiness [Veenhoven 1999]). Seligman (1990) argues that one necessary condition for meaning is the attachment to something larger than the self, and the larger that entity, the more meaning people can derive: 'The self, to put it another way, is a very poor site for meaning'. Schwartz (2000) says that individual autonomy and self-determination can become excessive, and freedom experienced as 'a kind of tyranny'. Twenge (2000), in reporting large increases (about one standard deviation) in anxiety and neuroticism in children and college students in the US between the 1950s and 1990s, links the rise to lower social connectedness and higher environmental threat (fear of crime, AIDS etc.), both of which, she says, stem from increasing individualism and freedom; economic factors such as unemployment and poverty seem not to be involved.

Baumeister and Leary (1995) argue that a need to belong is a fundamental human motivation: humans have 'a pervasive drive to form and maintain at least a minimum quantity of lasting, positive, and significant interpersonal relationships'. In a wide-ranging literature review, they show that there are multiple links between the need to belong and cognitive processes, emotional patterns, behavioural responses and health and well-being. 'The desire for interpersonal attachment may well be one of the most far-reaching and integrative constructs currently available to understand human nature.' Baumeister and Leary suggest that the 'belongingness' hypothesis could help psychology recover from the challenge posed by 'cultural materialism', with its assumption that human culture is shaped primarily by economic needs and opportunities, and so should be analysed with reference to economic causes.

The importance of values emerges in a cross-national study by Halpern (2001) of the relationships between crime and values, social trust and inequality. He found that tolerance for a set of 'materially self-interested' attitudes – like keeping something you've found, lying in your own interest, or cheating at tax – was higher in men, younger people, larger cities, and had increased over time, mirroring patterns of criminal offending. These self-interested values were also found to be statistically associated with crime victimisation rates at the national level. Inequality and social trust did not have fully independent relationships with victimisation rates, but were conditional on the prevalent values of society. Thus inequality *per se* was only modestly associated with higher crime, 'but when it occurs in societies that are characterised by high levels of self-interested values then its effects become more pronounced'.

Thus this mainly psychological literature challenges social epidemiology's narrow emphasis on structural factors, especially inequality. It also generally supports the validity and legitimacy of 'traditional' or universal values in terms of their benefits to well-being. In contrast, several of the defining characteristics of modern Western culture would appear, on the basis of the research evidence, to be harmful to well-being through their influence on values, goals, expectations, meaning and belonging.

Young people's health and well-being

Like the psychological literature on well-being, the sociological literature on late-modernity and post-modernity also offers a marked difference to the dominant epidemiological emphasis on socio-economic inequality. Again, there is little reference to this work in the social determinants literature. Postmodern scholarship focuses much more on the cultural qualities of contemporary life and the ways in which these qualities are closely intertwined with structural changes in the family, work and education, but not necessarily with inequality.

Furlong and Cartmel (1997a, 1997b, pp 65–81), drawing on the work of influential writers like Beck and Giddens, examined the extent to which the health risks faced by young people (in Britain) reflected traditional inequalities. They concluded that while many of the health risks encountered by young people were still differentially distributed along the lines of class and gender, 'the processes of individualisation, coupled with the stress which develops out of uncertain transitional outcomes, have implications for the health of all young people' (Furlong and Cartmel 1997b). In particular, 'the protraction and desequencing of youth transitions have had a negative impact on young people's mental health'.

Furlong and Cartmel describe the increased sources of stress 'which stem from the unpredictable nature of life in high modernity'. These include the ongoing sense of doubt, the heightened sense of insecurity, the increased feelings of risk and uncertainty, and the lack of clear frames of reference that mark young people's world today. While traditional forms of inequality remain, even young people from privileged social backgrounds worry about failure and the uncertainty surrounding their future. Conversely, those from disadvantaged backgrounds may feel that the risks they face are personal and individual rather than structural and collective.

Young people's health and well-being are important to understanding the social determinants of health for several reasons. One is the 'life-course' dimension of social influences on health, which emphasises the importance to later health of developmental stages and transition points from before birth to adulthood. These can make young people particularly vulnerable to social effects. Also, they have, generally speaking, yet to experience the health outcomes of long-term, degenerative biological processes associated with diseases such as heart disease, stroke and cancer.

Rates of psychosocial disorders among young people have risen since World War II in almost all developed countries (Rutter and Smith, 1995). These disorders include drug abuse, crime, depression and suicidal behaviour. The rise in suicide among young males has been a striking feature of these trends, with some countries, including Australia and New Zealand, showing more than a three-fold increase in suicide rates among males aged 15–24 (figure 4.4), and a more recent rise in males 25–39 (Cantor et al. 2000). The increase in suicide is despite the reduced lethality of suicide attempts over recent decades because of developments such as safer pharmaceutical drugs and better intensive-care medical technologies (which would have particularly affected suicide rates among women, who are more likely than men to attempt suicide and to use less fatal means).

Blum et al. (2000) found in a study of US high school students (years 7–12), that while some risk behaviours appeared to be more common among some groups of young people, demographic factors did not predict risk behaviours well. Race/ethnicity, income and family

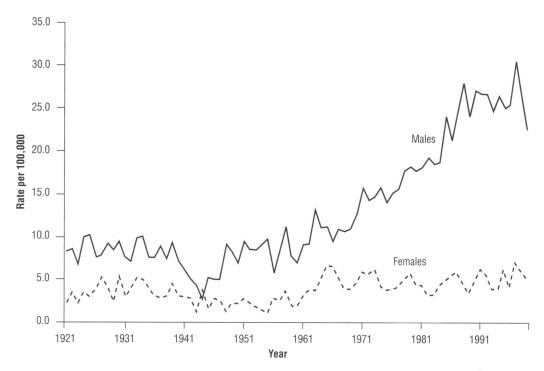

Figure 4.4 Youth suicide in Australia, 1921–99, males and females aged 15–24

Notes: Rates are aged-adjusted using the 1991 Australian population; the peak in 1997 is partly a data artefact, as may be the fall in 1999; the dip in male rates during World War II is at least partly a data artefact.

Source: National Injury Surveillance Unit, Australian Institute of Health and Welfare, using source data provided by the Australian Bureau of Statistics.

structure together explained no more than 10% of the variance in each of five risk behaviours – cigarette smoking, alcohol use, involvement with violence, suicidal thoughts or attempts and sexual intercourse – among younger adolescents, and no more than 7% among older youths. They caution that highlighting group differences runs 'a high risk of building our interventions on variables that are not amenable to change' and, even if they were, 'would not significantly alter behavioural outcomes'.

In a major review, Rutter and Smith (1995, pp 782–808) say that, to a large extent, finding causal explanations of the increases in psychosocial disorder among young people 'remains a project for the future'. However, they regard as unlikely several popular explanations for the trends, such as social disadvantage, inequality and unemployment (although these can be associated with disorder at an individual level). More likely explanations include: family conflict and break-up; increased expectations and individualism; and changes in adolescent transitions (in particular, the emergence of a youth culture that isolates young people from adults and increases peer group influence; more tension between dependence and autonomy; and more romantic relationship breakdowns among young people).

Rutter and Smith call for, among other things, further investigation of the theory that shifts in moral concepts and values are among the causes of increased psychosocial disorder. They note, in particular, 'the shift towards individualistic values, the increasing emphasis on self-realisation and fulfilment, and the consequent rise in expectations'. My own analysis of rising rates of psychosocial problems among young people has also focused on their cultural roots and young people's vulnerability to the failure of modern Western culture to provide, using Corin's words, adequate 'webs of meaning' that frame 'the way people locate themselves within the world, perceive the world, and behave in it' (Eckersley 1993, 1995, 1998b).

In a recent ecological study, I examined statistical associations between youth suicide rates in developed nations and 32 socio-economic and cultural variables (Eckersley and Dear, in press). Male youth suicide rates were positively correlated with several measures of individualism, including personal freedom and control. For females, the correlations were positive but in only one instance significant. Both male youth suicide and individualism were negatively correlated with older people's sense of parental duty (it is 'parents' duty is to do their best for their children even at the expense of their own well-being'). Correlations between suicide and other possibly relevant cultural variables – including tolerance of suicide, belief in God and national pride – were not significant. Nor was there a significant correlation between suicide rates and any of the socio-economic variables including divorce, poverty, youth unemployment and income inequality.

The interpretation of these findings is by no means clear-cut. Given other positive correlations, including between individualism and happiness, health and life satisfaction, the findings could suggest that suicide rises as life gets better (see Barber 2001, for an articulation of this view). However, taking into account possible cultural differences in survey responses and the broad context of young people's well-being today – especially the lack of evidence of any increase in overall happiness and the evidence of increasing psychological distress and disturbance that affect a substantial proportion of young people (Eckersley 1998b, 2001) – I believe it is more likely that the results reflect a failure of Western societies to provide appropriate sites or sources of social identity and attachment, and, conversely, a tendency to promote false expectations of individual freedom and autonomy.

Interpreted this way, the findings support Durkheim's theory that suicide is associated with a weakening of social cohesion, a failure of society to integrate the individual, as already discussed (Durkheim 1970). Individualism could impact on youth suicide through its effect on specific social institutions and functions, such as the family and child-rearing, as suggested by the negative correlation between parental duty and both youth suicide and individualism. However, its effects may go further than this. Western societies – and some more than others – may be taking individualism to the point where it can become more broadly dysfunctional – to society and the individual (perhaps especially males, because of gender differences in construing the self as independent or interdependent). In other words, these societies are promoting a cultural norm of personal autonomy that is unrealistic, unattainable or otherwise inappropriate. They project images and raise expectations of virtually unrestrained individual freedom, choice and opportunity, and of the happiness these qualities are supposed to deliver, which bear increasingly less resemblance to psychological and social realities.

My discussion of the health effects of cultural factors has focused largely on psychological health and well-being, where the impacts are most obvious. In recent years, health authorities have become more aware of the importance of mental illness to population health and well-being. This recognition has been associated with the development of new measures of disability, allowing researchers to move beyond mortality rates in assessing the burden of disease. Measured in terms of both disability and death (disability-adjusted life years or DALYs), psychiatric conditions, including depression, accounted for 23% of the disease burden in high-income countries in 1998, compared to 18% for heart disease and 15% for cancers (World Health Organization 1999). In the global ranking of disease burden, major depression is projected to rise from fourth in 1990 to second in 2020 (Murray and Lopez 1996). A psychosocial theory of health suggests the impacts of culture extend to physical health.

Conclusion

This analysis has highlighted the importance of exploring cultural influences in seeking to understand the social determinants of health and well-being – not just socio-economic factors such as inequality. It suggests cultural changes can amplify or moderate the health impact of inequality – that is, an increase or decrease in health inequalities is not necessarily due to a change in socio-economic gradients. It also indicates that cultural changes could impact on health quite independently of socio-economic factors. In particular, I have emphasised the ways in which key features of Western culture can jeopardise the personal, social and spiritual relationships and certainties that are crucial to well-being.

There are several significant implications of the analysis. Health inequalities may be due in part to differences within populations in cultural factors such as the orientation and congruence of values and goals, at both individual and group levels. These may or may not be associated with structural factors. Also, the social factors that most influence health differences within populations (ie, contribute to health inequalities) may not be the same factors that most influence health over time.

In arguing that defining cultural changes in Western societies pose risks to human health and well-being, I have to acknowledge that, despite these hazards, mortality rates continue to fall and life expectancies to rise. There are several possible explanations for this paradox: the analysis underestimates people's psychological adaptability and resilience; it exaggerates the cultural dangers, relative to cultural benefits to health and well-being; the harm is offset by increasing benefits in other domains of life, such as health care, nutrition and education; the risks to health are mainly of a non-lethal kind, and are more likely to be reflected in rates of chronic illness, especially psychosocial disorders; there are lags between the cultural changes and their life-threatening consequences to health (suicide excepted); and a combination of these reasons. A combination of offsetting benefits, non-lethal risks and lag effects is the most plausible explanation why the impact of cultural change is not more apparent in health status in Australia and other Western nations. We need to bear in mind that death, however much social epidemiology focuses on it, represents only one dimension of health and well-being.

The broader view of the social determinants of health presented here has profound political significance. The implications of socio-economic inequalities in health are serious enough, but they are relatively easily addressed through, for example, conventional policies for correcting or compensating for these inequalities. Acknowledging important cultural influences on health and well-being, on the other hand, means we need to re-evaluate the entire Western worldview and its values, goals and priorities.

Further Reading

Corin, E 1994, The social and cultural matrix of health and disease, in Evans, R G, Barer, M L & Marmor, T R (Eds), Why Are Some People Healthy and Others Not? The determinants of health of populations, Aldine de Gruyter, New York.
  – *A valuable review of the epidemiological literature on cultural influences on health.*
Hays, S 1994, Structure and agency and the sticky problem of culture, Sociological Theory 12 (1): 57–72.
  – *An insightful exploration of the separation of culture and social structure and why it matters.*
Campbell, DT 1975, On the conflicts between biological and social evolution and between psychology and moral tradition, American Psychologist, December: 1103–26.
  – *Based on a presidential address to the American Psychological Association, a fascinating look at the origins of moral values and the relationship between modern science and religious tradition.*

Part B
Explaining health inequalities

5

A general model of the social origins of health and well-being

Jake M. Najman

Whether we compare groups within a society, across national borders or over time, the findings are similar: health varies and reflects different social, economic and political realities. Not only are the social origins of health substantial and persistent, but they offer the greatest prospect for improvements in population health. Of course, health needs differ according to social and physical location, and health problems are variably responsive to prevailing social, cultural and political forces. Different social and physical environments variably lead to particular health outcomes. While we know a great deal about the impact of the social and physical environment on health, much remains to be learnt, especially about the policies and programs that could improve the health of the population.

A review of some key findings provides the basis upon which assertions about the social origins of health rely.

Major socio-economic inequalities in mortality are observed in every country that collects relevant data. These inequalities are noted for most major causes of death, across almost all age groups, and persist over time. They are observed in the weight of children at birth (lower socio-economic status groups have lower birthweights) and in the mental and emotional health of children as early as five years of age (Najman et al. 2000). As early in life as it is possible to gather reliable and valid data, children from lower socio-economic status groups have lower IQ scores and higher rates of developmental problems (Najman et al. 2000). There is compelling evidence that, for many, these health and developmental inequalities start before birth and lead via a number of pathways to poorer adult health (Najman et al. 2002). The magnitude (and occasionally direction) of these socio-economically determined health inequalities may change as social conditions change. For example, the mortality gap between upper and lower socio-economic groups seems to be increasing in countries that manifest increasing economic inequalities (Marmot 1999).

There are major health inequalities associated with religious affiliation. Whether religious affiliation is measured by membership of a particular group (eg, Mormons, Seventh Day Adventists) or by the degree to which a person participates in religious activities (frequent attenders versus occasional attenders), the evidence indicates that the more religious have a substantial health advantage (McEvoy and Land 1981; Lyon et al. 1994; Grundmann 1992). What is remarkable here is not the existence of a health advantage for the more religiously committed and devout, but its magnitude. For a number of major causes of death, the age-adjusted mortality ratios (eg, for lung cancer, heart disease) are as little as half those observed in a less devout group in similar socio-economic circumstances. Interestingly, there are few, if any, health differences when mainstream religious groups are compared (Catholics versus Protestants). As Mormon and Seventh Day Adventist religious groups have developed relatively recently, their members can be taken to have the same biological/constitutional characteristics as people in the surrounding community. The health advantage of the devout must be largely attributable to social factors. Of course, this leaves unresolved the determination of the causal factors that connect religious observance and health. Does membership of a minority and devout religious group confer emotional benefits, or a healthier lifestyle, or perhaps a combination of the two? Is devoutness a precondition for adopting a healthier lifestyle?

Gender differences in mortality are well known and documented (Lopez and Ruzicka 1983). To some extent, these inequalities are attributable to biological factors. For example, comparatively very few women die of heart disease before the age of 50. Of greater interest is the extent to which the gap in life expectancy and mortality rates between men and women has been changing over time. In the United States at the beginning of the 20th century, women outlived men by about two years. By the late 1970s, this had increased to almost eight years (Metropolitan Life Insurance Company 1980, p 2). In Australia in the early part of the 20th century, women outlived men by about three years. By the 1970s, this gap had grown to about seven years. The gap has since begun to diminish and is now a little below six years (Australian Institute of Health and Welfare 2000, p 342). Such dramatic and relatively short-term shifts in life expectancy can only be attributed to social origins – our constitutional make-up simply does not vary greatly in the short term. It is likely that these changing mortality differentials largely reflect male and female changes in lifestyle since the beginning of the century.

Marital status is a major indicator of health inequalities. For the same age groups, married persons are much less likely to die than those widowed or divorced (Johnson et al. 2000). Widowhood and divorce may have a greater impact on the health of men (Cheung 2000). Selection and protection might equally explain marital status inequalities in mortality. According to a selection interpretation, the healthiest (most fit) are selected for marriage – thus single persons and those divorced (both having higher mortality rates than the married) have worse health because they were less healthy early in their lives. This, of course, does not explain why the widowed generally have the highest mortality rate for most causes of death. In any event, studies which have controlled for the early health of those who marry, or do not marry, find similar health when comparing the different marital status groups, making the selection hypothesis less plausible (Ringback-Weitoft et al. 2000). Findings from the 1958 British birth cohort study that monitored levels of alcohol consumption in men and women before and after divorce indicate that there was a pronounced increase in alcohol use immediately following a marital breakdown (Power et al. 1999). Marriage arguably protects the health of those who remain married. Less clear are the mechanisms that lead to the health consequences of divorce, although a lower income and a less healthy lifestyle are likely to be parts of the causal pathway.

International comparisons point to mortality inequalities between countries that are apparently at similar levels of economic development. For example, the population of China and Cuba have life expectancies that are considerably better than other countries with a similar gross domestic product. The life expectancy of persons in China and Cuba approaches that of the developed countries (Najman 1989). The rapid and substantial decline in life expectancy (from age 15) of those living in Russia and the former Soviet Union since the late 1980s is persuasive evidence of the health consequences of economic and social decline (Marmot 1999, p 19). The caveat here is that while it is generally true that per capita income is a major predictor of life expectancy for low income countries, the marginal life expectancy benefits for the higher income countries are modest (World Bank 1993, p 34), raising the possibility that cultural, economic and political arrangements make a significant difference to the latter's health outcomes.

Woodward, Mathers and Tobias (Chapter 8, this volume) point out, in their comparison of the changing life expectancies in Australia and New Zealand, that New Zealand life expectancies exceeded those of Australia over the period 1960 to 1970. From the 1970s, however, Australian male and female life expectancies improved relative to the New Zealand rates and since the mid-1970s, the gap has grown to over a one-year life expectancy advantage for Australian men and women. This more rapid improvement in Australian life expectancies has been attributed to the increasing adoption of a Mediterranean diet within the Australian population.

Towards a general model of disease

How then do we account for these social variations in patterns of health and rates of death? Firstly, we must acknowledge the diversity of influences to be considered, as well as the different combinations of causes likely to be relevant to any specific disease condition. Sometimes, apparently differing causes turn out to be different ways of looking at the same causes or different points in the same causal sequence. Recognising this can simplify the delineation of a model. For example, smoking may lead to abnormalities of lung function, a step along the causal chain towards lung cancer. Poverty is associated with smoking, which, in turn, is predictive of lung function abnormalities. Poverty is associated with inequalities in social capital, with the uptake of cigarettes being directly attributed to lower levels of social capital. Particular studies which emphasise different single causes (eg, low social capital leads to lung cancer, smoking leads to lung cancer) may, in effect, be selecting different points in the same causal sequence related to the disease outcome.

Here, we might usefully think of causes that are closer to (and more distant from) a health outcome. Rather than conceptualising the causes of disease in binary terms (something is or is not a cause), we can more usefully think of causal pathways with some causes distant from the outcome, eg, poverty, others at an intermediate point, eg, cigarette smoking, and others proximate, eg, cellular abnormalities. It is important here to acknowledge the multiple levels of the social origins of disease.

Patterns of economic relations can influence health: for example, governments may discourage the consumption of healthier foods because vested interests lobby to limit relevant legislation; or, tobacco interests may curtail public health initiatives that would restrict the availability of tobacco products.

A comprehensive theory of disease needs to encompass very general phenomena associated with membership of particular national or other groups, and the consequences of this membership through to the way this membership produces cellular changes which precede diagnosable disease and death. Figure 5.1 presents a schematic representation of the different types of variables that are represented in studies linking the social origins of disease with their biological consequences. Some health problems clearly point to characteristics of the society as a whole. For example, there are higher rates of stomach cancer in Japan, very probably linked to the consumption of salted and/or cured foods. Rates of cigarette consumption may also be linked to the level of stomach cancer (Tominaga and Kuroishi 1997). By contrast, in countries like Australia and the United States, the rate of stomach cancer has declined dramatically as refrigeration has replaced other methods of preserving food. While rates of stomach cancer in Japan have also declined in line with the westernisation of their diet, the

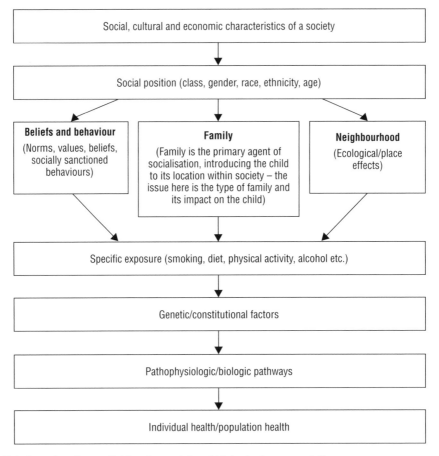

Figure 5.1 Causal pathways linking the social and biological causes of disease

higher rates of stomach cancer are likely to be a reflection of deeply entrenched cultural traditions associated with particular patterns of food consumption.

Social position is an important predictor of health. Both the social and economic characteristics of a society and social location of groups within that society are factors that influence health outcomes, partly because they involve particular beliefs, values and behaviours (figure 5.1). These behaviours may be adopted in a family context and reinforced within a geographic location. For example, the poor more often live in neighbourhoods with higher rates of crime, where less healthy lifestyles are more common and visible, and with lesser access to healthier foods. This in turn facilitates a set of specific behaviours, primarily to do with tobacco, diet, physical activity, sexual behaviour, alcohol consumption and the like. These specific behaviours (exposures) in turn lead to constitutional and biological changes that produce health outcomes. We argue here that the social and ecological are important but that they are filtered through specific exposures and biological pathways. Increasingly, the task of research is to identify the connections between the different levels of events that produce health outcomes. It is also pertinent to note that, the closer to the target health outcome one intervenes, the more immediate is likely to be the result. On the other hand, since the specific exposures are themselves a function of social and ecological contexts, they are likely to be resistant to change without changes in those contexts.

A general model of disease must encompass the timing of events that have health consequences. The health consequences of specific exposures will vary according to the duration and timing of exposure. This relationship need not be linear. Figure 5.2 illustrates the need to study exposures at different points in the life course and to recognise that the biological consequences of these exposures may differ depending upon when these exposures occur, as well as their duration and intensity. For some diseases, such as heart disease and some forms of cancer, there are exposures of 20 years or more before the health consequences become visible. With heart

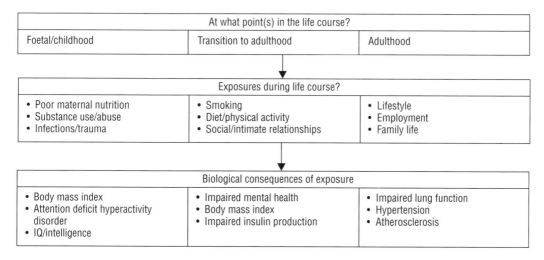

Figure 5.2 Exposures, timing and biological consequences

disease, assessments of 20-year-olds indicate the initial stages of atherosclerosis, yet the adverse health outcomes of these changes are generally not visible for another 20 or 30 years. This raises the general question of at what point in the life course the chronic diseases might first be observed were this information collected.

Biological or social origins of disease?

Finally, it is important to recognise the biological consequences of the social environment. While there may be value in distinguishing the biological basis of disease from its social causes, the biological and the social are, in practice, highly related. For example, a person's height is an indicator of that person's intelligence, ability and general health. Height here might be seen as a biological reality. However, from a social/structural perspective, it represents the outcome of a person's family history of nutrition and general living conditions. That is, the social environment influences physical development, which in turn influences an individual's capacity to take advantage of the environment in which he or she is located. Higher IQ in childhood is associated with a longer life expectancy (Whalley and Deary 2001). Whether this is because the social context within which a child is born and reared leads both to higher IQ and better health, or whether higher IQ itself leads to better health outcomes remains to be determined.

An individual's biological characteristics often are consequences of prior social environmental forces. How, for example, does one interpret the evidence of an association between body fat and a number of cancers (breast, prostate)? One can begin by acknowledging the believed carcinogenic effects of increased body fat. Increasing obesity is a characteristic of most Western societies: there is evidence of a societal increase in body fat, which has been described as of epidemic proportions in the economically developed countries. This is an indication of an increasing imbalance between energy input and energy expenditure. The most likely cause of this epidemic is reduced activity associated with more sedentary forms of work and recreation. A social change (decreased physical activity associated with the increasing access to electronic forms of work and passive recreation) here produces biological consequences (increased body fat), which may influence the course of particular diseases.

More attention now is given to biological changes to the foetus during pregnancy. Some behaviours or environmentally acquired infections produce biological changes to the foetus, which may have short-term and/or long-term health consequences. Of course, there are many events that might affect the developing foetus. These include toxic exposures at home or at work, potentially traumatic events experienced by the mother in pregnancy and the like. Here, the social and the environmental combine to produce what are potentially life-long biological consequences.

After birth, a child's nutrition and exposure to adverse environments, crowding, or infection may all significantly affect his or her biological make-up.

Distinction between the biological and the social causes of disease can be unhelpful. It can distract from the need to identify points in the causal sequence of disease that might serve as the basis for preventive programs. It would seem important to acknowledge the interaction between the biological and the social rather than to emphasise one or the other in pointing to the causes of particular diseases.

Foetal programming

The foetal programming theory argues that critical experiences/exposures that occur early in gestation can have life-long health consequences for the adult. Barker (1995), to whom this theory is largely attributed, argues that maternal undernutrition in pregnancy is a major factor which predicts subsequent disease in middle to late adulthood. According to Barker (1992, 1995) and his colleagues (Barker et al. 1993), a foetus adapts to poor maternal nutrition in pregnancy with a permanent change in physiology and metabolism. These changes in turn lead to increased rates of heart disease, stroke, diabetes and hypertension in adulthood. With around 40% of all deaths attributed to the above causes, this theory has a major place in discussions of the basis of the social origins of disease.

A body of evidence supports the notion of foetal programming. In one study, women in their 80s living in areas of England and Wales with high and low rates of cardiovascular mortality were asked to recall their diets when they were approaching the age at which a first pregnancy was a possibility. Those living in areas with a low rate of cardiovascular disease had had better access to a good and varied diet and lower fertility rates as youth (Ariouat and Barker 1993).

Of course, the foetal programming theory could be usefully extended to the idea that exposure to a variety of assaults/experiences during gestation has lifelong health consequences. There is now an extensive body of literature linking the health of a child to a variety of exposures during gestation, for example, cigarettes, illicit drugs, licit drugs (such as thalidomide), alcohol and so forth.

Nor are cardiovascular and cerebrovascular diseases the only major category of health impairment linked to poor maternal nutrition in pregnancy. The work of Ezra Susser examines the health consequences of maternal undernutrition for the child. This work is illustrative of the broadening of the foetal programming hypothesis to other than cardiovascular diseases. Susser's work linked records of data obtained about women who were pregnant before, during and after a particularly severe famine in Holland in 1944, and an examination of the mental health records of their children as 20-year-olds prior to their induction into army service in Holland in the 1960s. Susser and his colleagues found that those children born to mothers who experienced severe famine were more likely, some 20 years later, to have higher rates of minor and major psychiatric illness (Hoek, Brown and Susser 1998). The comparison group was of children who were born outside the period when the famine occurred. Interestingly, this study also found that inadequate maternal nutrition in pregnancy is associated with higher body mass index (in women) and higher rates of impaired lung function in adulthood (Ravelli et al. 1999; Lupuhaa et al. 2000). It does appear that inadequate nutrition and other experiences of the mother in pregnancy can have lifelong health consequences for the child.

The major criticism of the foetal programming view is that it fails to distinguish the impact of critical events in early pregnancy from subsequent experiences correlated with these early events on the one hand, and causally related to the health outcomes on the other. For example, mothers experiencing poor nutrition in pregnancy are more likely to be poor and, arguably, the health outcomes of interest are a consequence of a long history of poverty rather than specific undernutrition in pregnancy. Disentangling the impact of critical events in pregnancy from related and subsequent events is difficult. Certainly, evidence from studies of substance use in pregnancy (eg, thalidomide) and the work of Susser point to foetal programming as one possible causal pathway for subsequent disease, but the extent to which this pathway is causally implicated in a wide range of diseases remains unclear.

The life course and health

According to advocates of the life course view, health outcomes represent the accumulation of exposures over a period of time. The duration and intensity of exposure are important in determining health outcomes. Thus children who start smoking at a young age and smoke more cigarettes when they smoke are more likely to experience disease outcomes contingent upon this pattern of cigarette consumption. Similarly, longer exposures to poor diet, poverty, alcohol and/or a lack of exercise are all seen to be more strongly predictive of adverse health outcomes. Those who advocate a life course approach to understanding disease are primarily concerned with identifying circumstances, characteristics and exposures of those whose health is likely to be adversely affected. Exposures need not equally impact either on all people, or at all stages through the life cycle. A person who smokes heavily when young and then quits may be less likely to experience the adverse health consequences of smoking than is, say, a 60-year-old person who begins smoking and who has the risk of disease proportionally increased at a time when age-specific mortality rates are substantially higher.

While the foetal programming and life course approaches to understanding disease represent alternative explanations of what are sometimes similar outcomes, they are not necessarily conflicting ways of looking at the origins of disease. According to the foetal programming hypothesis, exposures occurring early in the development of the foetus and child have a greater impact than similar events occurring in the middle years of the life cycle. According to the life course view, the effects of exposures are possibly cumulative, with later exposures likely to be of greater significance. Both views acknowledge that they account for only a part of the disease burden. It is likely that, for most of the major causes of death, exposures in the foetal period and exposures during the life course act in a cumulative way to produce particular health outcomes.

The social origins and prevention

Understanding the pathways to disease provides both generic and specific guidelines for efforts to improve population health and longevity.

In industrialised nations, heart disease and stroke followed by lung cancer and breast cancer (in women) are the leading causes of death and arguably make the major contribution to the burden of disease. Here, it is interesting that only a few exposures are directly linked to these causes of death and that some of these exposures, for example smoking and diet, span more than one of these causes. If we are to improve the life expectancy of the population, we should address the major exposures before we attend to those that make a relatively minor impact.

The delineation of causal pathways suggests that health might be improved by interventions at different points: different types of policies and programs could be initiated at different points on a causal pathway, and such programs should be mutually supportive and reinforcing. If disease is the consequence of exposures from the foetal period to adulthood, then prevention programs might intervene at each point where disease impacts can be identified.

Rather than thinking in terms of specific initiatives to prevent disease, we might more usefully think about the characteristics of a society committed to improving population health. Such a society (see figure 5.3) would emphasise this in its national policies. Levels of inequality would be addressed at a national level. Availability of healthy and unhealthy products would, for example, be recognised through appropriate national policies. Groups experiencing the greatest health disadvantages would be identified, and policies would be initiated to reduce these disadvantages. Such policies would recognise the relationship between, say, knowledge and health or nutrition and health. Life-stage targets could begin with pregnancy and health promotion could be reinforced at various points in the life course.

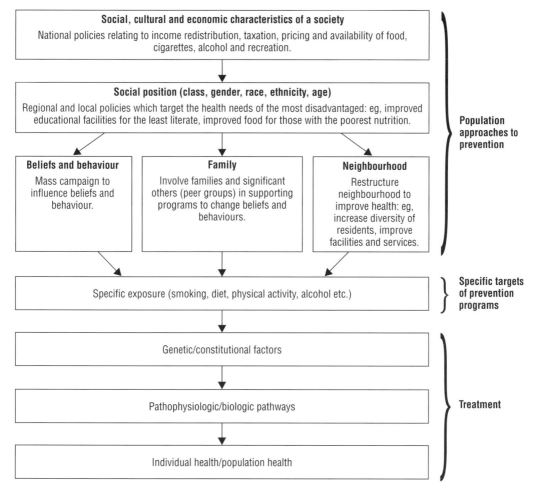

Figure 5.3 Causal pathways and health intervention policy

The health-promoting society will need to attend to national values and beliefs and the behaviours that flow from them. For example, as families remain the major force socialising the young, many health-enhancing policies may need to be implemented within the context of the family. Transformation of marriage and the family by ongoing demographic changes may present difficulties for policy implementation. Neither can existing neighbourhood effects be ignored: the way we physically arrange the environments in which people live has an impact on their subsequent health. In planning our cities (and our rural areas), we will need to think about the types of physical arrangements that produce the best health outcomes.

It is also important to acknowledge that treatment and compliance decisions may influence health outcomes. There is a considerable body of evidence on the relationship between treatment and the social context within which treatments are provided. For example, there is consistent evidence to indicate that about 50% of those who are prescribed treatments do not take these in the manner or quantity prescribed. There is evidence of considerable use of alternative therapies. What is clear is that these decisions and outcomes reflect the social world in which individuals are located, and understanding them is likely to be important in influencing the health outcomes of the population.

If we are to understand the basis of the health inequalities that exist in societies, we must begin by identifying the causal pathways that link social contexts with the biological bases of disease. The confusion created by numerous studies that treat the same phenomena using very different labels, or which emphasise different points along the causal pathway, needs to be addressed. Discussions of the 'causes' of health inequalities need to be disciplined by distinguishing those causes that have major impact from those that are of relatively minor significance. Disease prevention and health promotion need to become institutionalised within a mindset that transforms our way of thinking about population health. At all levels and through all sectors of decision-making the fundamental question should be, "What do we do to demonstrate that we are a health promoting society?" It is when we have addressed these tasks that we will be in a position to most effectively improve population health.

Further Reading

Amick, BC, Levine, S, Tarlov, AR and Chapman Walsh, D (Eds) 1995, *Society and Health*. Oxford University Press, New York.

Evans, RG Barer, ML and Marmor, TR (Eds) 1994, *Why Are Some People Healthy and Others Not: The determinants of health of populations*. De Gruyter, Berlin.

Keating, DP and Hertzman, C 1999, *Developmental Health and the Wealth of Nations*. Guilford Press, New York.

Shaw, M, Dorling, D, Gordon, D and Davey-Smith, G 1999, *The Widening Gap*. The Policy Press, University of Bristol.

6

Income inequality and health:
in search of fundamental causes

Gavin Turrell

Introduction

Despite the long-held myth of equality and egalitarianism, Australia is a socially and economically divided society: it was from the early days of white settlement (Connell 1977), it has been since (Western 1983; Baxter et al. 1991), it still is today (Fincher and Nieuwenhuysen 1998), and all indications are that it will continue to be so in the future (Megalogenis 2000). In fact, the socio-economic divisions within this country are predicted to widen (Kelly 2000; Steketee and Haslem 2000). Income inequality is a key indicator of this divide. Between 1982 and 1993/94, earnings and private income inequality increased in Australia, and while most of this increase was offset by government-initiated changes to the taxation and welfare systems (Harding 1997), Australia still has marked inequities in its distribution of income. One perspective on the extent of income inequality in Australia is illustrated in figure 6.1. These data indicate the share of total weekly income received by the poorest and richest 20% of families between 1994 and 1998. For each period, families in the bottom quintile of the income distribution received less than 4% of the total income going to Australian families, whereas those in the top quintile received just under 50%. This represents more than a 12-fold difference in share of the nation's income. The extent of Australia's income inequality has also been made apparent in recent international assessments that have shown that Australia is not far behind 'high' inequality countries such as the United States and Britain in terms of its level of income disparity (Smeeding and Gottschalk 1999).

The movement towards a more divided society is of concern, not only because of its inherent injustices and offence to moral sensibility, but also in light of studies showing that income inequality is bad for health. Since the mid-1980s, a growing body of epidemiological and public health research has demonstrated that morbidity and mortality risk is greatest in areas with high levels of income inequality. At present, our knowledge and understanding of how income distribution affects health is limited, although a number of explanations have been proposed. These include differential investment in human, physical and social infrastructure;

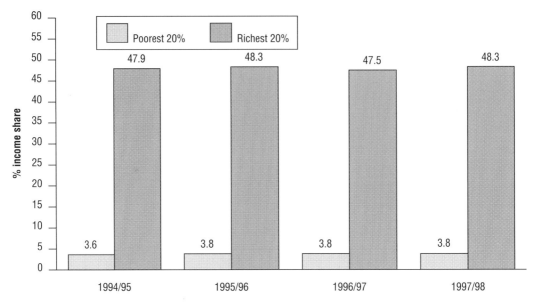

Figure 6.1 Percentage of total income received by the poorest and richest 20% of Australian families, 1994–8

Source: Australian Bureau of Statistics 1999.

psychosocial processes related to perceptions of one's position in the socio-economic hierarchy; and social cohesion. This chapter will argue that the relation between income inequality and health is ultimately a result of differential investments in people and places, which gives rise to economic and material disparities, and that psychosocial health and social cohesion are a consequence of these more fundamental structural features of society. Further, the chapter will argue that we should attend not only to links between income inequality and health, but also to how income inequality is generated and maintained, and whether and to what extent national governments should be trying to minimise the extent of income differentiation in society. A guiding rationale for this paper's argument is the belief that policy and intervention initiatives that help people deal with the consequences of income inequality (eg, psychosocial stress) rather than attacking the problem at its root (ie economic structure) are likely to have limited effects on health disparities at the population level.

What is income inequality?

Most studies investigating the link between income and health have to date conceptualised and measured income as a characteristic of an individual. Typically, individuals (which include families and households) are classified into discrete categories based on their levels of income, and the health status of these different income groups is compared. Studies examining the association between individual income and health show that income level is strongly related to mortality and morbidity risk, with the poor experiencing the highest mortality rates and lowest health status. These relationships have been demonstrated in the United States (Duncan 1996; McDonough et al. 1997; Pappas et al. 1993), Britain (Blaxter 1990; Ecob and Davey Smith 1999), many European countries (Martelin 1994) and Australia (Turrell and Mathers 2000; Saunders 1996; National Health Strategy 1992), and they have been observed for both males and females at every stage of the life-course (ie infancy, childhood and adolescence, adulthood, and old age).

While it is now well established that income at the individual level influences health, there emerged during the 1990s a new perspective about how income and health are related. This perspective, known as 'income inequality', focuses on the income properties of ecologic units such as countries, states, and neighbourhoods, and it views the health status of populations, population sub-groups, and individuals within these units as being affected by inequalities in the distribution of income. Put simply, health status is seen to be a function of the size of the gap between the incomes of the rich and the incomes of the poor: ecologic units with a more egalitarian income distribution will have a better health profile than units with large income inequalities. An income inequality perspective sees individual health as not necessarily (nor exclusively) being a consequence of individual characteristics, but rather, the social and economic characteristics of societies, environments and contexts inhabited by individuals.

Income inequality and health: how are they related?

For an overview of studies that have examined the relationship between income inequality and health, the studies are grouped into two broad categories: those that examine the relationship cross-nationally and those that examine it within a single country. This latter category is furthered divided into two sections: the first comprises studies that link income inequality with health measured at different levels of geographic aggregation (eg, states, counties, local government areas); and the second includes studies that assess the relationship on the basis of health measured at the individual level.

It is important to note that this discussion of income inequality and health is necessarily based on research conducted mainly in the United States and some other countries, but not Australia. To date, no known published Australian study has investigated the relationship between income inequality and health, and this represents a significant research and knowledge gap. In light of this, we need to reflect critically on the question of whether research findings from the US (and other countries) can be simply transplanted to the Australian context. For example, the factors that give rise to and sustain income inequality (eg, social, political, historical, and cultural forces) differ between Australia and the US, and structural features such as the economic segregation of the population are much more marked in America. Whether and to what extent income inequality and health are related in Australia awaits empirical verification. In the meantime, however, we are required to proceed on the basis of societal models that may be a poor fit *vis-à-vis* the Australian situation.

Cross-national studies

Early investigations of the relationship between income inequality and health focused on cross-country comparisons. (A detailed discussion of the available measures of income inequality has been provided by Creedy (1996) and Kawachi and Kennedy (1997a) and will not be described here.) The results of these studies are consistent in showing that that the extent of income inequality within a country is closely tied to its health profile. Rodgers (1979) examined the cross-sectional relationship between income inequality and infant mortality, life expectancy at birth and life expectancy at age five, on the basis of 56 rich and poor nations. Each measure of health was significantly correlated with the extent of income inequality after adjustments for gross national product (a measure of average income in each country). Le Grand (1987) examined the relationship between income inequality and average age at death across 17 developed countries and found that longevity was greatest in those nations with smaller income disparities. This association was independent of both gross domestic product and per capita expenditure on medical care: indeed these measures themselves were unrelated to average age at death. In a series of papers spanning the late 1980s to mid-1990s, Wilkinson corroborated these findings by showing that life expectancy was higher in developed countries with narrower income differentials, even after taking account of average income levels in each country (Wilkinson 1989, 1990, 1992a, 1992b, 1994a). Other cross-national comparisons indicating similar associations between income inequality and population health have been published by Flegg (1982), Waldmann (1992), Wennemo (1993), and Steckel (1995).

Wilkinson was also able to show that life expectancy and rates of mortality tended to change in response to increases or decreases in the extent of a country's inequality, suggesting that a causal link existed between inequality and health (Wilkinson 1989, 1992b). Similar evidence was earlier reported by Kehrer and Wolin (1979) who demonstrated that changes in the health of population sub-groups (particularly the most economically disadvantaged) responded to changes in income distribution. Support (albeit indirect) between income inequality and population health also comes from other observations made by Wilkinson (1994b). For example, despite the fact that most developed countries have witnessed increases in their absolute standard of living in recent decades, as well as overall improvements in health, this same period has been characterised by widening socio-economic health inequalities in some countries (Marmot and McDowall 1986; Pappas et al. 1993; Borrell et al. 1997). Wilkinson poses the possibility that these seemingly contradictory trends might be due to increases in income inequality which have also occurred in many developed societies in recent times (Smeeding and Gottschalk 1999; Massey 1996).

Taken together, the forgoing studies and observations suggest that the extent of income differentiation within a country is closely linked with a wide range of health outcomes. This evidence, however, has not gone uncontested, and a number of writers have raised questions about the validity and reliability of the data and methods used to draw inferences about the link between income inequality and health at the national level (Judge 1995; Saunders 1996). For example, Richard Wilkinson's early examination of the relationship between income inequality and health using cross-national data (1992a; 1992b) was the subject of intense criticism from other writers. Judge (1995) and Saunders (1996) claimed that Wilkinson's results could not be substantiated as they were based on erroneous data, inappropriate methods and selection bias. Wilkinson subsequently replied (1995) and the debate was later continued (see Judge et al. 1998; Wilkinson 1998b). Partly in response to this debate, researchers turned their focus from comparing across different countries to examining the relationship between income distribution and health within a single country.

Within-country studies (health measured at the ecologic level)

Studies investigating the relationship between income inequality and health on the basis of aggregated outcomes (eg, state mortality rates) have to date been conducted using data from the US, Canada, England/Britain, and Taiwan. For each country except Canada, similar findings have been reported, namely, that income inequality is significantly associated with mortality after adjusting for average income.

One of the first within-country studies examined the relationship between income inequality and age-adjusted mortality from all causes, low birth weight, and risk factors for the 50 US states (Kaplan GA et al. 1996). Significant correlations were found between income inequality and each health measure, and these relationships were largely unaffected by adjustments for state median income. Specifically, states with higher levels of income inequality had higher age-adjusted and age-specific mortality rates, and a greater proportion of low birthweight babies, smokers, and those who were classified as sedentary. A significant association was also found between income inequality and percentage change in age-adjusted mortality for the period 1980–90. States that were more unequal in 1980 had slower rates of mortality decline over the ensuing decade, lending further support to the possibility of a causal link. Further, moderate-to-strong correlations between income inequality were found for males and females for all deciles of the income distribution, although the associations were most marked for deciles below the 50th percentile. This finding suggested that inequality in the distribution of income adversely affected the health of the majority of the population, and not just the most socially and economically disadvantaged. Strategies that are directed at reducing disparities in the distribution of income, therefore, are likely to benefit most sections of the population and not exclusively the indigent or those living in straitened economic circumstances.

A second (and independent) study of the 50 US states examined income inequality and disease specific mortality (Kennedy et al. 1996). Significant associations were found with total mortality, infant mortality, heart disease, malignant neoplasms, and cerebrovascular disease. These associations were observed after taking account of state variations in poverty, median household income, household size, and smoking rates. Significant associations were also found between income inequality and mortality from potentially treatable causes of death, including infectious and hypertensive disease, tuberculosis and pneumonia, and bronchitis. Again, these relationships were unaffected by adjustment for poverty and prevalence of smoking. In a later study, these same authors tested the sensitivity of the relationship between income inequality and mortality by examining the association using six different indicators of inequality (Kawachi and Kennedy 1997a). All of the indicators were strongly correlated, and each was significantly associated with state-level mortality after adjusting for median income.

During 1996, the first study of relative inequality and health within Britain was published (Ben-Shlomo et al. 1996). This study did not focus on income inequality per se, but rather, examined the contribution of a small area's overall level of deprivation and variation in deprivation to mortality. As with its US counterparts, this study found that areas with greater disparities in economic deprivation had higher mortality rates. Importantly, however, this paper reported that the overall (or absolute) level of deprivation in an area was also related to health. Subsequent studies corroborated this finding. Lynch et al's (1998) study of 282 metropolitan areas of the US found that income inequality was strongly associated with age-adjusted and age-specific mortality after taking account of per capita income, median household size, and proportion of the population with incomes less than 200% of poverty. In addition, this study found that absolute income was significantly related with mortality independent of any shared association with income inequality. Studies by Stanistreet et al. (1999), Chiang (1999), Waitzman and Smith (1998), and Kahn et al. (1998) have reported similar patterns of association: that is, both income inequality (reflecting relative deprivation) and absolute income (reflecting average economic and material conditions in an area) are important for health.

A more recent examination of the relationship between income inequality and health investigated the association using cross-sectional data from the US and Canada (Ross et al. 2000). In keeping with earlier analyses, this study found a significant association between income inequality and state-level mortality rates for US infants, children and youth, and the working aged. However, no significant association between income inequality and mortality was found in Canada at either the province or metropolitan area level. This exception to an otherwise fairly consistent pattern of study findings is important for a number of reasons. First, it indicates that there is no universal or inevitable link between income inequality and health within a country. Second, it suggests that the US and Canada differ in ways that are important in terms of the pathways and processes linking income inequality and health. It may be that the extent of income inequality in the US has had a disproportionately detrimental effect on that country's social fabric, such that it is a less cohesive and a more divided society than Canada, and that this has had adverse consequences for people's psychosocial health (leading to poor physiological health). It is also possible that Canada's particular mix of social and economic policies, welfare provision, and resource allocation has served to offset, to some extent, earnings and private income inequality, and in so doing, minimised any negative impact of inequality on population health.

While the studies cited in this section have focused on the consequences of income inequality for population health, it needs to be mentioned that this is but one of a number of outcomes that have been linked with income inequality. Studies have shown that areas characterised by high levels of inequality also have above average rates of homicide (Szwarcwald et al. 1999) and other violent crime (Kawachi et al. 1999b; Wilkinson et al. 1998). Income inequality seems to be more than a configuration of factors that contribute specifi-cally to bad health: it also appears to reflect a more generalised condition of relative economic, social and material deprivation that produces a diverse range of negative outcomes and behaviours.

Within-country studies (health measured at the individual level)

Studies investigating the cross-national relationship between income inequality and health, and within-country studies examining this association based on health measured at the ecologic level, have provided valuable insights into how social and economic differentiation affects population health (and the health of sub-groups with these populations). However, these studies tell us very little (if anything) about how income inequality impacts on the health of individuals.

To date, only a small number of studies have examined the relationship between income inequality and individual health, and these have recently been reviewed by Wagstaff and van Doorslaer (2000). Overall, the results are mixed. A study by Kennedy et al. (1998) used a multi-level analysis to examine the relationship between income inequality and self-rated health for the 50 US states. They found that income inequality was significantly related to propensity to report health as 'fair' or 'poor' after taking into account individual-level (household) income, sex, race, smoking status, obesity, health insurance, health check in the past two years, household composition, and education. Specifically, after adjustment for these factors, individuals living in states with the greatest income inequality were 30% more likely to report their health as 'fair' or 'poor' than individuals living in states with the smallest income inequalities. On closer examination, however, the relationship between income inequality and health was contingent on one's personal income, with the strongest effects of income inequality being found among the low income group, and no effect being observed among the richest. In a later study, Soobader and LeClere (1999) reported significant associations between income inequality and self-rated health for white males aged 25–64 after adjusting for individual covariates and median income. This relationship, however, was dependent on the level of aggregation and level of income inequality: it was stronger and more consistent at higher levels of geographic aggregation (ie county rather than census tract), and it was evident only for men in high income inequality areas.

Other studies investigating the relationship between income inequality and individual health have failed to find any significant association. Daly et al. (1998) found no effect of income inequality on mortality for individuals aged 25 and over. Fiscella and Franks (1997) showed that income inequality was associated with individual all-cause mortality after adjusting for age, sex, and average community income; however, this relationship disappeared after adjusting for individual household income, and Mellor and Milyo (1999) found no association between income inequality and self-reported health using a population-based sample of 186,776 US adults aged 25–74.

The review by Wagstaff and van Doorslaer (2000) makes a significant contribution to our understanding of how income inequality impacts on health, and by critiquing the available literature and pointing to the limitations of the extant evidence, they have raised many questions and suggested new directions for future research. Importantly, Wagstaff and van Doorslaer's finding that the results of individual-level studies are mixed and inconclusive in no way threatens the more general thesis about income distribution and its relationship with health; rather, it serves to highlight the complexity and contingent nature of the association (eg, on levels of aggregation, position within the socio-economic hierarchy, extent of income inequality, and appropriate model specification).

Income inequality and health: why are they related?

An important challenge awaiting future research is the identification of the actual pathways and mechanisms that link income inequality and health. This section examines the three most widely discussed explanations: namely, psychosocial processes related to perceptions of relative disadvantage and position in the socio-economic hierarchy; social cohesion; and differential investment in structural, material and economic resources and human capital.

Psychosocial processes

All developed societies are characterised to a greater or lesser extent by the unequal distribution of income, wealth, and material resources (indeed, measures of income inequality represent a summary index of these disparities). Those at the bottom end of the socio-economic hierarchy are more likely to live on low incomes, work in hazardous and insecure jobs, reside in sub-standard housing in high-crime neighbourhoods, and lack the money necessary to buy healthy food or to improve the chances of upward social mobility of their offspring via better education. By contrast, their counterparts at the top end of the socio-economic distribution earn large incomes, work in more secure, rewarding jobs, reside in nice houses in safe and friendly neighbourhoods, enjoy healthy foods, and can ensure the intergenerational continuity of this advantage by sending their offspring to the best schools. Between these two positions are located the bulk of the population. Proponents of the psychosocial perspective argue that people will differentially perceive these inequalities, again depending on their socio-economic position, and that the interpretation and attachment of meaning to these inequalities may result in poorer mental health as indicated by elevated rates of stress, depression, hostility and hopelessness, and lowered self-esteem, coping and sense of control (Wilkinson 1996). Many different situations are likely to produce these adverse psychosocial responses. An unemployed person living on a low income, for example, may experience elevated rates of stress and anxiety about current personal disadvantage and prospects for the future. Others may be adversely affected by a more generalised response to wider societal inequality and all its associated injustices. Some may suffer poorer psychosocial well-being as a result of their self-positioning within the socio-economic hierarchy and consequent negative assessments of their ability to share in the opportunities, rewards and resources that are available to others. There are now a large number of studies that have examined the association between socio-economic position and psychosocial well-being and most show that these factors are positively correlated (Ross and Van Willigen 1997; Saunders 1998; Pincus and Callahan 1995; Taylor et al. 1997; Kaplan 1995; Kessler 1982).

Irrespective of how psychosocial morbidity is generated, its link with physiological health is conceptualised as operating through two main pathways, one direct and the other indirect. The direct link sees poorer psychosocial states such as stress and anxiety as negatively impacting on the endocrine and immune systems, which in turn produce adverse biologic reactions, such as hypertension, fibrin production, suppressed immune function, and adrenalin release. If sustained over long periods, these processes contribute to the onset and progression of chronic degenerative conditions such as cardiovascular disease. These types of pathways have been suggested in many studies (Anderson and Armstead 1995; Flinn and England 1997;

Chrousos et al. 1995; Carroll et al. 1997; Brunner 1997). The indirect link sees conditions such as stress and feelings of hopelessness as impacting on morbidity and mortality via health-related behaviours such as smoking, alcohol consumption and drug use. Again, the results of many studies lend support for this process. There is now a large literature showing links between socio-economic position and health-related behaviour, with those at lower levels of the socio-economic hierarchy being less likely to behave in ways that are conducive to better health (Turrell et al. 1999; Turrell and Mathers 2000; Lynch et al. 1997; Bennett 1995; Droomers et al. 1998).

In sum, psychosocial explanations of the relationship between income inequality and health see socioeconomic differences in health as arising primarily (although not exclusively) from the way people perceive, interpret and respond to inequality within their living environment (both proximate and distal). Environments with high levels of income inequality are likely to evoke more negative psychosocial responses from the population generally, and most particularly from those who experience the greatest disadvantage; and these responses, when mediated through health behaviours and psycho-neurological and biologic mechanisms, result in poorer health.

Social Cohesion

In recent times, evidence has emerged suggesting that high levels of income inequality are detrimental to social cohesiveness, which in turn has deleterious consequences for population health and individual health. Kawachi and Berkman (2000) refer to social cohesion as the 'extent of connectedness and solidarity among groups in society' (p 175). A critical determinant of this cohesiveness is the degree to which a society is endowed with stocks of social capital, defined by Putnam (1993) as 'features of social organisation such as trust, norms, and networks, that can improve the efficiency of society by facilitating coordinated actions' (p 167). A review of the literature pertaining to social cohesiveness and social capital suggests that cohesive societies are characterised by the following traits: high levels of trust, openness, and mutual tolerance; a willingness on the part of individuals and groups to participate fully in all aspects of civil life; close social ties and networks among individuals, and between individuals and the wider society; and the presence of associations and institutions that ensure the maintenance of democracy.

Wilkinson (1996a) has provided indirect support for the link between income inequality, social cohesiveness and health using historical case studies. In one, he showed how in wartime Britain, the extent of income inequality within the population narrowed, and that this was accompanied by greater social solidarity and cohesiveness and improvement in life expectancy. In another, he describes how the town of Roseto, Pennsylvania, was once considerably more cohesive than the surrounding towns, and that this was associated with a substantially lower mortality rate from coronary heart disease. The baseline differences in mortality between Roseto and the surrounding towns was not attributable to concomitant differences in heart disease risk factors such as smoking, diet, and obesity, as these were similar for all towns in the area. During the mid-1960s however, the town experienced rapid economic growth and a subsequent widening of income differences between the rich and poor. Within only a few years, Roseto experienced an increase in coronary disease deaths to a level similar to that of the surrounding areas.

A more formal and direct test of the link between income inequality, social cohesion and health was undertaken by Kawachi et al. (1997a). Using a cross-sectional ecologic study of US states, the authors operationalised two key concepts of social capital – civic trust and density of associational membership – and examined how these related to the distribution of income and all-cause and specific-cause mortality. They found that income inequality was strongly related to both social cohesion and health, and that social cohesion itself was significantly associated with mortality rates (all results were adjusted for age, state median income, and poverty). States with high levels of income inequality were characterised by low levels of social trust and group membership and high levels of total mortality, infant mortality and death due to heart disease, malignant neoplasms and cerebrovascular disease. In addition, states with low levels of social trust and group membership exhibited higher mortality. A regression path analysis revealed that social cohesion (or more particularly, disinvestments in cohesion) constituted a major pathway through which income inequality impacted on population health.

In a recent test of the influence of social cohesion on health, Kawachi et al. (1999c) undertook a contextual analysis based on a sample of 167,259 individuals residing in 39 US states. Specifically, the study examined whether social capital – measured using state-level indicators of civic trust, perceptions of reciprocity, and membership of voluntary organisations – influenced self-rated health at the individual level after adjustment for age, sex, race, health insurance coverage, health check-up in the last two years, obesity, smoking status, household income, education level, and living arrangement. The key issue being examined here was whether the social cohesiveness of an individual's lived environment exerted a measurable effect on individual health separate from the sociodemographic and risk-factor characteristics of the individuals themselves. The results of bivariate analyses indicated that states with low social capital also had a higher proportion of residents who reported their health as 'fair' or 'poor'. After adjustment for the individual-level variables, the relationship between social capital and self-rated health was attenuated, but remained statistically significant. States characterised as low trust, low reciprocity and low group membership were 44%, 48% and 22% more likely to have residents who rated their health as 'fair' or 'poor' respectively.

To date, no other known studies have examined the link between income inequality, social cohesion and health, so confirmation of the findings of Kawachi et al. (1997(a)) and Kawachi et al. (1999c) in other contexts and countries is not possible at present. Despite this, their results are highly suggestive, and when considered in light of less direct evidence and case studies cited by Wilkinson (1996), present the possibility that an unequal distribution of income does contribute to a more individuated and less communitarian society with negative consequences for health.

The establishment of an association between income inequality, social cohesion and health tells us very little about how and why these factors are related. How do disruptions to the social fabric by high levels of income inequality impact on health? Answering this question is difficult in the absence of 'hard' data; however, the two main proponents of the social cohesion perspective (Kawachi and Wilkinson) present a number of potential links.

Composition effects

We need to remain open to the possibility that the ecologic relationship between social cohesion and health is not truly reflecting the direct impact of environmental contexts per se, but rather, is due to a disproportionate concentration of isolated and unsupported individuals living in areas characterised by low social cohesion (ie a composition effect). Studies investigating the relationship between social networks and health at the individual level consistently show that well-integrated persons with dense and extensive networks (friends and family), who can call on others for support (financial, emotional, instrumental), have better health than their more isolated and less-integrated counterparts (Berkman and Breslow 1983; Berkman and Glass 2000; Seeman 1996). The findings reported by Kawachi et al. (1997a) and Kawachi et al. (1999c) may in fact be capturing this strong association between social networks and health at the individual level, and not, as is presumed, broad ecologic effects due to the cohesiveness of the social fabric. The most appropriate way of addressing issues relating to contextual versus compositional effects is via multilevel models that include data on both ecologic units and individuals. To date, no known study has used this approach to examine the association between social cohesion and health, thus the relative contribution of contextual and compositional effects is unknown.

Health-related behaviour

As was suggested earlier, a cohesive society (or any other ecologic unit) is characterised by shared norms, high levels of trust, and a general consensus about what constitutes 'appropriate' practices as these pertain to the benefit of individuals and society as a whole. Kawachi et al. (1999c) and Kawachi and Berkman (2000) have suggested that this 'moral' dimension of a cohesive society can act to shape and circumscribe behaviour in ways that produce positive health outcomes. For example, societies that value health are likely to positively sanction some processes (eg, physical activity) while negatively sanctioning behaviours that are inconsistent with this value such as public drinking and adolescent smoking. The flip-side of this position is that members of societies with low levels of social cohesion and a less binding moral order are more likely to tolerate health-damaging behaviours and less likely to take civic action in response to these practices.

Actions of 'appropriable' organisations

Socially cohesive communities are more likely to produce what Coleman (1990) calls 'appropriable' organisations that promote activities of benefit to the community and can also act to prevent the occurrence of things that are considered inconsistent with what the community values and deems important for quality of life. For example, voluntary groups, parents and citizens' groups and other social organisations, which are more likely to be visible and active in cohesive and less divided settings, can operate and lobby to ensure that their community receives health-related resources such as transport links, recreation facilities and green spaces, while also fighting against potentially health-damaging actions such as government cut-backs to essential services, or private sector initiatives such as land development.

Psychosocial Well-being

Wilkinson (1996a) has suggested that socially cohesive communities may act to promote and protect the psychosocial well-being of its members, and that one indicator of this is low rates of chronic degenerative disease in communities with high levels of social capital. If we accept that cohesive societies are more likely to be characterised by high levels of social trust, reciprocity, and mutual concern for others, and that members of these societies perceive the wider environment as being non-threatening and safe, then this link seems plausible. Living in a socially cohesive setting is likely to be conducive to better psychosocial well-being (ie less stress, anxiety, and hopelessness). Moreover, in the event of adverse psychosocial responses occurring, cohesive contexts may be better able to provide various forms of support and hence minimise the short-term and longer-term negative health effects of these conditions.

To summarise, it seems likely that high levels of income inequality are adverse to social cohesiveness and social capital, and that this in turn has deleterious consequences for population health. While the exact pathways and mechanisms linking income distribution, cohesion and health remain to be identified and more fully elucidated, some of the effects are possibly mediated through health-related behaviours, the activities of social organisations, and psychosocial processes. For further discussion of these issues, see Wilkinson (1997a), and Kawachi and Kennedy (1997b).

Differential investment in structural and economic resources and human capital (neo-materialism)

The neo-material perspective views the relationship between income inequality and health as being a consequence of how society is structured and organised, and the extent to which governments invest in economic resources and human capital. Health inequalities that correspond to socio-economic inequalities are seen to originate primarily from the differential distribution of resources and capital, variations in exposure to adverse material and economic conditions at critical periods (eg, infancy and childhood), and accumulated negative experiences and exposures across the lifecourse (Lynch et al. 2000b). The neo-material perspective is 'new' in the sense that it sees human, physical and social infrastructure as not only affecting the health of the more disadvantaged sections of society, but also functioning to influence health at most points on the socio-economic spectrum.

While the term 'neo-materialism' has only recently entered the parlance of health inequalities researchers, some of the central arguments and claims of the neo-material perspective can be identified in studies that emphasise the importance of 'place' in people's health. To date, only a small number of studies have focused on the relationship between the structural, economic and physical features of an area and the health profile of its residents (Kaplan 1996; Macintyre et al. 1993). An important clarification needs to be made here. A large number of studies have compared the health profiles of individuals living in areas differing in their socio-economic status. Many studies have also linked the ecologic characteristics of areas (eg, percentage on low income, percentage unemployed) with summary health measures such as mortality and morbidity rates. Few studies, however, have compared areas in terms of such things as their transport services, road conditions, recreation facilities, levels of government investment, health infrastructure etc. and used these as the basis for investigating health differentials. An early (and now classic) investigation of this type compared the mortality profiles of residents living in a feder-ally-designated poverty area with residents in a non-poverty area, using a random sample of 1,811 US adults aged 35 and over (Haan, Kaplan and Camacho 1987). Residents in the poverty area (which, by definition, was materially and economically under-resourced) experienced a significantly higher mortality rate after adjustment for baseline health status, race, income, employment status, access to medical care, health income coverage, smoking, alcohol consump-tion, physical activity, body mass index, sleep patterns, social isolation, marital status, depression and personal uncertainty. Note, that the association between area and mortality existed after the effects of psychosocial factors, social networks and health-related behaviours were taken into account, suggesting that aspects of the broader socio-physical environment contributed to mor-tality differences between the areas. In a second study, Blaxter (1990) used the British 'Health and Lifestyle Survey' to examine the relative contributions of social circumstances and behav-iour to socio-economic variability in health. Based on an analysis of interactions among these factors, Blaxter concluded, 'if (social) circumstances are good, "healthy" behaviour appears to have a strong influence on health. If they are bad, then behaviours make rather little difference' (p 216). This conclusion is extremely important, for it suggests that not only are behaviours such as smoking and physical activity shaped by the wider social and economic context, but that these latter factors are the most fundamental in determining health outcomes. A similar conclusion was later reached in a Dutch study that examined the relative contribution of behavioural, economic, and material factors in explaining health inequalities (Stronks et al. 1996). Based on the results of their study, the authors concluded that 'our research demonstrated that behaviour is imbedded, for an important part, in structural conditions' (p 672).

In a position paper examining the influence of area characteristics on health, Macintyre et al. (1993) discuss a number of aspects of the physical, social and cultural environment that are likely to either promote or damage health depending on their presence or absence. The issues they consider include quality of air and water, housing, secure and non-hazardous employment, affordable and nutritious food, safe and healthy recreation, education, transport, street cleaning and lighting, policing, the presence of community organisations and health and welfare services, political and economic history, and perceptions of the area's reputation by residents, outsiders, and service or amenity planners and providers. The authors then go on to show how a number of these factors (recreation, transport, primary care facilities, and crime) contributed to health differences between areas even when individuals of the same socio-economic level were compared.

One of the strongest cases yet for the influence of structural/material factors on individual health was produced by Yen and Kaplan (1999), who examined the effect of neighbourhood social environment on 11-year risk of death. Specifically, they undertook a longitudinal multi-level analysis of the effects of area characteristics on mortality risk, using a combination of census and area-based data to estimate the contribution of area variations in death rates separate from the impact of individual-level factors. The neighbourhood level measures com-prised per capita income, percentage of white-collar employees, crowding, commercial stores per 1,000 population (pharmacy, beauty salon/barber, laundry/dry cleaners, supermarkets) and environment/housing (population, size of area, percentage of households renting, percentage of single family dwellings). Individual level measures comprised household income, education, race/ethnicity, smoking status, body mass index, alcohol consumption and perceived health status. The main finding of this study was that residents of neighbourhoods characterised by greater levels of economic and material disadvantage were 58% more likely to die during an 11-year follow-up than their counterparts in more advantaged areas. This result held after simultaneously adjusting for all individual-level measures. This finding strongly suggests that the quality of socio-physical contexts within which people live makes a measurable contribution to health independently of factors operating at the individual level.

Each of the foregoing studies, while not focusing on income inequality per se, is consistent with a neo-material perspective on health inequalities in that it emphasises (and demonstrates) that health is ultimately a consequence of social organisation and structure and levels of investment in community resources and human capital. The only known study to directly link income inequality, neo-material conditions and health has been produced by Kaplan GA et al. (1996). This study (described earlier) examined the income inequality–mortality relationship for the 50 US states, but in addition, investigated how income inequality related to a range of social indicators and markers of investments in human capital. The study found that states with greater inequality in the distribution of income (and an associated higher mortality rate), also had elevated rates of unemployment, incarceration, individuals receiving income assistance and food stamps, and persons who were medically uninsured. States with high levels of income inequality also spent a smaller proportion of funds on education and library books per capita, and had poorer educational outcomes including lower rates of high school completion, and worse proficiency in reading and mathematics. When considering the broader implications of their results, the authors suggest that:

> While there may be higher rates of adverse psychosocial outcomes in states with high inequality these may only be a reflection of the greater difficulties in life that are caused by the structural characteristics that distinguish between states with high and low inequality. From a prevention point of view, it may be more important to deal with these structural features than their psychosocial consequences (Kaplan GA et al. 1996, p 1002).

This conclusion is entirely consistent with the position adopted in this chapter. Neo-material factors are the most fundamental determinants of health, and psychosocial processes, health behaviours and social cohesion, while representing important mediating mechanisms and pathways, are ultimately a product of these more primary factors. In the section that follows, a conceptual model is presented that offers a plausible explanation for how each of these factors, mechanisms and pathways interrelate, and how they influence population health and contribute to health inequalities.

Income inequality and health: what is the likely fundamental cause?

Studies investigating the cross-country association between income inequality and health have found that nations with large disparities in their distribution of income have poorer health profiles than nations with a narrower income gap between the rich and the poor. These associations were observed even after taking account of differences in average income between countries. Researchers investigating the relationship between income inequality and health within the same country have presented a similar picture: populations in areas with high levels of income inequality tend to have poorer health than populations in areas where the distribution of income is more equitable (although Canada is a notable exception. See Ross et al. 2000). Again, these associations have been found even though adjustments were made for differences in mean incomes and poverty levels between areas, and income (and other) differences between individuals.

Two issues emerge from the results of these cross-country and within-country studies. First, their findings strongly suggest that contexts and environments are important for health, and that these broader ecologic factors influence health over-and-above the characteristics of the individuals who live in these contexts and environments. Second, the fact that we still observe strong associations between income inequality and health after statistically adjusting for area and individual-level income suggests that this association is capturing *something* other than the effects of income per se. The question of what this 'something' is has become the focus of a growing debate and discussion in the public health and epidemiological literature. At present however, we don't know why and how the distribution of income affects health, or what it represents in terms of broader contextual influences: it is clearly a marker or surrogate for something, but for what? According to Wilkinson, Kawachi and others, the relationship between income distribution and health reflects the independent and interdependent influences of social cohesion and psychosocial processes, whereas Kaplan, Lynch and others argue that it is more likely an indicator of differential investment in physical, economic and material resources and human capital. Evidence and arguments pertaining to each of these positions was reviewed in the previous section of this chapter.

In this section, an attempt is made to draw together the three perspectives and incorporate them within a broader conceptual framework (figure 6.2), showing how each possibly relates to the others, and how all are crucially important for health. Despite their inherent limitations, frameworks such as the one proposed here can inform and guide future research by identifying knowledge gaps and suggesting new directions. They can also help researchers differentiate between factors that confound and factors that 'explain' associations (ie form part of the pathway). Distinguishing between these two types of factors is as much a conceptual issue as it is a statistical one. These frameworks also serve a useful heuristic purpose in terms of policy and interventions, as they provide a macro-view of the ordering of the likely influences and how these interact, thus suggesting entry points for action.

The framework explicitly assumes that the relationship between income inequality and health is capturing elements of each of the three suggested explanations; however, the model proposes that these elements differ in their 'distance' from health, and that some factors are more fundamental than others. Moreover, while the model represents only one of many possible interpretations of how income inequality and health are related, most of its proposed links can be supported by empirical evidence (some of which was cited and reviewed earlier). Other links have *prima facie* plausibility but await empirical verification.

The central argument encapsulated by the framework is as follows. Income inequality differences between areas reflect (or are a marker for) differential investment in an area's human, physical, health and social infrastructure, which over time results in area differences

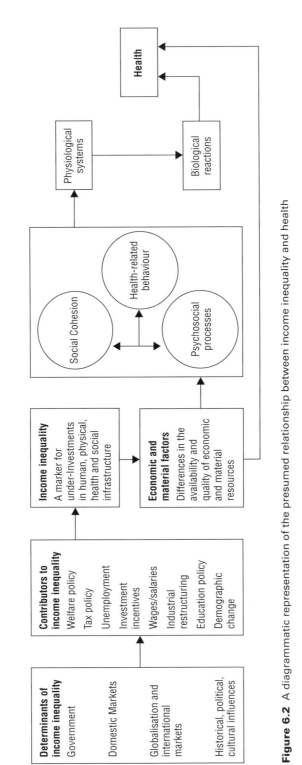

Figure 6.2 A diagrammatic representation of the presumed relationship between income inequality and health

in the availability and quality of economic and material resources (housing, schools, transport, health care facilities), which in turn influences social cohesion, psychosocial well-being, and health-related behaviours. These processes, when mediated ultimately through physiological systems and biologic reactions, impact on health. This series of pathways and mechanisms is entirely consistent with our current understanding of the aetiology of chronic degenerative disease in developed countries and of why populations and sub-groups within the population differ in their experience of these conditions (Brunner 1996; Marmot and Mustard 1994).

Under-investment in an area's resources, infrastructure and capital, and the subsequent economic and material disadvantage stemming from this, are also likely to have more direct and immediate health consequences via such things as accidents and injury and exposure to workplace hazards. The arrow directly linking resources and health represents this path. The model also caters for Wilkinson's (1996a) interpretation of how relative deprivation impacts on psychosocial well-being. It is the differential investments between areas which gives rise to the inequality that individuals then internalise, cognitively process, and negatively react to. Lynch et al. (2000b) have argued similarly: 'The structural, political, and economic processes that generate inequality exist before their effects are experienced at the individual level' (p 1202).

A further explicit claim made in this framework is that economic and material resources that flow from investments and capital inputs are fundamental to the whole process, and that these act to shape and circumscribe the degree of social cohesion as well as the psychosocial well-being and health-related behaviours of individuals. It is difficult to conceptualise these links as operating in any other order sufficient to substantially influence the health of populations and their sub-groups. Certainly, we can conceive of scenarios where people's psychosocial states and behaviours influence their socio-economic status (and hence access to economic and material resources), but this is unlikely to account for even a small part of the strongly graded associations between socio-economic position and health that have been found in numerous studies (Power et al. 1996; Blane et al. 1993). The ordering of influences in this framework is also consistent with the findings of studies that examine the relative contributions of economic, material and behavioural factors to health (Blaxter 1990; Stronks et al. 1996). More broadly, the framework's flow and composition are in accordance with current thinking and theories about the determinants of population health (Marmot and Wilkinson 1999; Blane et al. 1996; Evans et al. 1994).

Finally, as the framework makes clear, the degree of income inequality in a society is itself influenced by more upstream factors (eg, welfare, taxation, wages and salaries, education policy) and these are in turn determined to varying degrees by governments, domestic markets, globalisation and international forces, and broader historical, political and cultural influences. In the final section of this chapter, these issues, and their implications for population health, are examined in more detail.

Reducing income inequalities: implications for population health and health inequalities

Socio-economic differences in health, and population health more broadly, are closely linked to income inequality. As has been demonstrated in this chapter, large disparities in the distribution

Table 6.1 Some suggested mechanisms and processes contributing to income inequality

Authors	Factors contributing to income inequality
Morris, Bernhardt and Handcock 1994	• Emergence of a service economy and subsequent rising demand for skilled and educated labour (highly paid), associated with a 'stagnant' pool of low-skilled, poorly educated workers on low incomes • Disproportionate growth in both low-wage and high-wage jobs and a shrinking group of middle-class workers
Waitzman and Smith 1998	• Changes in investment patterns and industrial restructuring • Move from a manufacturing/industry-based economy to one based on service provision and technology, resulting in an increased demand for high skills and education, and consequent shifts in rewards • Division of the labour market into high-paying jobs for professional, technical and managerial workers, and an increase in low-paying service jobs with little opportunity for security and advancement (working poor)
Lynch et al. 1998	• Differential monetary returns on education and skills • Wage restraint pressures • Differential economic returns on capital compared with labour
Muntaner and Lynch 1999	• A shift towards a service sector economy that generates both high-wage and low-wage jobs, and declines in middle-wage jobs • The segmentation of the labour market • A steady increase in the demand for skilled workers relative to unskilled workers • The internationalisation of financial markets and the relative decline in manufacturing jobs • Technological change • Decline in union density and influence • Political decisions relating to taxation that promote an 'investor capitalism' strategy of low wages and high capital return
Wilkinson 1999b	• Changing industrial structure • Education policy • Declining power of trade unions and the influence of new technology • Development of 'winner-take-all' markets • Changing household structure (eg, increased numbers of single-parent households and elderly not living with younger generation)
Coburn 2000	• Rise of market-oriented (neoliberal) regimes and the subsequent undermining of the welfare state • Loss of influence of labour unions and other organisations opposed to the strict application of market mechanisms

of income have been associated with high levels of all-cause and specific-cause mortality, poorer self-rated health and risk factor profiles, and adverse social outcomes such as high rates of homicide, violent crime and imprisonment. These findings lead inexorably to the question of what can be done to reduce income differences within a society, and what role can and should governments play in facilitating this process.

Studies investigating the relationship between income inequality and health have focused largely on describing the association and addressing attendant methodological issues, as well as proposing (and where possible testing) some suggested explanations. Very few public health researchers or epidemiologists have examined the more fundamental (and arguably equally important) question of what generates income inequality in the first place. To date, research and debate around this issue has been confined largely to the economics and political economy literature, although there are a number of notable recent exceptions (Coburn 2000; Muntaner and Lynch 1999; Muntaner et al. 1999). Clearly, this topic deserves greater attention, as it would seem crucial to better understanding the genesis of health inequalities and the development of policies and strategies to redress them (Lynch 2000).

What gives rise to income inequality, and how it is sustained and/or changed over time, is complex, not completely understood, and is the subject of ongoing investigation. Given this, only a brief sketch of the main issues will be provided here. At the most macro level, income inequality is the result of historical, social, and economic forces played out thorough such things as globalisation, political ideology, class relations, domestic and international markets, and welfare state dynamics. In discussions focusing on the significance of income inequality for population health, a number of writers have identified some of the more specific mechanisms and processes that are a consequence of these broader forces that contribute to income disparities. These are summarised in table 6.1. They suggest many ways in which governments can lessen the extent of income inequality in society (eg, progressive taxation, income maintenance for low-income individuals and families, improved access to education and training, job creation, and structural adjustment programs), and given the now strong evidence linking income distribution and health, there is ample justification for them to do so. A number of studies and reports have examined ways of reducing income inequality with a view to improving health (Andrain 1998; Shaw et al. 1999; Gordon 2000).

Reducing income inequality calls for greater and more equitable investments across areas in terms of physical, social and economic infrastructure, underpinned by an explicit acknowledgment that such measures are ultimately investments in population health. Relatedly, governments need to recognise that public policy is health policy writ large, and that all new policy initiatives should be carefully assessed in terms of the extent to which they might exacerbate income inequalities in the future (Kaplan GA et al. 1996). Further, a focus on more equitably distributing income must not be seen as conflicting with policies aimed at poverty eradication: indeed, 'policies that are directed at either poverty reduction or income inequality are not likely to be achieved in the absence of the other' (Fiscella and Franks 1997, p 1726).

In recent decades, we have witnessed in many developed countries (including Australia) an undermining of the welfare state and a concomitant rise in neoliberal political doctrine, which together, have acted as a countervailing force against attempts at a more equitable distribution of income. Coburn (2000, p 138) has characterised neoliberal philosophy as follows:

• That markets are the best and most efficient allocators of resources in production and distribution.
• That societies are composed of autonomous individuals (producers and consumers) motivated chiefly or entirely by material or economic considerations.
• That competition is the major market vehicle for innovations.

Consistent with these tenets of neoliberalism has been the view of many governments that what is best for population health, and the health of the poor in particular, is overall economic growth: in short, improving the lot of the poor means enlarging the pie (Lynch and Kaplan 1997). Recent comments by Australia's Workplace Relations and Small Business Minister reflect this view:

> If we are to provide the social services we all want for the disadvantaged and aged; if we are to build new national infrastructure; if we are to better resource our schools, our health system, our law enforcement; if we are to redress disadvantage suffered by indigenous peoples – then we continuously need to build a more prosperous and competitive Australia. That must be the national goal. (Shanahan 2000)

Evidence from a variety of sources cautions against such an optimistic view of the contribution of continued economic growth to population health (Glyn and Miliband 1994). Studies have shown, for example, that overall economic growth does not necessarily nor inevitably help the poor (Cutler and Katz 1991). Other research has reported that economic growth is slowest in countries with high levels of income inequality (World Health Organisation 1998), and, as was noted at the beginning of this chapter, Australia is listed as not far behind the US and Britain in income inequality. Further, it is very likely that government-initiated attempts to increase economic growth (eg, via tax breaks, private sector investment initiatives, financial rewards for capital ventures) benefit population groups differentially, such that overall growth is accompanied by widening income inequalities (Danziger and Gottschalk, 1993).

Bringing about macro-level social and economic change (such as income redistribution) is clearly very difficult (Erickson 1992; Andrain 1998; National Advisory Committee on Health and Disability 1998), and some view it as a largely non-viable and unrealistic public health strategy (Syme 1998). Despite this, sufficient evidence now exists to suggest that the largest gains for public health, and the health of disadvantaged groups in particular, will accrue through strategies that result in a more equitable distribution of economic and material resources, both across geographic areas and among individuals who reside in those areas. This can be visually illustrated to some extent using a graph that plots the relation between individual-level income and health (figure 6.3). It should be noted that the relation between individual-level income and health does not completely specify or capture the relationship between income inequality and health at the ecologic level (Lynch et al. 2000b; Wolfson et al. 1999). In other words, they are probably reflecting largely different mechanisms and processes, although some degree of shared variation exists.

As is evident in figure 6.3, the shape of the relation between individual-level income and health is very often curvilinear, with the gradient being steep and near linear at low income levels, tapering quickly to a gentler slope at moderate to high income levels (Blaxter 1990; Turrell 2000; Backlund et al. 1996). Increments of income on the flatter section of the

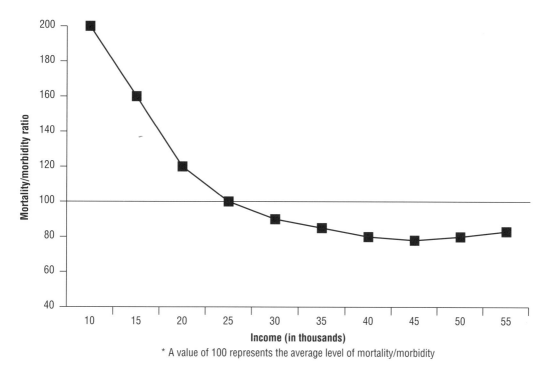

Figure 6.3 Health plotted against income, hypothetical example*

Note: * A value of 100 represents the average level of health.

curve often result in little, if any, additional health benefit. This curvilinear form implies that redistributing income and other economic and material resources from the rich to the poor will benefit the health of the poor far more than it will be detrimental to the health of the rich (Wilkinson 1990). In addition, it suggests that national mortality rates are strongly influenced by this patterning (Wilkinson 1992b). High mortality rates of the poor add disproportionately to a nation's overall mortality rate. Reducing this burden by distributing income more equally would therefore not only improve the health profile of the most disadvantaged groups, but also of the nation as a whole.

In closing this chapter, it would seem appropriate to comment further on the conceptual framework's implications for public health and the quality of the social fabric more generally. First, investments in human, physical, and social infrastructure are crucial both to individual and population health. These investments influence health via the economic and material environment they create, via the effect this environment has directly and via other mechanisms. These other mechanisms include social cohesion (or the lack of it) and psychosocial processes and the effect of these factors on health-related behaviour. Societies with a more equitable distribution of income are likely to be characterised as more socially cohesive as a consequence of being well endowed with stocks of social capital (Kawachi and Berkman 2000; Kawachi et al. 1997a; Kawachi and Kennedy 1997b), and this densely interconnected social fabric will act to promote and protect psychosocial well-being and minimise the likelihood of health-damaging behaviours.

During the last few decades in Australia and overseas, we have seen a rise in the youth suicide rate (Cantor et al. 1999) and a general decline in the psychosocial well-being of young people (Rutter and Smith 1995). Over the same period, we have witnessed an increase in levels of social and economic inequality, one indicator of which is the emergence in major urban areas of clearly defined concentrations of affluence and disadvantage (Australian Bureau of Statistics 1998c). If the conceptual framework accurately depicts reality, then these two trends are unlikely to be independent; rather, it would seem that the widening socio-economic gap in this country may have contributed to these adverse health trends among Australian youth. Further, despite marked improvements in overall level of health, Australia experienced increased socio-economic mortality inequalities between 1987 and 1997 for a number of the major contributors to total mortality, such as circulatory system disease and cancer (Turrell and Mathers 2001). Are these seemingly contradictory trends also due, as the framework would suggest, to an increase in Australia's relative inequality?

Lastly, a characteristic feature of more downstream approaches to tackling socio-economic health inequalities, such as health promotion and behavioural interventions, has been their limited success with disadvantaged groups (Whitehead 1995). It has also been suggested that these strategies have actually contributed to the widening of health disparities (Kawachi and Marmot 1998). Given that socio-economic health inequalities occur for most major causes of disease, attempts at addressing this large-scale problem using narrowly conceived and specific approaches would seem to be questionable in terms of their likely effect on health disparities at the population level. While health promotion and intervention obviously constitute an important part of any overall strategy to address health inequalities, the greatest gains (as the framework suggests) are likely to result from more fundamental change such as the narrowing of income differentials and economic and material improvements among the less advantaged sectors of the population.

Further Reading

Wilkinson, R G 1996a, Unhealthy Societies: The afflictions of inequality, Routledge, London.
 – *Examines the question 'Why are some societies healthier than others, and how does inequality affect health?'.*
Kawachi, I, Kennedy, B P and Wilkinson, R G (Eds) 1999b, Income Inequality and Health: The society and population health reader, The New York Press, New York.
 – *Brings together the most important (previously published) papers in the field of income inequality and health. It examines the question of why societies with greater income and social inequality have poorer health profiles than do more equal societies.*
Berkman, L F and Kawachi, I 2000, Social Epidemiology, Oxford University Press, New York.
 – *A collection of articles that provides the non-specialist reader with a clear exposition of social epidemiology and its main fields of study.*

7

Mediation of the effects of social and economic status on health and mortality: the roles of behaviour and constitution

Richard Taylor

Disease and mortality characterised by socioeconomic differentials

There is a wide range of diseases and causes of mortality that are differentially distributed by socioeconomic status. This is not surprising since most disease and premature mortality are due to environmental influences, and exposures differ according to social and economic position. The major causes of illness and premature death are usually grouped as:

- infections and diseases of the perinatal period;
- noncommunicable disease, particularly cardiovascular disease and cancer (especially lung and breast); and
- injuries, including suicide and homicide (Murray and Lopez 1997a, 1997b).

In contemporary developed countries, the major causes of premature mortality are related to noncommunicable disease and injury, and these conditions have the greatest effect on socioeconomic differentials in health status. Conditions selected for particular attention in this review are important causes of premature mortality and morbidity in Australia and other developed countries:

- coronary heart disease (CHD), still a major cause of death and disability;
- lung and breast cancer (the major causes of cancer death in males and females respectively); and
- suicide, now equal to deaths from motor vehicle accidents.

In general, socioeconomic differentials in health and mortality are a consequence of the differing occurrence and outcome of the mass diseases and conditions afflicting society. In Australia and other Western industrialised society near the end of the 20th century, higher mortality and morbidity in groups of lower socioeconomic status (SES) is principally accounted for (Taylor et al. 1992, Lawson and Black 1993, McMichael 1985) by:

- cardiovascular disease, especially CHD;
- cancer, especially lung cancer; and
- injuries, especially traffic accidents, suicide and occupational injuries.

These conditions are not unchartered territory, and explanations for socioeconomic differentials in their occurrence must encompass what is known of their biology and epidemiology, and their changes over time.

Requirements for explanations of SES differentials and health

Explanations for SES differentials in health and mortality must encompass a number of complex circumstances:

- Variation in the major diseases and conditions accounting for socioeconomic differentials in health over time and between populations. During the first half of the 20th century, SES differentials in health and mortality were mostly due to under-nutrition and infection (especially in infants and children), and this is still the case in many developing countries, but by the late-20th century, SES differentials were due mainly to differences in noncommunicable disease and injury in adults.
- Overall improvements in health and declines in mortality in the various socioeconomic strata. Mortality declined in all SES strata during the 20th century, and absolute differences narrowed, even though relative differences widened or did not decrease.
- Variation in the socioeconomic location of major conditions. This particularly applies to CHD which was formerly more common in upper SES groups in the first part of the 20th century (as it is now in many developing countries), then descended the social scale. It also applies to suicide.
- Biological and behavioural mechanisms. Considerable knowledge is available on the causes of major conditions responsible for premature mortality in contemporary developed countries and this needs to be integrated into explanatory frameworks.

Furthermore, explanations for SES differentials in health must incorporate all, or most, of the evidence available in a logically coherent framework without major contradictions.

'Constitutional' susceptibility theory

This explanation posits that people of lower SES are more susceptible to a whole range of diseases and conditions due to a nonspecific 'constitutional' weakness (Syme and Berkman 1976, Yen and Syme 1999). That is, there are not specific and different reasons why lower SES people contract particular conditions. One of the main reasons advanced to support this notion is that people of lower SES suffer from a wide range of ailments and perish prematurely from a wide range of conditions. Thus, it is argued, they are more likely to have a general susceptibility to disease and injury rather than a wide range of unconnected coincidental factors operating simultaneously as causes.

Three basic variants to this model relate to possible causality. Firstly, the most common contemporary view is that socioeconomic status affects health directly, not via individual risk factors but by activating disease mechanisms possibly due to the effects of psychosocial stress operating through immune and neuro-endocrine systems (Syme and Berkman 1976, Yen, and

Syme 1999) This is the so-called 'stress diathesis'. The second hypothesis is that many adult conditions are to a significant extent due to prenatal and perinatal influences (often associated with low birth weight), and adverse factors in early development are more common in those with lower socioeconomic status (Godfrey and Barker 2000, Frankel et al. 1996). The third hypothesis, more prominent 50 years ago, is that of genetic inferiority. Proponents of this view explain, within a Darwinian paradigm, why the lower classes were at the bottom and stayed there. The genetic hypothesis will not be further pursued here. Particular hypotheses have been associated with particular diseases and conditions since empirical research must at some stage bridge the gap between posited underlying causal influences, whether genetic or acquired, and the patho-physiology of disease.

These causal hypotheses have important implications for public health methods to control disease and improve health. Genetic and perinatal hypotheses imply that not much can be done because the die has been cast. However, for the next generation, there are implications involving eugenics (including gene manipulation), and antenatal and perinatal care to reduce low birth weight and associated factors. Needless to say, genetic explanations for mass diseases are very popular with geneticists and genetic researchers, and the antenatal/perinatal theories are very popular with paediatricians and obstetricians. For adults with innate and irreversible 'constitutional' susceptibility to disease, the only approach is early detection of environmental factors which interact with this susceptibility and 'aggressive' control in these unfortunate individuals. That is, healthy life styles are more necessary for some individuals than others. This approach is implied in much research that focuses on individual susceptibility, and ignores the structural (socioeconomic, environmental, cultural) determinants of health-related behaviour. Furthermore, evidence of effectiveness of mass screening to identify susceptible individuals would be required prior to implementation.

The implication of the theory of 'constitutional' susceptibility due to psychosocial stress is that prevention needs to be directed towards relief of psychological and social stress. Perhaps pharmacological intervention at the level of immune or neuro-endocrine mechanisms would be helpful, or mass medication with psychoactive drugs, or mass counselling. Most proposed interventions tend to focus on proximate associations of psychosocial stress related to the individual, family and work environment (including autonomy and 'control'), and how these could be manipulated to relieve stress. This approach does not usually connect with macro-economic and macro-social factors in any direct meaningful way. Furthermore, this theory does not consider, to any significant extent, health-related behaviours and risk factors, because, in its most developed form, it proposes that psychosocial stress works independently of these. Once it is proposed that psychosocial stress is an intermediary between socioeconomic status and health-related behaviours (diet, tobacco, alcohol, etc.), we then have a causal framework that is indistinguishable from behavioural risk factor models.

What is the evidence against nonspecific 'constitutional' susceptibility to disease as an explanation of socioeconomic differentials in health? First, while it is true for a wide range of diseases and conditions, that lower SES people suffer at higher rates than upper SES groups, this is not invariable: SES gradients are absent for many conditions and, for some conditions, upper SES groups have higher rates. For example, while SES gradients are evident for some cancers with higher rates in lower SES groups (especially lung cancer), gradients are absent for many other cancers, and for some cancers, incidence is higher in upper SES groups (Smith et al. 1996). Breast cancer is the most common cancer (apart from skin cancer), and the most common cause of cancer death in women in industrialised countries. Various studies have demonstrated that women of higher income, social class or education have higher rates of breast cancer incidence (Ewertz 1988a, 1988b; Kelsey 1993; van Loon et al. 1995; Barbone et al. 1996). Both individual and group studies have generally produced similar results. The SES gradient is most likely due to differences in education and occupation, and mediated by differing reproductive experience – upper SES women are older at first pregnancy and have fewer children. Diet may also be a factor. The higher incidence of breast cancer in upper SES women may not necessarily translate into higher mortality, because of greater compliance, easier access to mammographic screening, consequent earlier diagnosis and more effective treatment. These factors are also related to education.

If there were a general susceptibility to disease in lower SES groups, evidence of differentials for all conditions would be expected. More plausible is that there are particular explanations as to why certain conditions are more prominent in the various socioeconomic classes. Lung cancer is more common in lower SES groups because of greater exposure to tobacco smoking and probably occupational carcinogens. Breast cancer is more common in upper SES women because of reproductive factors, but, because of screening behaviour, this may not translate into higher mortality.

Second, the major causes of disease and premature mortality can move between social classes over time, and patterns may differ between developed and developing countries. The most important example here is CHD. Early in the 20th century, CHD was a disease principally of the wealthy and affected professionals and businessmen to a much greater extent than workers. This was documented in both the UK (Ryle and Russel 1949) and USA (Hedley 1939). Furthermore, the current situation in many under-developed countries is that the first to be affected by CHD are the wealthy – politicians, businessmen, bureaucrats, professionals. For example, Singh et al. (1997) showed higher CHD and associated risk factors in upper SES in rural India. With time, CHD descended the social scale and, since the 1960s, has been more common and has caused higher mortality in the lower SES groups than upper SES groups in industrialised countries, such as Australia (Dobson et al. 1985 McMichael 1989 Taylor et al. 1999).

How can a condition be due to a 'constitutional' weakness when it changes classes in such an adept manner? A more plausible explanation is that the wealthy were first to be affected by CHD because they did not have to undertake physical exercise to earn their living (and thus were sedentary) and were able to afford manufactured cigarettes and a plentiful diet high in animal fat. With continued economic development, an abundance of food and tobacco was available to all, including the lower SES strata, who also may have found solace in this consumption. At the same time, mechanisation significantly reduced the amount of physical work undertaken by those previously engaged in manual labour. The result was that the incidence of CHD became approximately equal across social classes. With dissemination of information on the relation of CHD to diet and exercise, and tobacco smoking, the upper SES changed their behaviour first because they had the education to appreciate the information and the control over their lives to change their consumption, as well as alternative outlets

as pleasurable activities. CHD risk behaviour changed eventuall[
coupled with improvements in treatment (especially of hype[
reduced, but more slowly and to a lesser extent in lower SES gr[
SES differentials. .

Suicide is another example. In Europe in the late 19th century, Du[
the highest suicide rates to occur in the highest social classes, and attributed th[
social regulation and integration of these groups (anomie). By the middle of the 20th centu[
investigators found the highest suicide rates to occur in both the highest and lowest SES groups
(Sainsbury 1955). However, by the latter part of the 20th century, the lowest SES groups were
committing suicide at higher rates than the highest SES groups (Monk 1987, Kreitman et al.
1991). And this was the case in NSW, Australia, 1985–1994 (Taylor et al. 1998). Again, how
can this be explained on the basis of a 'constitutional' susceptibility affecting those in the lowest
SES. Perhaps Durkheim's notion of anomie or normlessness is an explanatory framework which
can encompass these changes in suicide frequency through social classes over time.

Third, there is much known of the biology and epidemiology of the major causes of illness
and death in humans. It is not necessary to posit propositions such as general 'constitutional'
susceptibility when we know of the effects of exposures and behaviours which lead to the major
cardiovascular diseases, cancers and injuries. Specific and particular explanations drawn from
existing knowledge in most instances will account for differences in diseases and mortality
among various socioeconomic groups. Furthermore, particular explanations suggest the need for
adaptation of health promotion and prevention and control programs to those groups at highest
risk, as well as the amelioration of underlying social and economic conditions.

Accounting for disease and mortality differences among socioeconomic strata on the basis of risk factors

Some of the most important evidence brought forward to undermine the importance of biological risk factors in disease causation is that SES differences in disease incidence or mortality
cannot be fully 'explained' on the basis of measured risk factors; in some instances, only a
small part of the difference is 'explained' by risk factor differentials. The most important
example here is CHD, where most conventional studies demonstrate an inability to 'explain'
a significant proportion of the variance (deviance) in logistic regression equations of CHD
incidence or mortality (y variable) in individuals on their measured biological and behavioural risk factors (x variables). And furthermore, the differences in CHD among SES groups
cannot be fully accounted for on the basis of risk factors using these analyses.

This has led to hypotheses that there are important undiscovered risk factors and other
causal influences for CHD, which are yet to be discovered, and that other explanations must
be sought to explain a significant part of the difference in CHD among SES strata.

Regression dilution bias
First, it must be understood that the word 'explain', when employed in relation to variance (or
deviance) results from regression equations, is being used in a technical, statistical sense.

second, the most important under-appreciated factor in CHD research has been measurement error in many of the risk factors leading to 'regression dilution bias', which reduces the relative risks (odds ratios) towards the nul (1.00). Measurement problems can be a consequence of observer or instrument error, which may occur with measurement of blood pressure, serum cholesterol, and other physical factors, and subject reliability (eg, reporting of tobacco smoking). However, more importantly, measurement error is also a consequence of the fact that many biological and behavioural risk factors validly vary over time. Most epidemiological studies of CHD (the most important example of this sort of measurement error) have relied on very few measurements of risk factors to characterise individuals. Measurement error leads the estimated odds ratios in regression analyses to move towards the nul (1.00). Consequently, most conventional studies demonstrate an inability to 'explain' a significant proportion of the variance (deviance) in logistic regression equations of CHD incidence or mortality (y variable) in individuals on their measured biological and behavioural risk factors (x variables). And furthermore, the differences in CHD among SES groups cannot be fully accounted for on the basis of risk factors using these analyses.

Although 'regression dilution bias' has been known for quite some time, it is only during the 1990s that it has been taken into account in studies of cardiovascular disease epidemiology (Clarke et al. 1999), particularly for the effects of hypertension (MacMahon et al. 1990) and serum cholesterol (Law et al. 1994) on CHD and stroke, and salt intake on hypertension (Elliott et al.1996). It has been found that the effects of risk factors on disease are underestimated by 50–66% when uncorrected for regression dilution bias compared with the use of multiple measurements to characterise individuals.

Cumulative effects, lag times and proxy effects

The other important considerations in studies of causes of cardiovascular disease are the questions of cumulative and lag effects, and proxy effects.

CHD is a consequence of the cumulative effect of risk factors over an extended period, and thus even longitudinal studies, especially those which start in middle age, are unable properly to assess the period over which elevated risk factors have operated. Thus, individuals and groups may have different rates of CHD occurrence with risk factor levels which are not too dissimilar, because the duration of raised risk factors was longer in some than others; or had been higher in some and had been lower in others in the past.

Proxy effects relate to the fact that several measured risk factors are to some extent proxies for more precise causative influences. For example, serum cholesterol is a useful indicator of saturated fat intake, but there are more detailed and specific lipid profiles which correlate better with CHD.

Explanations for trends and differentials in coronary heart disease occurrence

Studies in Australia and elsewhere have demonstrated that differences in risk factor prevalence between sub-groups parallel differences in CHD occurrence (Dobson et al. 1985, Rose and Marmot 1981, Waters and Bennett 1995), and decline in CHD occurrence parallel reductions in risk factor prevalence (Hardes et al. 1985, Dobson 1987). Many studies of differentials and trends in CHD occurrence in the past have failed to explain a substantial part of the variation on the basis of measured risk factors for either SES (McMichael 1989, Marmot et al. 1978, Rose and Marmot 1981), ethnic (Armstrong et al. 1983) or geographic differences, or period trends (Dobson 1987, Beaglehole et al. 1989).

Several approaches have been employed since 1970 to account for the decline in CHD mortality in industrialised countries (where this has taken place) in terms of changes in population risk factors and treatment, in order to assess the effects of prevention and control efforts. These include: simple analysis of trend data with assumptions of effects of prevention and treatment; qualitative and semi-quantitative correlation of CHD mortality decline with changes in population risk factors or their proxies; application of predictive equations derived from cohort studies of individuals to populations; use of simulation models and synthetic cohorts; and direct imputation of changes in CHD from changes in risk factors in populations using data (corrected for 'regression dilution bias') from intervention trials and cohort studies. Using this last approach, Dobson et al. (1999) were able to account for almost all of the annual rate of decline in major CHD events (which reflects incidence) in the Hunter region of NSW, Australia, 1985–93 (ages 35–64 years) on the basis of declines in population mean serum cholesterol, mean diastolic blood pressure, and tobacco smoking prevalence (each contributing around one-third). Changes in risk factors also explained the mortality reduction in CHD mortality in Iceland (both sexes, ages 45–64 years) over 1981–86 (Sigfusson et al. 1991), and in Finland, changes in blood pressure, smoking and serum cholesterol explained 75% of the CHD mortality decline over 1972–1992 (Vartiainen et al. 1994).

Direct effects of psychosocial stress

As previously noted, psychosocial stress has been invoked as a direct cause of illness and premature mortality in order to explain some of the differences among social strata. One variant of this model is that which has already been discussed: psychosocial stress leads to a 'constitutional' weakness and susceptibility to disease, possibly via effects on the immune and neuro-humoral systems. Another variant is that psychosocial stress leads to specific diseases through specific physiological mechanisms, particularly neuro-humoral. For example, various causes of psychological and social stress lead to CHD quite independent of risk factors such as diet and exercise, and tobacco smoking. This is certainly a celebrated example, since CHD was widely regarded as due to stress (in the upper classes) in the mid-20th century (Ryle and Russel 1949). It is thus interesting to see the (direct) stress hypothesis disinterred, but as an explanation for higher mortality in the lower classes at the end of the century.

It has been reported that psychosocial circumstances at work, encompassed by the term 'job control', can account for the differences in male CHD incidence among (Whitehall) civil service grades that is not 'explained' (in a regression equation) by difference in risk factors (Marmot et al. 1997a). The conclusion made is that 'job control' is a specific 'toxic component' (Marmot et al. 1997b) that is a direct proximate risk factor for CHD. There are several other publications that relate to this and similar work. Although there may be speculation, the biological basis of such an association has not yet been ascertained.

An alternative explanation of these findings is that 'job control' is another measure of socioeconomic status, and perhaps superior to employment grade in some ways, and it is not surprising that this variable will result in decreases in the odds ratios for grade when entered into a regression equation with it. After all, autonomy and control over one's life are important characteristics of socioeconomic status as indicated by education, income and occupation. This explanation is posited by White (1997) in a comment on the article by Marmot et al. (1997a). Furthermore, job stress is most likely correlated with CHD risk factors as well as employment grade, and the effects of this multi-collinearity of predictor variables in the model may lead to incorrect conclusions that 'job control' is an independent risk factor.

Furthermore, it is not easy to explain the impressive declines in CHD since 1970 in industrialised countries, including in lower SES groups, on the basis of amelioration of psychosocial stress.

Conclusion

Concerning 'constitutional' susceptibility theory, it is noted that: SES gradients are absent for many conditions; SES gradients vary over time and between populations; and there are important diseases that are, or were, more common in upper SES groups. Furthermore, cogent explanations for SES gradients for particular conditions (or groups of conditions) are available, and these are important in design of prevention and control programs.

In relation to explanation of disease on the basis of biological and behavioural risk factors, it is noted that statistical models that 'explain' variance (deviance) in individual case–control or cohort studies often systematically under-estimate the effects of risk factors because of measurement difficulties; this has been labelled 'regression dilution bias'. Furthermore, information from intervention trials indicate that almost all the decline in mortality and disease in populations can be accounted for on the basis of the reduction in risk factors or treatment.

Concerning the direct effects of psychosocial stress, it is noted that 'job control' is a measure of socioeconomic status and that in a regression equation it may well reduce the effect of other status measures (such as employment grade), as well as leading to multi-collinearity of predictor variables. Furthermore, although various neuro-endocrine and immunological changes have been linked to psychosocial stress, such changes have not been established to be major causes of disease.

It is concluded that there is little evidence to support the propositions examined. The explanations for SES differentials in health and mortality are of considerable importance in the design of prevention and control programs to reduce differentials. Incorrect formulations are a threat to public health.

Further Reading

MacMahon, S, Peto, R, Cutler, J, Collins, R, Sorlie, P, Neaton, J, Abbott, R, Godwin, J, Dyer, A, Stamler, J 1990, Blood pressure, stroke, and coronary heart disease, Part 1, prolonged differences in blood pressure: prospective observational studies corrected for the regression dilution bias, Lancet 335(8692): 765–74.

– *The first major article which demonstrated the extent to which the effects of risk factors on coronary heart disease have been systematically under-estimated in cohort studies because of inadequate numbers of measurements leading to 'regression dilution bias'.*

Dobson, A J, McElduff, P, Heller, R, Alexander, H, Colley, P, D'Este, K 1999, Changing patterns of coronary heart disease in the Hunter region of New South Wales, Australia, Journal of Clinical Epidemiology 52(8): 761–71.

– *Shows that the decline in coronary heart disease in the Hunter region over a decade can be entirely accounted for by decreases in population risk factors (adjusted for 'regression dilution bias') and treatment interventions.*

– *These studies do not support the idea that there is a significant amount of unexplained variability in studies of coronary heart disease in relation to the classical modifiable risk factors (cholesterol, hypertension, smoking).*

8
Migrants, money and margarine:
possible explanations for Australia–New Zealand mortality differences

Alistair Woodward, Colin Mathers and Martin Tobias

Introduction

In the past, international comparisons have been treated as a useful starting point for studies of the social determinants of health, but that is all. In fact, they have rather more to offer. For a start, national populations provide a natural unit of observation to tackle some of the biggest and most important questions in public health. These are questions such as:

- Why are mortality rates falling so consistently in most parts of the world, in virtually all age groups?
- What distinguishes the exceptions to this general pattern?
- Who or what deserves credit for the improvements (and the blame for the exceptional declines in life expectancy)?

Comparisons between countries also serve a unique bench-marking function, indicating what could, plausibly, be achieved if the performance of comparable countries was emulated.

Ecological studies have often been a source of hypotheses about the causes of disease, exploiting the fact that variations in behaviour and environment between countries tend to be greater than variations within countries. These hypotheses have typically involved risk factors for disease measured at the level of individuals. However, the causes of disease that are 'social' are, by definition, characteristics of groups rather than individuals and in some instances, are characteristics of whole countries. (Examples include taxation policies and occupational health legislation.) Here, international comparisons provide the only means of studying directly the association between social circumstances and health outcomes. The same approach may be taken to analyse interventions that are implemented nation-wide, such as the introduction of co-payments in health care (Schoen 2000) or the relation between distributive income policies and health inequalities (Kunst 1997).

Australia and New Zealand are obvious candidates for comparison: despite extreme variations in geography, the societies have much in common. Donald Horne suggested that 'in one sense no country except New Zealand can be compared with Australia: these are the only two "Western" nations that are strategically part of Asia' (Horne 1966). They share a history of

British colonial settlement, and have inherited language, culture and public institutions from a common stock. However, there are also important differences between the two in population make-up, natural resources and political arrangements. As the connections with Britain have loosened, the contrasts between Australia and New Zealand have become more marked. Reasons for this divergence include different patterns of migration and economic development, the assertion of indigenous cultures (that have little in common apart from a history of dispossession) and global flows of capital and human resources. One would think that this mix of similarities and differences made fertile material for comparisons. Yet relatively little has been written, in the health field, that contrasts the experience of the two countries, with the exception of studies of heart disease based on the MONICA project (Hobbs et al. 1991). Detailed comparisons are made more frequently with European countries, or North America.

The purpose of this paper is to examine the health status of Australians and New Zealanders, and to explore reasons for the differences that are apparent. We rely principally on mortality rates since these are readily available, directly comparable and reliable, but acknowledge their limitations as measures of population health. The comparison raises two questions:
- Why do Australia and New Zealand differ at present?
- Why have they followed different trends over time?

The second question is the more difficult and more interesting one.

Current differences

In nearly all respects, the health of Australians is, on average, better than that of New Zealanders. For a start, Australians live longer. In 1996, life expectancy at birth in New Zealand was 79.6 years for females, and 74.3 years for males (Statistics New Zealand 1998). The corresponding figures for Australians were 81.0 years (females) and 75.4 years (males) (Australian Institute of Health and Welfare 1999). A difference of just over a year in life expectancy may seem relatively trivial for an individual, but represents a substantial loss of years of life for a population. To illustrate the magnitude of the effect: in New Zealand, deaths due to unintentional injury reduce life expectancy at birth by 'just' 1.1 years (Ministry of Health 2000). If all smoking-related deaths were avoided, life expectancy at birth would rise by roughly the same amount as the difference between Australian and New Zealand life expectancies for females: 1.5–2 years (Bronnum-Hansen and Juel 2000).

Lifestyle risk factors

What explains the difference in life expectancy? Mortality for most specific causes of death is generally higher in New Zealand than Australia. (Cirrhosis of the liver and skin cancer are two exceptions to the general pattern.) Heart disease, the most common cause of death in both countries, contributes about 54% of the overall difference in mortality for males, and 28% for females. There are differences between the two countries in so-called lifestyle factors, consistent with the mortality differences. For example, the New Zealand diet contains high levels of saturated fats. In 1995, New Zealanders ate more butter and meat fats per person than anyone else in the OECD. In that year, the New Zealand food supply was ranked first in the OECD in terms of the thrombogenic index, third by the atherogenic index and second in terms of the proportion of energy from animal origin (Laugesen and Swinburn 2000a). In the mid-90s, butter consumption in New Zealand was about 8.2 kg per person per year, compared with 3.1 kg per person in Australia. It has been estimated that this difference, combined with historically higher smoking rates amongst women (smoking prevalence has differed little between Australian and New Zealand men) may explain between half and two-thirds of the New Zealand excess of coronary deaths. (Laugesen 1998 unpublished)

Economic circumstances

New Zealand and Australia are, by global standards, both affluent countries, well past the 'shoulder' in graphs that compare average national wealth with health measures such as life expectancy. Cross-sectional comparisons show a steep increase in life expectancy with increasing national wealth, to a point equivalent with roughly US$5000 gross national product (GNP) per person, and then a marked flattening of the curve. However the line is not absolutely flat at higher levels of gross domestic product (GDP). An analysis of data around 1993 from all countries with a gross domestic product over US$10,000 (adjusted for purchasing power parity) found a correlation between GDP per person and life expectancy at birth of 0.51 (P = 0.003) (Lynch et al. 2000b). Such an association would 'explain' about a third of the difference between life expectancy in New Zealand and Australia (in the mid-1990s, GDP per person in Australia was approximately 25% greater than in New Zealand) (Statistics New Zealand 2000).

Health services

How do Australia and New Zealand compare in terms of their economic investments in health services? Among economically developed countries, there is little relationship between expenditure on health services and population health outcomes such as life expectancy at birth (Wilkinson 1996b). Yet, a stronger relationship exists between *variations* in health expenditure between countries and *variations* in life expectancy. Such a comparison may be helpful in ranking countries according to the relative efficiency of their health sectors (ie the returns yielded by health investment) and in identifying suitable models for more detailed analysis.

We extracted data on health expenditure (public plus private) and GDP (both in purchasing power parity dollars per capita), and life expectancy, for 1996 for 22 OECD countries (excluding Turkey) from the OECD Health Statistics 1999 Database. An ordinary least squares regression model was developed to predict health expenditure from GDP. (Health expenditure (in purchasing power parity dollars per capita) = 0.1107 x GDP (in purchasing power parity dollars per capita) – 543.6; R^2 = 59%, t_{21} = 5.47, p = <0.001.) For each country, the proportional deviation from predicted health expenditure was then calculated. Similarly, the deviation from expected life expectancy at birth for each country was calculated as the difference from the OECD mean (all data relate to 1996).

Countries in the lower right quadrant of figure 8.1 spend more than predicted on health, yet achieve lower life expectancy than predicted. This group of poorly performing countries includes the USA and Germany. Countries in the upper right quadrant also spend more than predicted on health, but receive a return for this in terms of better than expected health outcomes. This group includes Australia, Canada, Sweden and the Netherlands. Countries in the lower left quadrant spend less than predicted on health and do less well in terms of life expectancy. It is here that we find New Zealand (which spends slightly less on health than expected, and achieves a life expectancy in line with this), along with the UK. Finally, there are countries which spend less than predicted on health, yet manage to achieve better health outcomes than expected (ie countries falling into the upper left quadrant of figure 8.1). This group includes Norway and most notably Japan.

This analysis suggests that New Zealand is achieving reasonably good returns on its investment in health. At the same time, the data for the UK show that similar health outcomes could be achieved with less expenditure, and the examples of Norway and Australia

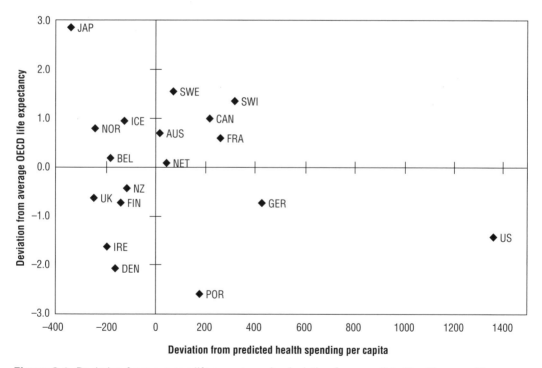

Figure 8.1 Deviation from average life expectancy by deviation from predicted health expenditure, selected OECD countries, 1996

Notes: AUS Australia, BEL Belgium, CAN Canada, DEN Denmark, FIN Finland, FRA France, GER Germany, ICE Iceland, IRE Ireland, JAP Japan, NET Netherlands, NOR Norway, NZ New Zealand, POR Portugal, SWE Sweden, SWI Switzerland, UK United Kingdom, US United States.

suggest that even better outcomes could be possible with little or no increase in relative expenditure on health.

The model is clearly simplistic. Health inputs are grossed up to total expenditure, irrespective of variations in the proportions going to health promotion and disease prevention rather than treatment and rehabilitation services (also, no account is taken of other structural and organisational variations in health service funding and delivery, nor of differences in the inflation rates of health sector prices relative to other prices in the countries compared). Also, standardisation of the health expenditure data across countries – unlike the GDP or life expectancy data – may not be complete, so making fair comparisons difficult.

Similarly, health outcome is measured as life expectancy, so neglecting the quality of life dimension. While health expectancy would be a more comprehensive outcome measure, data are not available for all countries. No adjustment is made for time lags between investment in health services and return on investment. Nor is the relationship deconfounded for factors other than health expenditure that are also related both to GDP and to life expectancy (eg, culture). In fact, if a regression model is fitted to the data, variation in health expenditure is found to account for just under 20% of the variation in life expectancy. If only socio-economically and culturally similar countries are compared, the relative influence of health expenditure compared with other factors is likely to be greater than this, however.

Ethnicity

Comparisons of averages may be misleading, since good health is not shared evenly, in either country. Consider, for example, the experience of Maori in New Zealand and Aboriginals and Torres Strait Islanders in Australia.

The breakdown of mortality data by ethnicity is subject to errors, ranging from incomplete ascertainment of deaths to variations in coding between numerators and denominators. Mortality amongst Aboriginals, for instance, is reported variably between States and is thought to be under-estimated overall (Australian Bureau of Statistics & Australian Institute

Table 8.1 Life expectancy at birth for indigenous and non-indigenous populations, Australia and New Zealand, 1996

	AUSTRALIA		NEW ZEALAND	
	Nonindigenous (97.9% of national population)	**Aboriginal & TSI (2.1%)**	**NonMaori (85.5%)**	**Maori (14.5%)**
Male	75.6	56.9	75.3	67.2
Female	81.3	61.7	80.6	71.6

Note: The life expectancy figures for Aboriginal and Torres Strait Islanders are based on data from 1991–1996.

References: Australian Institute of Health and Welfare (1999); Statistics New Zealand (1998).

of Health and Welfare 1999). In New Zealand, changes in the way ethnicity has been coded make it difficult to compare Maori mortality after 1996 with previous rates (Ministry of Health 2000a). Even so, the poor health of these groups is apparent. The gap between indigenous and nonindigenous life expectancies is wider in Australia than in New Zealand; a comparison that is worth examining in its own right. Kunitz (1994) has shown that international comparisons of the health of indigenous peoples throw a different light on the causes of high mortality than comparisons within countries. On the other hand, Aboriginals make up a much smaller fraction of the national population than do Maori. If Aboriginals were present in similar proportions, life expectancy in Australia would overall be approximately 1.5 years *less* than in New Zealand.

Can the poor health of Maori and Aboriginal peoples be explained in terms of the traditional social determinants? Some argue that 'ethnicity' cannot be separated meaningfully from social, economic, historical and behavioural circumstances (Kaufman and Cooper 1999). If this were true, it would be a serious matter for epidemiologists, since much of the quantitative work on social determinants of health assumes that factors such as ethnicity and occupational status can be partitioned out. The debate hinges on how broadly causes are defined (Krieger and Smith 2000). But it seems to us that all attempts to estimate attribution and preventability are thought experiments requiring an imaginative leap from what is to what might be, and analysis of ethnicity is no different in kind.

We know of no relevant data in Australia, but it appears that factors such as income, occupation and education explain only part of the disadvantage experienced by Maori. For example, within categories of deprivation measured by the New Zealand Deprivation Index (NZDep), a census-based summary of social deprivation at the small area level (Crampton et al. 2000), Maori mortality rates are higher than nonMaori.

Moreover, although it is not shown in figure 8.2, Maori are over-represented in the high-deprivation areas and under-represented in the most affluent parts of the country. In 1991, 50% of Maori lived in the most deprived parts of the country (NZDep deciles 9 and 10) compared to 15% of other ethnic groups (Blakely et al. 2000). Plainly, there must be important prior causes in a sequence leading to material disadvantage and poor health. Moreover, the balance of deprivation and other factors associated with ethnicity may vary between age groups and between birth cohorts. Analysis of 1991–4 mortality rates using NZDep shows a much stronger effect of ethnicity than deprivation amongst men and women over 55, and the reverse for children and young adults (Blakely et al. 2001). This may be an artefact of the way ethnicity is assigned. But more likely the variation by age reflects cohort effects, varying ability of the New Zealand Deprivation Index to capture accurately socio-economic status at different ages, or cumulative effects of social factors over a lifetime. To understand the pattern shown in figure 8.2 may require a wider view of the social causes of illness than is usually taken in public health. Pervasive and long-standing features of Australian and New Zealand society must be acting to disadvantage indigenous peoples so severely and comprehensively.

Explanations, like causes, can be constructed at different levels. One could say that the present difference between the health status of Australians and New Zealanders is largely due to poor health of indigenous peoples. If Maori and Aboriginals and Torres Strait Islanders

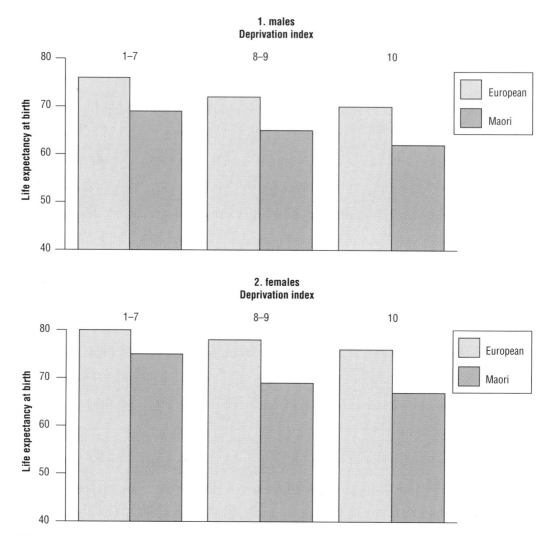

Figure 8.2 Life expectancy by ethnicity, gender and socio-economic status, 1996–7

Note: Units on the deprivation index are deciles. 1 = least deprived 10% of small areas; 10 = most deprived 10% of small areas. NonMaori nonEuropean are excluded from this analysis. (Effectively, this means excluding Pacific Islanders, who are concentrated in the most deprived categories and Asian migrants who make up relatively small numbers overall.)

Source: NZDep96.

experienced the same longevity as their compatriots, the difference in life expectancy between New Zealand and Australia would shrink by almost two-thirds. This does not explain the mechanisms by which ethnicity influences mortality, nor the 'upstream' factors that give ethnicity its particular salience. What is more, the causes of current differences may not be the same as those responsible for changes over time, as will be seen in the next section of the paper.

Different trends

Australians haven't always lived longer than New Zealanders. Indeed, until the 1970s, life expectancy was greater in New Zealand than in Australia.

In figure 8.3, change in life expectancy at birth is charted for Australia and New Zealand, from 1961 to 1998. For both males and females it appears that the two countries followed similar flat (no change) trajectories until around 1970, when life expectancy began to improve, but at a faster rate in Australia than New Zealand. This period of divergence

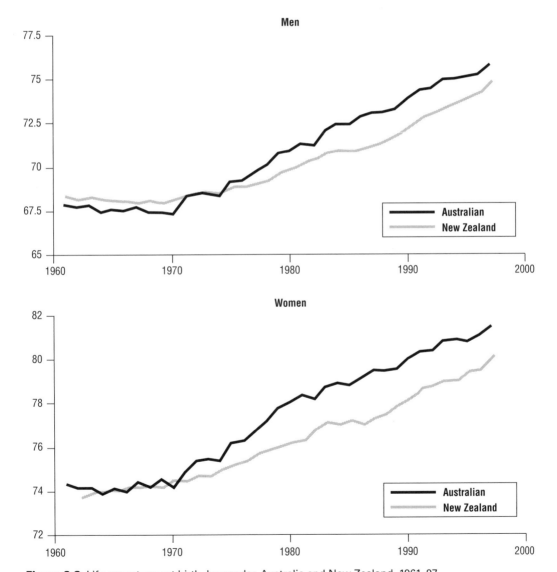

Figure 8.3 Life expectancy at birth, by gender, Australia and New Zealand, 1961–97

lasted for about a decade and from the early 1980s onwards the two countries have tracked more or less in parallel, but with Australia enjoying a margin of two to three percentage points.

This mortality 'crossover' cannot be explained by the poorer health of Maori and Aboriginals, since times series show the same transition for nonMaori as for the total population.

Indeed, during the period that New Zealand slipped behind Australia, Maori life expectancy was improving at its fastest rate ever.

This pattern is driven by mortality in middle age and later life as might be expected, since this is when most deaths occur. (Trends in infant mortality are very similar overall.) The changes observed in coronary mortality match closely the trends for all deaths. The turn-around in the coronary heart disease epidemic occurred at about the same time in both countries, but the decline in heart deaths was much sharper, initially, in Australia. Amongst the other major causes of mortality, stroke deaths show a very similar mortality crossover to that seen with coronary heart disease. Trends in cancer deaths have a different pattern. Mortality from this cause has been consistently higher in New Zealand than Australia, especially amongst women, and this may be explained in large part by smoking rates (Laugesen and Swinburn 2000b).

Figures 8.2 and 8.3 raise two questions. First, why is mortality falling, year after year, in a pattern common to most developed countries? Second, why did the course of decline differ in Australia and New Zealand? The answer to the first question is not self-evident. Materialist explanations for the fall in mortality in earlier times (eg, the 19th and first half of the 20th centuries) are less convincing when applied to recent trends (Wilkinson 1996). For example, the long term trend of declining child mortality world-wide has been surprisingly resistant to economic setbacks, even in the most vulnerable countries (Murray and Chen 1993).

We focus here on the related, but more circumscribed comparison of Australia and New Zealand, and suggest five possible explanations for the mortality crossover: artefact; changes in the compositions of the two populations; health care factors; individual risk factors ('lifestyle'); and, social and economic conditions.

Artefact seems most unlikely as an explanation – in Australia and New Zealand, national mortality statistics are based on death registrations, recorded in a standard fashion for a very high proportion of all deaths, and high quality population censuses. While there may be variations in the coding of cause of death, it is difficult to imagine that the difference in overall mortality could be caused by error.

Migration

Change in the make-up of the population appears a more attractive explanation, since there were substantial changes in both countries in the second half of the 20th century. In New Zealand, the proportion of the population labelled as European fell from 93.3% in 1951 to 81.3% in 1991(Easton 1997).This group included chiefly persons of British origin. Maori increased from 6.0% to 11.3% of the population (noting that the method of assigning Maori ethnicity changed over time also). In relative terms, the biggest increase was in the proportion

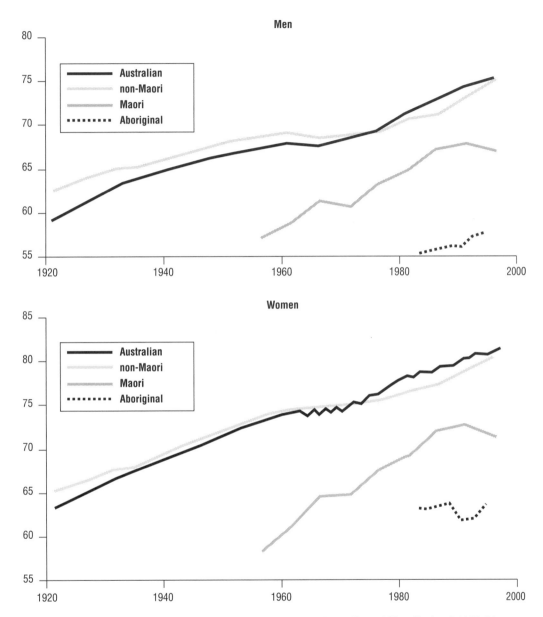

Figure 8.4 Life expectancy at birth, by ethnicity and gender, Australia and New Zealand, 1920–99

Notes:
1   There were major changes in the classification of ethnicity in New Zealand in 1996, so that trends in mortality since that time cannot be compared confidently with earlier series (New Zealand Ministry of Health 2000).
2   In New Zealand, Maori and nonMaori mortality were distinguished only from 1956 onwards.
3   In this graph, 'Australian' includes the total national population.
4   Aboriginal life expectancy is estimated from data obtained in a sample of states. There are no comprehensive national data available (Australian Bureau of Statistics & Australian Institute of Health and Welfare 1999).

of the population of Pacific Island ethnicity (increasing from 0.2% to 4.4%). The Australian population changed also, but in different ways. Over roughly the same time period (1947 to 1988), the proportion of the population of British or Irish ethnic origin fell from 89.8% to 74.6%, due to increases in residents from northern Europe (5.7% to 7.3%), eastern Europe (0.6% to 3.9%) and southern Europe (1.5% to 7.4%) (Wooden et al. 1994).

To what extent might these changes, which were due both to migration and to natural population growth, have affected the rate of mortality decline in Australia and New Zealand? A full answer would require a detailed analysis of mortality by length of residence, taking account of flows of migrants into and out of the two countries, and variations in age structures of the different groups. However, at first glance, it seems plausible that migration could have played a part in setting mortality decline on different trajectories in the two countries. The fastest growing sections of the New Zealand population were Maori and Pacific Islanders, groups that in general have higher levels of mortality than the New Zealand average (table 1). Across the Tasman on the other hand, several of the new settler groups are conspicuous for their much better than average levels of health. The most striking example is persons of southern European origin. Mortality rates are usually a little lower than the national average for migrants, at least in the first years of residence, due to the health selection effects that apply. But in the 1980s, persons born in southern Europe had mortality rates that were substantially lower than the Australian population overall, and these rates converged only very slowly on the national average with increasing duration of residence in Australia (Powles and Gifford 1990).

After the Second World War, migrants from Italy, Greece and other parts of southern Europe played a part in changing for the better Australian lifestyles. For example, the increasing popularity of Mediterranean-style diets and changes in social drinking patterns brought health benefits to the whole population. But the arrival of long-lived migrants also had a direct effect on national mortality. The numbers of newcomers were relatively small, but sufficient to account for a sizeable fraction of the inter-country difference in life expectancy.

In the simplest of terms, an increase from 1.5% to 7.5% of a sub-group with mortality two-thirds the national average would lower overall mortality by 2%. Taking New Zealand life tables for 1995–7, we re-calculated life expectancies after reducing mortality rates in each age group by 2%. The effect was to increase life expectancy at birth by 0.26 years for males, and 0.24 years for females. The changes in Australia would be slightly less given the lower mortality in that country, but as a rough guide, one could say that life expectancy in Australia in the 1990s was about 0.2–0.25 years higher than it would have been if the proportion of the population contributed by migrants from southern Europe had remained as it was in the 1940s. This represents around 15–20% of the present difference between New Zealand and Australia. Such calculations are crude approximations only, but suggest that the influence of migration on health trends in New Zealand and Australia warrants closer attention. Included in a more detailed analysis should be population movements across the Tasman. Since the first European settlements, there have been considerable flows of migrants between the two countries, particularly from east to west. About 400,000 New Zealanders are now resident in Australia.

Health care

Health care would be a possible explanation of between country differences in mortality if there were effective treatments to common, otherwise lethal conditions that were applied on a wide scale in Australia, but not in New Zealand. In general, measures of health service activity explain a small fraction of the variation in health status between developed countries (Mackenbach et al. 1994). Even so-called amenable causes of death are more closely related in international comparisons to social and economic factors than to levels of medical provision. There is evidence from the 1980s onwards that survival following a myocardial infarct may be worse in New Zealand (Hobbs et al. 1991). Lower rates of surgical and intensive medical intervention may play a part, but the difference between the two countries has been most marked for out of hospital deaths. However, it is not clear that the same pattern applied at the time Australian and New Zealand mortality rates diverged. A study of survival following myocardial infarction and stroke in the late 1970s reported similar case fatality rates in Australia and New Zealand (Beaglehole et al. 1986). Overall, the decline in coronary mortality in the 1970s in both countries was more likely due to changes in disease incidence than case fatality (Beaglehole et al. 1997).

Risk factors

What behaviours or life style factors could explain these changes? Smoking rates followed rather similar patterns in the two countries following the Second World War, although smoking rates have remained a little higher amongst NZ women (with particularly high rates amongst Maori women). Differences in diets have been more marked. Since the 1960s, there have been significant changes in dietary patterns in both countries, and in particular a decline in consumption of saturated fats. In Australia, butter intake fell from about 8 kg per person in 1974 to less than 3 kg per head in 1996 (John Goss, personal communication). New Zealand has been slower to make the change from dairy fats to vegetable oils. The New Zealand dairy industry is extraordinarily productive, and relatively cheap, high-fat dairy products have always been widely available. (Milk was subsidised until the late 1970s; margarine was available only on medical prescription until earlier in that decade.) More detailed calculations are needed to estimate the effect of these differences in risk factor levels on coronary mortality. While the interval between exposure to high-fat diets and development of disease is thought to be relatively long (decades perhaps) (Law and Wald 1999), there may be a much quicker response to a reduction in risk factor levels (Zatonski et al. 1998).

Changes in diet, smoking and other 'risk' behaviours may have contributed to the slower fall in coronary mortality in New Zealand, but these remain insufficient, on their own, as explanations of the overall mortality pattern. The reason is that the timing and direction of the change in mortality were the same for causes of death that do not share the same behavioural risk factors. A crossover occurred for injury deaths, for instance, at the same time as coronary mortality. One possible explanation for such a pattern is that there were influential 'upstream' factors, in the social and economic environment that affected mortality as a general phenomenon.

Social and economic changes

It is striking how closely New Zealand's economic performance matches its international rankings in population health. Immediately after World War II, New Zealand did as well as Australia, or better, on most economic indicators. Until the 1960s, GNP per head was higher in New Zealand than Australia. But at the end of that decade in New Zealand, there was a sharp fall in the terms of trade and a loss of traditional markets for agricultural exports, preceding Britain's formal entry into the European Economic Community in 1972. The oil shocks of the early 1970s also had a severe impact on economic activity. Australia of course was subject to the same external forces, but enjoyed a greater diversity of raw resources and a much stronger manufacturing base. A similar pattern is apparent also when New Zealand is compared to OECD per capita GDP: a slow decline (in relative terms) from the 1950s, but the sharpest fall occurring in the 1960s and 1970s (Easton 1997).

There is no doubt that the New Zealand economy fared poorly by comparison at the same time mortality tipped to the advantage of Australia. But have conditions been so adverse that they could cause these changes in death rates? In absolute terms, the differentials were modest, but it may be that the nature of the change was at least as important as the size of the New Zealand decline.

In the mid-1970s, New Zealand began a period of rapid social change, swinging from the 'Think Big' extravagances of the Muldoon era to the abrupt winding down of public services by Roger Douglas and colleagues (Easton 1997). Australia moved in similar directions, but more slowly. There were incremental shifts in areas such as benefits, employment and public utilities, rather than relatively sudden changes of direction. As an example, the telecommunications industry was privatised in New Zealand by the early 1990s, but not until the end of the decade in Australia. Not only was the speed of change greater in New Zealand, but in some respects, New Zealand had more to lose. For instance, since the 1940s, there had been almost no unemployment in New Zealand (Statistics New Zealand 1998). When employment services for job-seekers were established in the 1970s, senior staff had to be recruited from Australia: there were few locals with relevant experience.

Is the timing right to explain the mortality crossover in terms of social and economic changes? Figure 8.5 suggests that it may be: the deterioration in New Zealand Gross Domestic Product relative to Australia follows a similar pattern to the change in mortality, with a lag period of about five years. The experience of Eastern Europe in the 1990s showed that deteriorating social conditions can have an almost immediate effect on national mortality rates, and not just for causes of death such as injury that are recognised to have short latencies (Zatonski et al. 1998, Leon et al. 1997). But how relevant is this to New Zealand's much milder social distress? Economic measures such as GDP are crude measures of prosperity, and little is known about the mechanisms by which economic activity is translated into health outcomes. Education, employment and household income are all possible linking variables. So are intangible and important characteristics of community life, such as inclusiveness and trust. Unfortunately, we know of no data that would enable comparisons to be made between New Zealand and Australia.

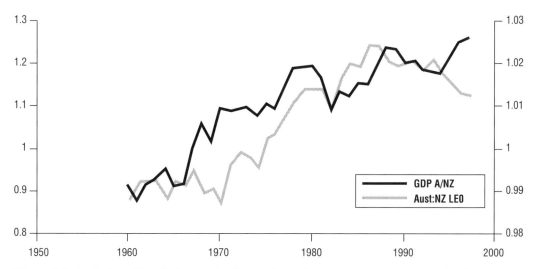

Figure 8.5 Australia to New Zealand ratio of gross domestic product per capita and male life expectancy at birth, 1961–97

Note: Ratio of gross domestic product per capita is based on purchasing power parity dollars and is shown on the left-hand vertical axis. The ratio of male life expectancy at birth (LEO) is on the right-hand axis.

Sources of information are World Bank, OECD.

Other aspects of international comparisons

Is life expectancy (combined with, preferably, an allowance for the quality of life) the best measure of progress in public health? The problem is that gains in the number (and quality) of years lived may come at too high a price. Based on present patterns of consumption, economic growth cannot be sustained indefinitely. There are signs already (climate change, diminishing biodiversity) that the demands on global support systems are excessive. If mortality decline at any cost is not a viable indicator of progress, perhaps we should adopt measures of doing better with less. Average years of life per dollar of national economic activity has been suggested as one possible index (Hertzman and Wilkinson 1996). There is little to separate Australia and New Zealand by this measure, which shows diminishing health returns per unit GDP as economies have grown.

Finally, a reflection on two issues that are discussed in depth elsewhere in this book: income inequalities, and the merits of a 'life course' approach to health determinants. The trends in income inequalities in Australia and New Zealand do not fit with the diverging paths of national mortality. Through the 1970s and 1980s, the degree of inequality in incomes increased in both countries, but until the 1990s, New Zealand fared rather better (that is, had less unequal distribution of incomes). Second, the dramatic improvement in life expectancy that was seen in both countries in the early 70s, although it was more marked in Australia than in New Zealand, applied to all age groups. As shown here, similar trends were observed for coronary mortality (affecting predominantly middle-aged and older people) and injury (including many deaths amongst young adults). This pattern is much more likely to result from exposures affecting all members of the population at roughly the same time, whatever their age, than from exposures that relate to particular birth cohorts.

Conclusions

Comparisons between Australia and New Zealand are a rich source of questions and hypotheses. They underline the importance of differences between ethnic groups in any consideration of health inequalities. From a parochial perspective, one could say that New Zealand is unlikely to recover parity with Australia in the mortality rankings until inequalities between Maori and nonMaori are reduced. Likewise, the appalling health of Aborigines should not be overlooked in any comparison of national averages. However, the determinants of change may well differ from the causes of present differences. It is unlikely in our view that health care and individual lifestyle factors explain the trends in mortality in the two countries. It is tempting to attribute a role to the substantial social and economic changes that were occurring in New Zealand at the same time as the mortality crossover. A better understanding of present differences and trends requires formal analysis of the impact of factors such as migration and dietary changes. Comparisons based on cohort life expectancies may identify effects overlooked in the present, cross-sectional analyses. It would be instructive to focus on vulnerable sub-groups (such as low income families) who are more sensitive to economic and social changes. Health status measures other than mortality would broaden the scope of the comparisons – at present there are some measures (such as disability-free life expectancy) that permit cross-sectional comparisons, but no times series data. Further analyses might include comparisons of New Zealand with individual Australian states (variations in life expectancy between states are greater than the difference between Australia and New Zealand), and extending the number of countries included.

Further Reading

Kunitz, S J 1994, Disease and Social Diversity: The European impact on the health of non-Europeans, Oxford University Press, New York.
  – *Compares the response to colonisation of indigenous peoples in Australia, New Zealand and other countries around the Pacific, and explores reasons for the marked differentials in health status within and between countries.*
Kelsey, J 1995, The New Zealand Experiment: A world model for structural adjustment, Auckland University Press.
  – *A provocative analysis of the economic changes in New Zealand from 1984 onwards, which proceeded on a substantially different path from policies in Australia at the same time and had major impacts on employment, income, social services and other basic determinants of population health.*

9

Income, income inequality and health in New Zealand

Philippa Howden-Chapman and Des O'Dea

Inequalities in health have to be seen against a background of economic inequality. (Atkinson 1999, p 283).

Introduction

Compared to other OECD countries, New Zealand moved particularly rapidly in deregulating its economy in the 1980s, undertaking far-reaching social and economic reforms, and having the fastest growth in income inequality (Statistics New Zealand 1999). Income inequality rose most notably in New Zealand in the late 1980s during a major economic recession, but it did not fall during the subsequent economic expansion in the mid-1990s (O'Dea 2000). Thus the increase in income inequality appears to have been driven by structural changes to New Zealand society, which persisted after the economic recession.

There is some agreement among researchers about the reasons for about half the increase in income inequality; the reasons for the remaining increase in inequality are less easily identified. Changes in the 1980s to the taxation system appear to have been regressive, although removing tax loopholes and increasing company tax may have partially offset this effect. The rise in unemployment from the late 1980s contributed, but the most significant factor appears to have been the increase in income inequality among the employed as shown by the widening income differentials by occupation, education and hours of work.

At a household level, there has also been a reduction in the number of households where a bread-winner supports another adult and children, resulting in an increase in work-rich households, where both adults work and work-poor households where no adults are in paid employment (Callister 1998). There has also been a change in household composition, with the growth of sole parent households and older households without children. During the late eighties' recession, more people relied on government benefits as a source of income

(Stephens and Waldegrave 1996). In 1991, the Government reduced welfare benefits, which also had some impact, though small, on income inequality (Statistics New Zealand 1999).

In consequence of these changes, income inequality has increased in New Zealand over the past two decades. Middle-income families have fallen in number relative to both lower-income and higher-income families. Over the period 1986 to 1996, household disposable incomes actually fell in real terms in most deciles, but increased substantially in the top two deciles. Low-income households lost proportionately less of their income than those in the middle-income range (Statistics New Zealand 1999), but were often more vulnerable to begin with. It has to be remembered however, that households move up and down the income distribution, and the low-income households at the starting point are not identical to those at the end-point.

In this chapter, we first develop a conceptual framework. While broader political and economic influences can exacerbate income inequality, this chapter has a narrower focus that begins with income inequality. However, we recognise that income inequality is a manifestation of background historical, political, cultural and economic factors that have far-reaching consequences in the fabric of daily life (Lynch 2000). After discussing the model, we then briefly analyse the literature, looking first at the association between income levels and health and second at the debate on income inequality as a determinant of health. We test our framework by looking at two data sources: the 1996/97 New Zealand Health Survey and the 1996 New Zealand Census. Results are first presented for household income and health and then for average household income and income inequality. We discuss these results in the light of the international literature and the implications for policy.

A conceptual framework

To consider the place of income and income inequality in relation to health we have adopted the normative framework of Amartya Sen (1999). Here, well-being consists of a set of intrinsically valuable, interrelated *functionings* such as having adequate food, avoiding premature mortality, having a satisfying job, having self respect, being respected and being happy.

While these functionings are very general and to a large extent cross-cultural, they are manifest in culturally specific ways. For example, to explain the importance of people being able 'to appear in public without shame', Sen gives an example taken from Adam Smith (1776). Leather shoes were a necessity for women in England, but not in Scotland – or New Zealand – because in Scotland, the lowest order of women could go barefooted without discredit, while in England, this would be a matter for shame. Everybody needs to be able to leave their house and appear in public without feeling self-consciously embarrassed about their clothing, but the commodities they need to do so will vary across cultures (Sugden 1993). Similarly 'taking part in the life of the community' was identified in New Zealand's Royal Commission (1988) as essential to health and well-being.

According to Sen, individuals vary in their opportunities or *capabilities* to achieve these valuable functionings and one of the factors that restricts their freedom at a societal level is income inequality. The appropriate way to function in a society such as New Zealand is determined by the opportunities available to individuals and how they are positioned relative to others.

Extending this framework, the dispersion of income may act as a proxy for the influence of various income-facilitated functionings on health and subsequently on mortality (see figure 9.1). (Note that in order to focus on socioeconomic determinants we have omitted from the diagram such other important determinants of health as genetic inheritance, and environmental and cultural factors.) The individual's place within the income distribution is postulated to be an important determinant of premature mortality for the individual. The distribution of socio-economic status can be changed by structural means such as progressive taxation and, in the longer term, redistribution of educational opportunities.

Economic inequality provides an incentive for effort. Extending this argument, it is often maintained that a reasonably high degree of economic inequality is good for growth, and that a degree of inequity now means that everyone is better off in the long run. The counter-argument is that excessive inequality is not only inequitable but inefficient, because it may inhibit economic growth by reducing investment incentives to borrow by the poor, as well as leading to lower health status and increasing economic and political instability (Aghion et al. 1999). There is some support for this in empirical studies based on cross-country regressions, which have found a negative correlation between the average rate of growth and measures of inequality (Benabou 1996).

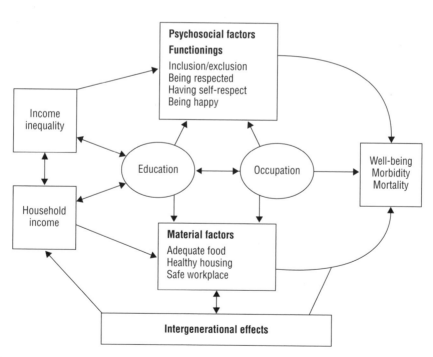

Figure 9.1 A model of the relationship between household income, income inequality and health

The choice of income as a measure of socioeconomic status

Income is just one indicator of 'socioeconomic status' (SES), but is strongly correlated with others such as education and occupation and may be a better predictor of health status than any other SES indicator (Davis et al. 1997). However, comparative studies have found that the ranking of countries in relation to income and health inequalities is not necessarily similar to ranking by education and occupational class (Cavelaars et al. 1998). This suggests that although measures of socioeconomic status are usually highly correlated, they are also partly independent determinants of health. In the framework adopted here, income and income inequality are considered to have effects on health independent of the effects of education and occupational class on health (see figure 9.1).

One methodological problem is that income is influenced by age (Berkman and Macintyre 1997) unlike educational attainment, which is relatively static through adulthood. Income commonly follows an 'inverted U' profile during the years of working life, falling sharply in retirement.

A brief summary of the literature

The association between income level and health

Almost every study of the links between income and health has shown that those on lower incomes have poorer health, after appropriate age-standardisation (Mathers 1994; Kawachi and Kennedy 1997b, Kawachi et al. 1999c; Wilson and Daly 1997). Analyses of data from the 1996/97 New Zealand Health Survey and the 1996 New Zealand Census have shown this holds for all the usual measures of health outcome, including morbidity, disability, perceived health status and mortality (NZ Ministry of Health 1999; Howden-Chapman and Tobias 2000).

The relationship between income and health is nonlinear, being much less pronounced at higher income levels (Ecob and Davey Smith 1999; Wilkinson 1998a). This relationship applies to nations as well as families. Hales et al. (1999) in a recent paper on cross-country comparisons of infant mortality found infant mortality was strongly associated with per capita gross national product (GNP) for poorer countries, but for countries above a certain income level, the impact of increasing per capita income is either weak or nonexistent.

The suggestion is that the relationship between income and a measure such as life expectancy is 'concave' when graphed. At levels of extreme poverty, the slope is very steep, at low to moderate income levels the slope is less steep, but at higher income levels, there appears to be no decrease, and several studies have shown a slight increase in ill-health (Blaxter 1990, pp 69–74) and mortality (Kitagawa and Hauser 1973). However, this last result needs substantiation (Backlund et al. 1996).

This sort of relationship between income and life expectancy has potentially important policy consequences for population health. The implication is that the redistribution of income from the top income brackets to those worse off could improve the overall health of the population presuming there is a causal link, direct or indirect, from income to health (Contoyannis and Forster 1999).

The debate on 'income inequality' as a determinant of health

'The capabilities of people to function in a particular society are significantly influenced by the living standards of others' (Atkinson 1999, p 284).

It is not only the income of individuals and households that has been linked to health, but also the distribution of income across the community. A lively debate in the international literature has emerged between those who consider that cross-national research on the effect of income distribution on mortality (Rogers 1979; Waldman 1992; Wennemo 1993; Hales et al. 1999; Wagstaff 2000) has shown a reasonably clear and stable cross-sectional relationship (Wilkinson 1992; Wilkinson 1996a; Kennedy et al. 1996; Kaplan GA et al. 1996; Kawachi et al. 1999c) and those who remain sceptical, both about the strength (Judge 1995) and the underlying causal explanation (Saunders 1997). This debate has intensified as the relation between income inequality and health has been explored in smaller jurisdictional units in the USA, such as at the state-level (Kawachi et al. 1999c), metropolitan areas (Ross et al. 2000) and neighbourhoods (Wilson and Daly 1997). It appears that the impact of the distribution of income inequality is more robust for larger population units than for counties (Fiscella and Franks 1997) or metropolitan areas (Blakely and Kawachi 2000).

The claim that relative income is a key determinant of health inequality remains controversial. One attack has been on the statistical measures used, including the choice of inequality measure and of income concept and the use or not of equivalence scales (Judge 1995). In response, Kawachi and Kennedy (1997) tested the relationship of six different income inequality indicators to mortality in the 50 US states. They showed that all measures were highly correlated with each other and all were strongly associated with mortality, even after adjustment for median income and poverty.

Another line of attack points to the methodological difficulties of using 'ecological' (community) variables to predict individual outcomes. Gravelle (1998) illustrates with a simple model in which individual mortality (or morbidity) is assumed to depend solely on income, and is inversely related to income, and finally – the crucial point – as income rises mortality falls, but does so at a declining rate. That is, the relationship of ill health to income is not linear but is curved towards the origin. It is then easy to show, graphically or mathematically, that any increase in dispersion of the income distribution about the current average leads to a deterioration in population health. This is because the worsening in health of those whose income position has deteriorated exceeds the health gains of those whose income position has improved. However, Wolfson et al. (1999) in an empirical investigation found that the 'Gravelle mechanism' could not 'entirely or substantially' explain the observed association between income inequality and mortality for the 50 US states.

Fiscella and Franks (1997) analysed USA longitudinal survey data for some 105 counties or combined counties, covering over 13,000 adults. They found that community income inequality showed a significant association with subsequent community mortality, and with individual mortality after adjustment for age, sex, and mean income in the community of residence. However, after adjusting for individual household incomes, the association with mortality was lost.

Kennedy et al. (1998) in their large US multi-level study involving 205,000 individuals, came to contrary conclusions supported by considerably more statistical power. They found that, after controlling for personal characteristics and household income, differences in state income inequality still had a significant effect on self-rated health. Self-rated health is known to be a good predictor of mortality. The authors also questioned some methodological points in the work of Fiscella and Franks, including the truncation of income data at the $25,000 level, possibly resulting in under-estimation of the true degree of inequality.

Clearly, the debate is not yet concluded, although the latest results do appear to favour the hypothesis of 'relative income' having an effect on health outcomes independent of 'absolute income'. However, the mechanism by which the community variable of income inequality influences individual health outcomes is not yet fully explained.

In recent papers, Kawachi and others (1997a; 1999c) have argued for the importance to population health of 'social capital' – those features of social organisation which 'facilitate cooperation for mutual benefit' – and that income inequality is one factor which helps determine the level of social capital. Three pathways were proposed in the 1999 paper by which social capital might influence individual health. These were, first, by promoting the diffusion of health information, and encouraging or imposing healthy norms of behaviour; second, by increasing access to local services and agencies; and finally by influencing the health of individuals via psychosocial processes. The earlier 1997 paper examined data for 39 states of the USA, including constructed 'social capital' survey variables. The authors' conclusion was that,

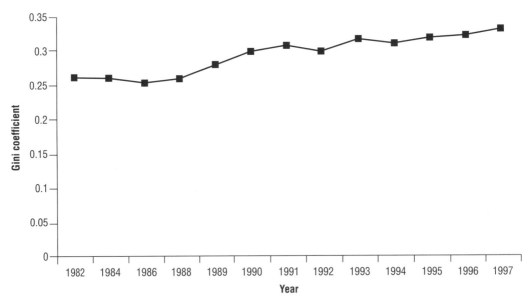

Figure 9.2 Growth in New Zealand's income inequality, 1982–97 equivalent disposable household income

Note: The increase appears to have been more rapid than that in other developed economies (see figure 9.3).

Source: Statistics New Zealand 1999, p 100.

'These data support the notion that income inequality leads to increased mortality via disinvestment in social capital.' A census community-based measure of social capital developed in New Zealand, based on the extent of volunteering outside the home, has also shown a significant relationship between the level of social organisation and mortality, even after controlling for average household income and income inequality (Howden-Chapman 2001).

Income inequality in New Zealand

An analysis of the New Zealand situation is timely, because income inequality in New Zealand has risen markedly since the mid-1980s, as figure 9.2 shows (Statistics New Zealand 1999).

It is not only for New Zealand as a whole that income inequality has grown – income inequality across regions has also increased. The gap in incomes between Auckland and Wellington cities and the rest of the country has grown in recent years, while the relative position of some regions (particularly Northland) has slipped (Martin 1999).

Associated with the recent increase in income inequality in New Zealand, and the increase in ethnic income differentials, there is also a correlation between increasing Maori unemployment and Maori male mortality in the period following the mid-1980s economic restructuring (Brown 1999).

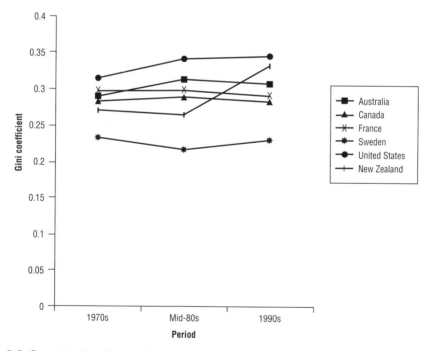

Figure 9.3 Growth in New Zealand's income inequality, relative to other countries, 1970s–1990s equivalent disposable household income

Source: Statistics New Zealand 1999, p 94.

The influence of gender, age, and ethnicity on income ranking

The place of individual New Zealanders in the income distribution is influenced by gender, age and ethnicity. Women are over-represented at the lower end of the income distribution, because on average, they earn less than men, are more likely to be sole parents and they live longer. Conversely, men are more likely to be earning higher incomes. Older people – 65 and over – are strongly concentrated in the second and third household income (equivalised) quintiles.

Children also are grouped more to the lower end. This is partly for 'life-cycle' reasons. Parents with dependent children tend to be at a stage of their working life where incomes have not yet peaked, and the presence of young children often restricts income-earning opportunities, particularly for the mother. There is also, however, an ethnic dimension to the concentration of children in lower-income households. Maori, Pacific Islanders, and the 'Other' ethnic group are over-represented in the lower income quintiles, and under-represented in the top quintiles. This is particularly so for children, in part a reflection of the relatively young age structure of the Maori and Pacific populations.

There appears to be a significant difference in the income distribution between 'sole Maori' (those specifying NZ Maori but not any other ethnic group) in response to the survey question, and 'mixed Maori' (those specifying more than one ethnic group, including Maori). 'Sole Maori' group are poorer, on average, than 'mixed Maori'. The sample numbers on which this comparison is based are small, but the result is consistent with some other evidence (Callister 1996).

The two data sources

Two sets of results follow, drawn from *Social Inequalities in Health* (Howden-Chapman and Tobias 2000). The first analyses data from a nationwide health survey (only some specimen results are given here); the second analyses regional differences using census data.

For both, gross household income was used as the measure of income, which includes benefits, pensions and market income, measured prior to the deduction of taxes. Although in practice, individuals do not necessarily have access to the income of other family members in the same house (Fleming 1997), household income is likely to be a better indicator of the well-being of household or family members than the income of any one household member. The household income measure is 'equivalised', that is adjusted to take account of household size. A larger household needs a larger income to have the same standard of living as a small household. The adjustment is made using an equivalence scale; in this report, the Luxembourg Income Study (0.5) equivalence scale is used (Atkinson et al. 1995).

Household income and health
The data for this part of the analysis come from the 1996/97 New Zealand Health Survey (NZHS), and the associated Nutrition Survey (NNS). Estimates were weighted to take account of the stratified random sample, with 'over-sampling' of Maori and the differential

nonresponse by population sub-groups. Individuals under 65 were classified from the NZHS data-set into 'equivalent gross household income' quintiles, numbered from 1, for the lowest income grouping, to 5, for the highest income group. Proportions and averages are compared across these five income quintiles, and all results were age-adjusted. The overall survey non-response proportion was 18.8%. The results are confined to those aged under 65. In addition, they are standardised for differences in age composition in each income quintile.

Regional average household income, and income inequality
The data source is the 1996 census of population and dwellings. Measures of average household income and of income inequality (the Gini coefficient) were constructed for each of 27 regions. Regional populations ranged from about 30,000 (King Country and the West Coast) to 400,000 (North-West Auckland and Canterbury).

The results

Household income and health
Only a small selection of the results derived from the NZ Health Survey and the original analyses are discussed here, and fewer still charted. The key dependent measures we consider are self-assessed health, behavioural risk factors, and service utilisation.

Self-assessed health
The survey asked respondents to give a self-assessment of their health state on a five-step scale from *poor* to *excellent*. This was used to calculate the 'self-assessed health' percentages in figure 9.4. The proportions of those who assess their state of health as either *very good* or *excellent* are higher for those in the higher income brackets, with the differences statistically significant. The same was found for summary SF-36 'mental' and 'physical' scores. The one exception is the physical score for females, for which the difference between top and bottom just fails to be statistically significant at the five per cent probability level.

Disability
Disability prevalence decreases with income for both men and women, but as figure 9.5 shows, the difference between bottom and top quintiles is statistically significant at the five per cent probability level only in the case of men.

Behavioural Risk Factors
Three behavioural risk factors were analysed: smoking; alcohol abuse; and obesity (body mass index > 30). For women, the three risk factors are all more prevalent in the lower income quintiles, and the differences over the income range are highly statistically significant for all three.

   As figure 9.6 shows, the proportion of men smoking also decreases significantly as

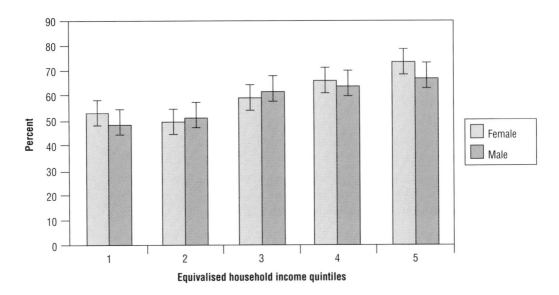

Figure 9.4 Percentage of adults assessing their health *excellent* or *very good*, by equivalised household income quintiles

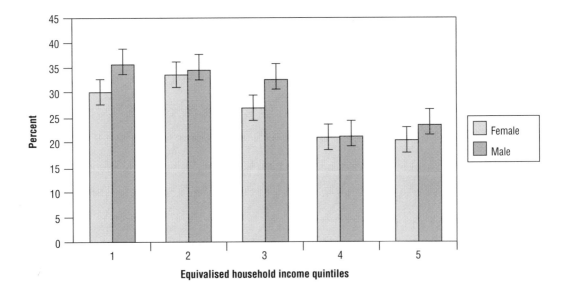

Figure 9.5 Percentage of adults reporting disability, by equivalised household income quintiles

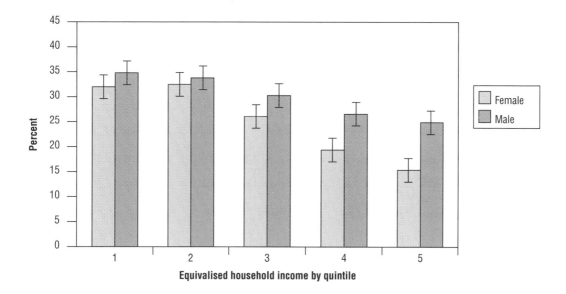

Figure 9.6 Percentage of adults who smoke, by income quintile

income increases, but the gradient is less steep than for women. Hazardous usage patterns for alcohol consumption appear to increase, however, with increasing income. While obesity falls in the middle quintiles it rises in the top decile group, although the difference between bottom and top quintiles is not significant. These results for men contain some hint of the possible U-shaped relationship between income and health discussed in Wilkinson (1992). It is not just low incomes, but the highest incomes that can also be associated with life-styles that increase 'health risk'.

Health services utilisation

Two factors, offsetting each other, can be expected to influence the relationship between income and health services utilisation. First, to the extent that those in lower income groups are those with greater 'need', their utilisation would be expected to be higher. Against this, higher income groups might have greater income-induced demand for health services, and be better placed to overcome any barriers to access such as cost by making out-of-pocket payments or taking out private health insurance.

Utilisation of general practitioner services is measured by the proportion of people reporting fewer than three visits or fewer than six visits in the past 12 months. For dental services, it is measured by at least one visit to a dentist or dental nurse in the past 12 months.

The proportion of people visiting the general practitioner six or more times in a 12-month period is higher in the lower income quintiles, but as figure 9.7 shows, visits to a dentist increase with income.

For both men and women, higher income is related to less use of hospital services in the last 12 months. The pattern for hospital admissions is less clear. There seems a definite downwards trend for males with income, but not for females. Possibly, this is because many female admissions are connected with childbirth, rather than illness.

Maori score lower than nonMaori on all measures of 'health state', and have a higher proportion with disability. The differences are strongly significant for the comparison of Maori women with nonMaori women, but not quite so clear-cut for men. The income gradients found for the entire population are also apparent for both Maori and nonMaori.

There is a clearly higher prevalence of risky behaviours for Maori as compared with nonMaori, at all income levels. Proportions smoking and with hazardous usage patterns for alcohol are significantly higher overall. The trends with income for Maori are similar to those already discussed for the whole population; although the relatively small numbers of Maori in the survey mean that the trends are not always statistically significant, more especially for the hazardous use of alcohol. Analysing Maori separately from nonMaori men makes the upwards trend in hazardous alcohol use with income by nonMaori males more clearly apparent.

Regional average household income, and income inequality

We turn now to an examination of regional differences in income, and health outcomes. In this section, mortality is measured by the standardised mortality ratios (SMRs) for 27 New Zealand regions defined by the Ministry of Health (1998). Averages over the five-year period 1990 to 1994 have been used, as the annual SMRs vary considerably from year to year for the smaller regions. Hospitalisation is measured by the standardised discharge ratios (SDRs) from the same source. These have been averaged over the three years 1994/95 to 1996/97.

The income measures, derived from 1996 census data are gross, that is pre-tax, and included income from all sources. After household incomes were equivalised as described earlier

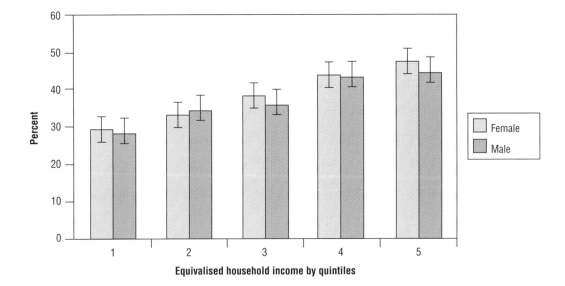

Figure 9.7 Percentage of adults who visited dentist or dental nurse in last 12 months, by income quintile

in this chapter, average income and a measure of income inequality, the Gini coefficient, were then calculated for this 'equivalent household income' data. Both averages and Gini coefficients were in terms of individuals. That is, each person in the household was assigned the equivalent income of that household, and then averages and Gini coefficients calculated for individual persons. The results for each region were age standardised to All New Zealand age-group proportions. The standardisation made little difference, however, to the Gini coefficients.

Income and Ethnicity

Europeans have household incomes on average five to six per cent higher than the overall average. The average for both Maori and Pacific people is less than 80% of the NZ average, while the 'Other' group has an average income of 86% of the NZ average (see table 9.1 and figure 9.8).

Table 9.1 includes two measures of income inequality. Whereas 40.7% of respondents have an equivalent income less than $27,500, this increases to 54% for Maori, and over 50% for the other two ethnic groups.

The Gini coefficients measure income inequality *within* each ethnic group. On this basis, income inequality is moderately higher for Maori and Pacific Islanders than for Europeans, and substantially higher for the 'Other' ethnic group.

Income measures, by region

Wellington has by a good margin the highest income, followed by Auckland City and then other areas in the Auckland, Wellington-Hutt and Waikato regions. Auckland City has, however, the highest measure of income inequality.

To what extent are regional differences in mortality and hospitalisation explainable by, or at least associated with, regional differences in average income? Scatter-diagrams show an apparent inverse relationship for both SMRs and SDRs with average income. Are differences in mortality and hospitalisation between regions additionally associated with differences in

Table 9.1 Household income measures from 1996 census, by ethnic group in New Zealand

Ethnic group	% responding	Income average	Gini coefficient	% less than $27,500
European	88.0	$44,337	0.366	36.5
NZ Maori	74.5	$32,429	0.376	54.1
Pacific people	62.0	$32,899	0.373	50.7
Other	74.5	$35,867	0.434	50.5
Total	84.0	$41,745	0.377	40.7

Note: Numbers are for individuals, in terms of equivalent gross household income, age-adjusted.

'Equivalent income' dollars are not real dollars – in this case, the proportions show those persons whose 'economic well-being' is less than that of a 'two-person' household with total income of $27,500.

The bigger the Gini coefficient is, the more unequally income is distributed.

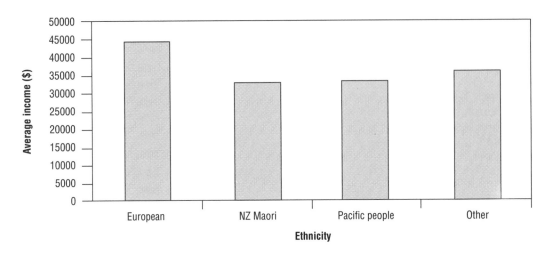

Figure 9.8 Average equivalent household income per person, by ethnic group, 1996 census, for those households reporting income, age adjusted

income inequality? That is, do regions with a more unequal income distribution also tend to have worse health outcomes, after controlling for differences in average income?

Table 9.2 gives the results from log-linear regressions of regional SMRs, and SDRs, on the census income variables derived for this report. All data were expressed as regional ratios to the New Zealand average, set at unity. The age-standardised income variables used here give a slightly better fit than nonstandardised income variables for mortality, though a marginally less good fit for hospital discharge rates.

Results for each are given first for just the one explanatory variable – average income (equivalised household income). The results are similar for mortality and hospitalisation. The coefficients show that a one per cent increase in average regional income is associated with a fall on average of 0.32% in mortality and 0.57% in hospitalisation. The association in both cases is highly significant with the probabilities (the 'p values') of such results occurring by chance being very low at 0.0004 and 0.0003, well below the commonly used criterion of 0.05 for statistical significance. Nearly 40% of the variation between regions is explained for both mortality and hospitalisation by differences in average regional incomes.

Results are then given for regressions of SMRs/SDRs on two variables – average income, and income inequality (the Gini coefficient). The result is a better fit than that for income alone, with the adjusted R^2 increasing to nearly 50% for both mortality and hospitalisation. The 'average income' effect is stronger than the inequality effect, in a statistical sense, but the contribution of the Gini coefficient is also statistically significant in both cases, at the 95% confidence level. A one per cent increase in the Gini coefficient corresponds to a 0.60% increase in mortality and a 1.06% increase in hospitalisation. Overall nearly half of the regional variation in mortality and hospitalisation rates is explained by the combination of regional average income and regional income inequality.

Table 9.2 Regional mortality and hospitalisation regressed on regional measures of average income and income inequality

Mortality (standardised mortality ratios)	Constant	Coefficient	Probability value	Adjusted R²
(i) Regressed on single variable – Average income	0.00	−0.32	0.0004	0.37
(ii) Regressed on two variables – Average income and Income inequality	0.02	−0.36	0.0001	0.46
Gini coefficient		0.60	0.0309	

Hospitalisation (standardised discharge ratios)	Constant	Coefficient	Probability value	Adjusted R²
(i) Regressed on single variable – Average income	0.00	−0.57	0.0003	0.39
(ii) Regressed on two variables – Average income and Income inequality	0.03	−0.66	0.0000	0.48
Gini coefficient		1.06	0.0309	

Note: All income measures are based on equivalent gross 1996 census household income, age-adjusted, each individual in the household then being assumed to have this household income. Standardised mortality ratios are averaged over the five years 1990 to 1994. Standardised discharge ratios are averaged over the three years 1994/5 to 1996/7. Regressions are log-linear.

We conclude from these regional analyses that differences in mortality, and in hospital admission rates, between geographical regions are associated with differences in average income. Regions with lower average household incomes tend to have higher mortality and higher admission rates. In addition, but independently, mortality and hospitalisation differences are also associated with differences in income inequality. Regions with a more unequal distribution of income tend to have higher mortality and higher admission rates, after controlling for differences in average income.

There are however two statistical caveats about these results. The outcome variables, SDRs and SMRs, are based on 'indirect' standardisation rather than 'direct' (Ministry of Health 1998). 'Indirect standardisation' applies national age/gender rates to regional populations for comparison with actual regional outcomes. It is preferable in general to 'direct standardisation' in which regional age/gender specific rates are applied to the national, or other standard, population. This is because it is less sensitive to extreme variations in the regional specific rates. However, it does mean that regional differences in population structure could account for some of the variation in the indirectly standardised SMRs and SDRs used here; and that the results here should be tested for robustness using directly standardised rates.

The second caveat concerns the possible influence of ethnicity. It is apparent that some regions with high mortality and hospitalisation rates are also regions with high proportions of Maori population, such as Eastern Bay of Plenty and Tairawhiti. Changes in ethnicity defini- tions in recent years have made more complicated the task of deriving standardised 'ethnic' measures of mortality and other health outcomes. The simple addition of a 'proportion Maori' variable to the equations tabulated above does indicate, however, the importance of ethnicity, particularly for hospital discharges, and suggests that some at least of the association between income inequality and health outcomes is connected with differences in ethnic composition of regional populations. Further work is needed on the influence of ethnicity on regional health outcomes.

Discussion

The results in this chapter are generally similar to international evidence. For example, the 1992 Australian National Health Strategy report, also using health survey data, found that people with low family incomes reported more disability and chronic illness, greater morbidity, and more days of reduced activity due to illness. Lower income groups made more use of hospital services and general practitioners (but not dentists), but these differentials tended to become statistically insignificant in multivariate analyses when current health state was allowed for. Multivariate analysis showed that even when the higher prevalence of known risk factors for low-income earners was accounted for, they still had poorer health status. Other factors associated with higher mortality or poorer health included being single or part of a single parent family.

The impact of income on health is significant. The level of personal and household income in society could have a direct effect on individual's health, for example through enabling people to buy adequate food, appropriate housing and private health care. The distri- bution of relative income could have an indirect effect, through psychosocial mechanisms, such as being less inclined to vote and thus being marginalised in redistributive political processes (Blakely, Kennedy and Kawachi 2001).

The literature increasingly supports this model. A US study (McDonough et al. 1997), based on longitudinal survey data over the period 1968 to 1989, found that income level was a strong predictor of mortality, especially for persons under the age of 65. Persistent low income was a particularly powerful predictor of mortality risk, and, for middle-income individ- uals, income instability was also important. All these effects persisted after adjustment for education and initial health status – evidence against the 'selective mobility' hypothesis.

There is a strong association between a community having a low average income and it also having poor health outcomes. Numerous cross-regional or cross-national studies over the years have shown this association. Poor countries in general have poor health outcomes and higher mortality. It has, however, been observed that this association at country level holds strongly only up to a certain level of per capita income – about US$4,000 in the early 1990s (Wilkinson 1996a).

At sub-national level, the results in this study show that differentials in health outcomes persist even when national income is high. Either lower than average income causes poor health outcomes, or low income is associated with other factors that cause poor health outcomes. As mentioned above, studies elsewhere (National Health Strategy, 1992) show that for individuals, this result persists after controlling for known risk factors, and also that longitudinal data suggests that it persists after controlling for initial health status (McDonough et al. 1997).

As well as providing evidence that absolute income at a national or community level has an impact on health, our results perhaps provide support for Wilkinson's (1996) hypothesis about the impact of relative income inequality. In addition to the influence of the level of personal income on an individual's health, or the level of average income on a community's health, the *spread* of income in a community also possibly influences the health of individuals. More precisely, the hypothesis is that the greater the income inequality in a community, the worse on average is the average health outcome, and further, that this result is independent of the effect of income level on health outcomes. That is, 'relative income' matters as well as 'absolute income'. Wilkinson (1997b) in discussing possible mechanisms claimed that compared with the influence of material circumstances, the psychosocial effects of social position account for the larger part of health inequalities. That is, he downplayed the effect of income on health, *vis-à-vis* the effect of income inequality.

Wilkinson's hypothesis could be labelled the 'strong' version of the hypothesis as against the 'weak' version postulated by Gravelle (1998) whereby an increase in income inequality leads to poorer health outcomes, but the poorer outcomes are caused by changes in individuals' incomes resulting from the change in income inequality, rather than by income inequality itself directly influencing health outcomes. The two alternatives are potentially testable against each other where individual data on income level and health outcomes are available in addition to community data. In our research, which looked at income inequality at a regional level, we showed that both income inequality and average household income had an association with mortality and hospitalisation.

The dynamics of income distribution complicate any interpretation (Creedy 1997; Hyslop 2000). Cross-sectional data only enable us to draw conclusions from a 'snapshot' picture of current income, which ideally should be supplemented with data on income over a lifetime. Also, one generation's income affects opportunities and hence health outcomes of the next generation. Nonetheless, our data suggest that income inequality in New Zealand could have a significant impact on mortality and hospitalisation, over and above the impact of the level of household income.

There are clear-cut ethnic differences for some but not all outcomes. For instance, Maori have in general a lower percentage than nonMaori in each income quintile rating their health as *very good* or *excellent*. And the fact that Maori are also disproportionately concentrated in the lower income quintiles increases the frequency with which Maori self-assessed their health state as low.

We have not included any measures in this chapter from the fruitful area of health expectancy, the difference between the length and quality of life. An examination of health expectancy in New Zealand between 1981 and 1991 found that adjusting for health status narrowed the gender gap, but widened socioeconomic and ethnic differentials (Davis et al. 1999). Similar results have been found in Australia, UK and USA.

Policy implications

Can the negative impact of social and economic inequality on health be reduced by income redistribution? Would changes in income alone have an effect on health outcomes without changes in other mediating factors such as education and occupational status? Our analyses cannot answer these questions. If the model in figure 9.1 is correct, however, redistribution of income would affect the health and well-being of the population.

Even in a 'pared back' welfare state, governments have the power to redistribute as well as distribute resources. Through benefits and other elements of the social wage, governments have come to play a major role in the distribution of family disposable incomes. Governments also have considerable moral authority to influence social norms about fairness. For example, the newly elected Labour/Alliance Government in New Zealand expected ministerial staff to take salary cuts when their contracts came up for renewal and commented critically on the large salaries of television personalities.

The distinguished British economist Atkinson would probably approve. Commenting recently on the Acheson report, he highlighted the role of governments in reducing inequalities:

> I do not believe that the governments are totally without power. In particular, the distribution of economic outcomes is considerably influenced by national government policy. Government and social judgements affect the labour market, where differentials are not simply a matter of supply and demand. Income inequality is not only the result of widening earnings dispersion, but also reflects the direct effect of the government budget, which accounted for the sharp and unparalleled rise in the Gini coefficient in the UK in the 1980s. Countries which have maintained, or even strengthened, their welfare states have not seen the same rise in poverty as in the UK.
>
> ... In my view, the economic constraints on redistribution are exaggerated. Politicians have more room to manoeuvre than they like to admit (1999, p 287).

However, redistribution of income or wealth is unlikely to be sufficient when the main source of inequality does not just lie in the distribution of wealth, but in the social and institutional arrangements that give access to health-promoting environments. Amartya Sen has pointed out:

> It is important to distinguish between income as a unit in which to measure inequality and income as the vehicle of inequality reduction. Even if inequality in capabilities is well measured in terms of equivalent incomes, it does not follow that transferring income would be the best way to counteract the observed inequality (p 84).

Herein lies the difficulty for policy. Income alone will not compensate the disabled person who needs a higher level of income to participate (Sen 1999). The economic incentives inherent in different institutions' arrangements may still perpetuate inequalities even if individual incomes are equivalised. For example, Maori professionals, with tertiary education, still earn significantly less than nonMaori professionals (Davis et al. 1997), a phenomenon common to minority ethnic groups and not peculiar to New Zealand (Loury 1977; Menchek 1993).

There is a role for suitably designed redistribution policies in enhancing aggregate health. The existence of diminishing returns has important implications for health policy. It suggests that if income tax is more progressive, the very poor may benefit without any impact on the health of the rich. The model explored by Backlund et al. (1996) supports this conclusion on the basis that differences in mortality may primarily be a function of income at the low end of the socioeconomic continuum, and a function of education at the higher end.

Policies that result in low-income households having more economic resources should reduce health inequalities. Such policies could include economic policies that further reduce unemployment over the longer term, tax and benefit redistribution policies in general and policies redressing ethnic or gender-based inequities. Such policies are desirable both from the health perspective, and from the wider perspective of social justice. Some support for this view comes from Canadian research, which compared the relation between mortality and income inequality in Canada and the USA at the metropolitan area level. In a combined model, income inequality was a significant explanatory variable for all age groups, except for elderly people, but there was a lack of a significant association within Canada. The authors concluded that the potential impact of income inequality on health may be blunted by the different ways in which social and economic resources are distributed in Canada and the USA (Ross et al. 2000).

It would be claiming too much, however, to say that redistributive policies on their own will eliminate the social gradients in health. It is apparent that these gradients have complex socioeconomic causes, as shown for example by their persistence in relatively egalitarian Scandinavian societies (Martikainen and Valkonen 1999). While the average rates of ill health and premature mortality rates in Europe have the expected north/south gradient, the steepness of the social gradient for health inequalities also differs depending on government policies, though not always consistently across all age groups or according to the 'ill-health' country rankings. For example, while Sweden had small income-related inequalities compared with education and occupation, Sweden and Norway had larger inequalities than most other countries in both morbidity and mortality, whereas Switzerland and Spain had smaller-than-average inequalities in both outcomes (Mackenbach et al. 1997). As the authors conclude, such findings suggest that welfare policies can affect one dimension of social inequalities in health, such as income-related inequalities, while leaving others relatively untouched. The pattern of social inequalities and health may differ depending on the policy interventions that have been adopted, eg, government benefits, employment policies, regulation or affirmative action plans.

For developed countries, reducing income inequality by lifting the incomes of the poor appears to be a more effective strategy for lowering mortality rates – including infant mortality – than increasing average incomes. At this stage, the evidence on the links between income inequality and health is strongly suggestive, but the 'transmission mechanism' requires further elaboration and empirical research. Sen's ideas as described in this paper appear fruitful and should be able to be tested in further research. This should be a priority for social research looking at the impact of the pathways between income and income inequality on health.

Acknowledgements

The authors would like to thank Ralph Chapman and an anonymous reviewer for valuable comments.

Further Reading

Atkinson, A B 1999, Income inequality in the UK, Health Economics 8: 283–8.
 – *A leading figure in the economics of income inequality, Atkinson in this essay advocates a shift to policies aimed at reducing inequality.*
Graham, H (Ed.) 2001, Understanding Health Inequalities, Open University Press, Buckingham.
 – *Useful results of the British research funded under the Health Variations Program by the UK Economic and Social Research Council.*
Howden-Chapman, P & Tobias, M (Eds) 2000, Social Inequalities and Health: New Zealand 2000, Ministry of Health, Wellington.
 – *First monitoring report of social and economic determinants of health in New Zealand.*
Kawachi, I, Kennedy, B & Wilkinson, R 1999c, Society and Population Health Reader: Income inequality and health, The New Press, New York.
 – *A volume of readings including all the important papers on the topic up to the late 1990s by key contributors to the field.*
Sen, A 1999, Development as Freedom, Oxford University Press, Oxford.
 – *A cogent analysis of the philosophical issues around the concept of inequality by the Nobel Prize winning economist.*

10

Equity in access to health care

Stephen Duckett

There is now extensive literature documenting significant inequality in health status associated with a person's different place in Australian society. The starkest differences are revealed in comparing the health status of indigenous Australians to nonindigenous Australians. However, a series of publications from the Australian Institute of Health and Welfare (AIHW), the National Health Strategy and academic authors has demonstrated the existence of health inequalities in Australia on a range of dimensions. There is some theoretical debate about the causal factors associated with the inequalities. A major contributor to recent work in this area is Wilkinson (1996a) who argues that it is not social disadvantage, per se, which is associated with poor health but rather the extent of social inequality (but see Saunders 1996 and Judge et al. 1998 for critiques of Wilkinson's argument).

The role of the health system in promoting health and curing ill health is self-evident, but, as with health status, the health care system may involve significant inequality. The US work by Anderson, Aday and colleagues at the University of Chicago has pioneered one aspect of this area, namely analyses of differential use of health services. The model used by Anderson and colleagues has evolved over time (Andersen 1995), and the emerging model involves environmental factors (including the functioning of the health care system); population characteristics (including predisposing characteristics, enabling resources, and need); and health behaviour (including personal health services and use of health services). These factors lead to outcomes (in perceived health status, clinically measured health status and consumer satisfaction).

Different models of the impact of the health system on health status will obviously lead to different conclusions about the mutability of the health system's role in addressing differential health status. The Chicago work made some initial assumptions about the mutability of various factors, and in this context, it is important to recognise that social structure was seen as relatively immutable.

This paper focuses on the extent to which barriers to access to health services might be inequitable. Ensuring access and facilitating health service utilisation is not, of course, the only way the health system might respond to health inequalities. Changing the focus of health promotion programs might also lead to reduction in inequity (Duckett 1998).

Barriers to access to health care

The structure and function of the health care services can impact on health status in a number of ways. First, different structures in the health system will have a differential impact on access to health care. Second, the way the health system works for particular individuals or groups of individuals may impact on the outcomes of care following treatment, eg, if a provider cannot understand a client/patient because of inadequate interpreter services, outcomes could be compromised.

The most significant development in terms of equity of access was obviously Scotton and Deeble's work in the late 1960s. Their work provided the academic underpinning for the introduction of universal health insurance to address financial barriers to access and ensure equity in financing (see Scotton and Macdonald 1993 for an account of the processes involved in this; McClelland and Scotton 1998 for Medicare and equity). The election of the Whitlam Labor government in 1972 led to the introduction of Medibank in 1975. The introduction of Medibank was fiercely contested, and the policy direction was then progressively reversed by the Fraser governments over the period 1975 to 1981 (Duckett 1984). Medibank's successor, Medicare, commenced in 1984 following the election of the Hawke Labor government the previous year. Unlike the overt whittling away under the Fraser Liberal government, the Howard Liberal government has not directly reversed any of Medicare's key fundamentals, and there is now bipartisan agreement as to the importance of ensuring universal access to medical care through removing financial barriers to access in the health care system.

Access to general practitioner services is now available without significant financial barriers as demonstrated by the generally fairly high level of bulk billing, although levels of bulk billing are lower in rural areas. Direct billing, more commonly known as bulk billing, has increased each year since the introduction of Medicare and now stands at 72.2% for all services across Australia. Overall, 81.7% of all medical services are charged at or below the schedule fee. Figure 10.1 shows the growth in direct billing for general practitioner attendances.

This high rate of direct billing for general practitioner attendances is an important means of ensuring that consumers do not face financial barriers to access to primary medical care. The estimated rate of general practitioner direct billing in 1999/2000 is 79%, down from a peak of 80.6% in 1996/97. However, direct billing rates are not as high in all areas of medical practice. Figure 10.2 shows the level of direct billing and observance of the schedule fee by type of service.

It can be seen that while general practitioner services have a very high level of bulk billing (79.2%) and a similarly high level of schedule fee observance, less than one-third of specialist attendances are direct billed. There are similarly low bulk billing and schedule fee observance rates for obstetrics, anaesthetics and for surgical operations. Consumers have a choice about whether to use private surgeons for these in-hospital services (such as operations)

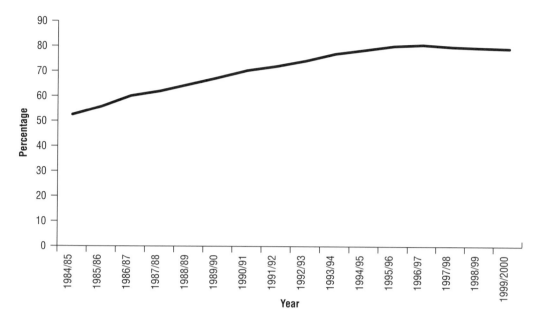

Figure 10.1 Percentage of general practitioner attendances bulk billed, 1984/5 to 1999/2000

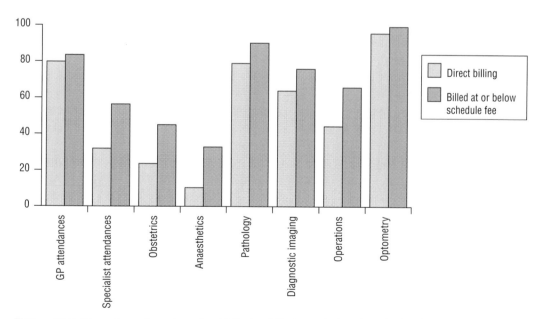

Figure 10.2 Percentage of services direct billed or billed at or below the schedule fee, by type, 1999/2000

or the alternative of surgery through hospital Medicare arrangements. However, for noninpatient specialist services, the low level of bulk billing and schedule fee observance appears to affect access for people with low incomes (Scott 1997) and is a matter of concern, especially as hospitals reduce their provision of specialist outpatient services.

Public provision of allied health and dental services is very limited, and hence, people needing these services, which are not covered by Medicare, either require ancillary health insurance or face out-of-pocket costs. As a result, it is not surprising that higher-income groups have better access to services such as dental, physiotherapy and chiropractic (Schofield 1999).

The situation for dental services is a particular concern. The abolition of the Commonwealth Dental Health Program in 1996, 'saving' $100m annually, ended the only systematic national program in this area, leaving provision for low-income people to the vagaries of differential state policies (Lewis 2000). In 1998/99, $603m of dental benefits were paid by health insurance organisations under ancillary insurance tables. The existence of the 30% Commonwealth Private Health Insurance Rebate means that the Commonwealth now effectively spends over $180m annually supporting dental services, almost twice the cost of the Commonwealth Dental Health Program. Because prevalence of health insurance is greater with greater levels of income (Cameron et al. 1988; Cameron and Trivedi 1991; Willcox 1991, Burrows et al. 1993; Australian Bureau of Statistics 1994; Cameron and McCallum 1996; Hopkins and Kidd 1996; Schofield 1997), this new dental health support is much more inequitable than the pre-existing Commonwealth Dental Health Program.

Access to public hospitals without financial barriers is guaranteed. Financial barriers to access to medical services, especially general practitioner services, are minimised through Medicare bulk billing. The absence of financial barriers to inpatient care does not, however, guarantee equity: consultation times for consumers with lower socio-economic status are shorter than for high-status consumers (Wiggers and Sanson-Fisher 1997; Martin et al. 1997), and there may be differences in the quality of care provided. There are also still financial barriers to access to specialist services (Scott 1997).

An important aspect of financial barriers is the differential access to timely care. Baume (1995) has demonstrated that there are significant waiting times in gaining access to private surgeons, but the most publicly debated issue in this area remains waiting times for elective surgery in public hospitals. This is despite a significant reduction in waiting times for the most urgent surgery in Victoria and other states (Street and Duckett 1996).

The heavier the reliance on private sources in the funding of health care, the more regressive and inequitable financing of care will be. Compared to other OECD countries, Australia relies relatively heavily on private sources of funding for health care. In 1997, 31% of health expenditure in Australia was from private sources (health insurance premiums or out-of-pockets), relative to 24% in Ireland and New Zealand, and 15% in the UK. Private funding is inherently inequitable, partly because of the fixed premiums for health insurance (Wagstaff et al. 1999). On average, Australian households spent $32.47 per week on medical care and health expenses according to the most recent household expenditure survey in 1998/99 (Australian Bureau of Statistics 2000a). This represented about 3.7% of average household income. The distribution of consumer payments (whether through health insurance or as out-of-pockets) is inequitable with lower income consumers paying proportionally substantially more (almost 10%

of income) compared with those on higher incomes (see figure 10.3). Further, the regressive nature of health spending appears to have worsened between 1993/94 and 1998/99 with lower income groups paying a higher proportion of their income for health care in the more recent survey.

Although households in the highest income quintile spent more per week on medical care and health expenditure in 1998/99 ($52.91) than the poorest 20% of households ($17.21), in percentage terms, poorer households spent 10.8% of income compared to the 2.7% of household income for the wealthiest 20% of households.

A significant proportion of household health expenditure is for health insurance, representing average expenditure of $5.46 per week (3.4% of household expenditure) in low-income households compared to $20.18 per week (1% of expenditure) in higher-income households. Health insurance premiums are not income related, which inevitably means they represent a higher proportion of income for the low-income insured. The increasing average weekly payment reflects the higher prevalence of health insurance in higher-income households.

Traditionally, private contributions in the Australian health sector have been used for four main purposes:

- To buy additional amenity (such as single rooms, improved food choices, etc.).
- To buy enhanced consumer control principally via 'choice of doctor'. A very important component of marketing private health insurance has been that health insurance allows 'free choice of doctor', ie consumers could elect to be treated by specialists known to them or who have a history of treating them. Obviously, in emergency situations, such a choice is illusory.

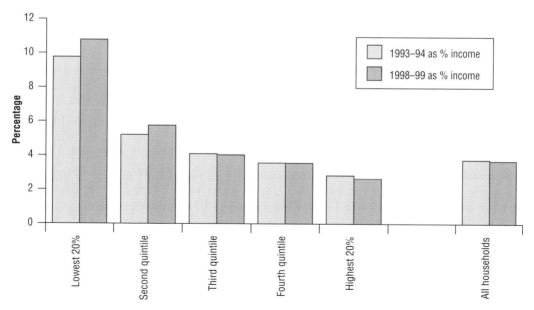

Figure 10.3 Percentage of household income spent on medical care and health expenses, 1993/4 and 1998/9

- To buy improved timeliness of care. Private health insurance allows consumers to be treated at a private hospital where operations or other admissions can be scheduled at the patient's or doctor's convenience rather than the facility's. This is especially the case for elective surgery where there are often significant waiting lists in the public sector.
- To buy a wider scope of services. The differential scope can be of two kinds. First, consumers may access care that would not reach treatment thresholds within the public sector because of resource constraints or that may be unavailable because it may not be cost effective. Second, they may access therapies, such as chiropractic and naturopathy, not traditionally covered by public sector arrangements.

There can be little objection to consumers using private funds for some of these purposes (such as improved amenity). However, to the extent that the private sector provides consumers with an opportunity to bypass waiting lists and other public sector constraints (and this is one of the marketing claims for private insurance), then it is anomalous that there should be a public subsidy, which the rebate effectively provides and hence increases inequity.

Other aspects of the health care system also evidence inequity. There are significant differences in access to health care (both primary care and hospital care) between urban and rural areas. Identification of the nature of the problem here is complex, as geographic equity is usually described relatively, eg, there are fewer doctors per 1000 population in rural Australia relative to urban areas.

Figure 10.4 shows trends in general practitioner:population ratios in urban and rural areas in Australia. The pattern of lower provision in smaller rural communities relative to larger rural centres is consistent with a previous study (Richardson et al. 1991) which found that the likelihood of general practitioner presence increased with town size and that there was a threshold effect for presence of other medical specialists. Brasure et al. (1999), in a US study, found a similar threshold effect and noted that the population increment needed to attract a second medical practitioner was less than required to attract the first. There has been a significant increase in general practitioner provision in both metropolitan and rural areas, with a higher ratio in capital cities relative to rural and remote areas. What is remarkable about this is that, although there is a perception of under-provision of general practitioners in rural areas and a significant focus of policy attention on access in rural and remote areas (Humphreys et al. 1997), the contemporary level of rural access is *above* the metropolitan level in 1984/85. As figure 10.4 shows, the general practitioner:population ratio has increased from the 1980s to 1990s.

Figure 10.4 does not show the distribution of medical practitioners within a single category such as small rural centres. Where in the past, most towns may have had one or two doctors, some now have three and others none. Towns with only one doctor are vulnerable to that doctor retiring or otherwise relocating, especially as community expectations of 24-hour access to the practitioner may conflict with the life-style expectations of doctors and their families.

Access to hospital services in rural communities is also perceived to be a problem, in part because of the need to travel significant distances to gain access to specialist services. In a sense, this is almost inevitable as super-specialist services need to be concentrated to achieve economies of scale and expertise and are available in only a limited number of tertiary hospitals.

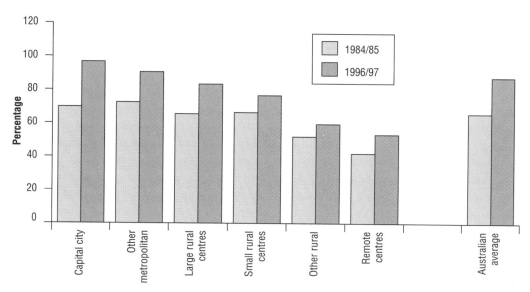

Figure 10.4 General practitioners per 100,000 population, 1984/5 to 1996/7

Infrastructure requirements even for more generalist hospital services are increasing, leading to the concentration of hospitals in the larger rural centres and closure of the smaller rural hospitals. However, small rural communities value their local hospital highly, largely because of the hospital's perceived role as a source of emergency care, and so rural hospital closures are hotly contested politically.

The further element of equity of access is the issue of racial barriers to access. Access issues here are complex. Deeble et al. (1998) have shown that health expenditure for indigenous populations is not too dissimilar to that for the nonindigenous population. But given the differences in health outcomes for Aboriginal people, there is an obvious case for greater levels of expenditure. Deeble estimated in an unpublished paper recently prepared for the Australian Medical Association that an increase of 27% in expenditure on Aboriginal health could be justified. This would mean that government expenditure for Aboriginals and Torres Strait Islander people would be about twice the nonindigenous average.

One potential effect of the health system on equity may be differential outcomes for different groups. However, there does not appear to be any evidence suggesting that, once a person is admitted to a hospital, technical quality of care is different based on socio-demographic factors.

Although the US stands out as the country with inequity built into the very structure of the health system because of the high proportion of uninsured, Australia still evidences substantial inequity in cross national surveys. Schoen et al. (2000) showed that 8% of Australians did not get needed care, compared with 14% in the US. The rate for people of below-average income was 12% in Australia and 20% in the US.

Conclusion

Despite the achievements of Medicare, the health care system can do more to promote equity. In terms of access to health care, Medicare has meant that most financial barriers to access have been removed. However, the system is still inequitable, and public patients are forced to wait for care while private patients receive a 30% subsidy (through the private health insurance rebate) to bypass the queues. People in the lowest income quintile spend a higher proportion of their income than people in higher income quintiles, a difference partly explained by spending on health insurance. A clear first step in promoting greater equity in the system would be a more equitable funding system, in particular, redirecting the health insurance rebate to improved public hospital provision. Improving public hospital provision would also help reduce the perception of people in low-income quintiles that private health insurance, which by nature is regressive, is a necessary purchase. Similarly, abolition of the ancillary insurance rebate could be used to fund a more targeted scheme providing access to dental care and other allied health services.

Addressing out-of-pocket costs is more problematic. One approach is to develop a 'participating doctor' scheme: under these arrangements, Medicare rebates would only be available to doctors who direct bill all their patients. Although such a scheme may introduce greater access in metropolitan areas, it is likely to founder in rural and regional centres. Some combination of increasing supply and enhancing opportunities for substitution, especially involving nurses, will be required in these areas.

Further Reading

National Health Strategy, 1992, Enough to make you sick: how income and environment affect health (Research Paper No. 1), National Health Strategy, Canberra.
  – *A somewhat dated but very comprehensive analysis of influences of income, family composition etc. on health status and health care utilisation.*
Lairson, D R, Hindson, P et al. 1995, Equity in health care in Australia, Social Science and Medicine 41(4): 475–82.
  – *Uses Kakwani index to measure equity of health care financing in Australia and compares it with other countries.*
Schofield, D 1999, Ancillary and specialist health services: The relationship between income, user rates and equity or access, Australian Journal of Social Issues 34(1): 79–96.
Schofield, D 2000, Public hospital expenditure: how is it divided between lower, middle and upper income groups? The Australian Economic Review 33(4): 303–16.
  – *Estimates utilisation rates for hospitals and other services by income quintiles. The hospital paper also compares results using different estimation approaches.*
Scott, M-A 1997, Equity in the distribution of health care in Australia, proceedings of the eighteenth Australian conference of health economists, A H Harris, Coffs Harbour, Australian Studies in Health Service Administration. 81: 319–58.
  – *Examines income gradients for various measures of health care utilisation.*

Part C
Social organisation and health

11

Human settlements:
health and the physical environment

Peter Newman

Introduction

The healthy cities movement is not new; it began in the late 19th century in response to industrial city slums. The problems of polluted water, filthy streets and fetid air, together with the lack of any natural parkland gave rise to modern town planning. The role of health professionals in this movement was very significant. This chapter will gather some perspective from the history of settlements before showing how we are facing a set of issues just as critical as those that faced the first industrial cities. It will try to show what those problems are and how some settlements are facing them. The role of health professionals in gaining acceptance of the required integrative approach will be stressed, as will the need for a sense of hope in these debates.

The physical environment of our cities presents a range of problems that concern health professionals: indoor air pollution, toxic chemicals in the workplace, industrial pollution, toxic site remediation, and so on. The focus of this chapter is on the physical environment as it relates to the transport and land use issues associated with the automobile. As with all physical environmental issues, we must consider their social and economic context.

Healthy cities in history

The health profession was a major factor in changing the nature of cities in the 19th century. The rapid growth of industrial cities meant that often, simple needs like separating water from waste (well known in every indigenous culture) were unmet. John Snow's 'discovery' that a sewage-contaminated well was causing cholera in London was said to have led to a burst of public health awareness in the late 1840s. Sewers were built, and public health approaches were adopted from that period but these improvements were outpaced by the growth of the cities and their polluting industries.

By the 1890s, the worst depression ever known had led to terrible poverty and crime throughout industrial cities. The air was full of the smoke and smells of the 'dark satanic mills'. People crowded into tenements, and all the services were overwhelmed. Garbage filled the streets, and epidemics raged through the slums.

The social, economic and environmental problems of the cities dominated political and academic agendas. In response, the resulting 'hygiene' movement spread through the developed world's cities.

Doctors and public health authorities commanded the field of urban affairs as they sought simultaneous cures for the social and health problems of the cities. The solutions? Reduce overcrowding, banish industries to other areas and bring parks into the city. But, it was all explained in terms of health (Boyer 1983). As Kostoff says, 'Hygiene was a prime concern – fresh air, light, washable clothes, and floors polished with beeswax which was said to generate "health-giving ozone"' (1991, p 201). The movement was simultaneously a moral crusade to provide education and jobs for the poor as well as a better physical environment.

This movement had direct links to the 'garden city' movement and thus to town planning. The main breakthrough was the use of infrastructure for transport, water, sewerage and power in linear corridors. The 'transit city' was based on trams and trains that spread the cities out, but with the necessary urbanity of a 'walkable' centre around the train station or the tramline (Newman and Kenworthy 1999). The solutions were slowly applied, and the old industrial city was gradually cleaned up.

The seeds of many of our 21st century problems with automobile dependence were sown in the processes set up to alleviate those from the late 19th century. Both low-density development and segregated land use, which are at the base of auto-dependence, express the underlying shift from a creative, design-oriented process to one that turned the planning process into the routine application of engineering-based rules to build cities around cars. There are many cities today that did not go down the path of the Automobile City, but like Stockholm or Singapore, they continue to use the Transit City design solution of corridors with dense centres strung together along the train lines like beads on a string. However, these cities are rare, and most have gone the way of the car with endless suburbs and heavy traffic going in all directions. The problem is that the justification for building around the car was provided by health professionals who targeted density and mixed land use as the health problem.

Density

A century ago, it was common to claim that 'density of population beyond a certain point results in disorder, vice and disease' (Moore 1909). The fact that it was the unemployed who were forced into crowded tenements was not seen as relevant to the causes of social disorder, ill health and vice. The problem was simply too many people.

Despite numerous studies since, no serious sociological link between high density, ill health and social disorder has been demonstrated (see Newman and Hogan 1981); crime today seems to be more linked to low density (Newman and Kenworthy 1989). Nevertheless, there is a strong planning tradition of preventing density getting too high, in order to prevent social evils and have a more 'healthy' community. Engineering-based rules are thus created in many cities to reduce density no matter what. That these cities tend nearly all to be in the

Anglo-Celtic world suggests some kind of cultural basis to this anti-density fervour. The motto of the English Town and Country Planning Association (the garden city movement's NGO) was 'Nothing gained by overcrowding', and this has dominated town planning in the English-speaking world for over 100 years. The result has been that town-planning rules have been religiously applied to restrict density in British-American town planning traditions for most of the 20th century.

The physical health link to density was part of the 'scientific' rationale. Its basis was the theory of 'miasma'. Miasma was thought to be the noxious emanations that floated in the air and caused disease; they were dissipated by a 'healthy supply of clean air' and by absorption into trees (Boyer 1983). If there were too many people, then, there was too much miasma.

Even today, town planning literature and regulations are full of references to space increasing health. This is despite a century of experience that shows the vast majority of infections that lead to urban epidemics come from contaminated water, not air, and fairly clear evidence that rural health levels are worse than urban levels (eg, Newman et al. 1996). The extremely high-density cities of Hong Kong, Tokyo and Singapore have managed to achieve freedom from epidemic diseases, while maintaining densities that are much higher than in the 19th century. However, they have reduced the number of people per room and per bed; this poverty-relief factor seems to be more important than population density, as long as water quality is managed. Hong Kong with a density of 300 people per hectare (20 times higher than Australian cities) has one of the highest life expectancies and lowest infant mortality rates in the world.

Density will always be a controversial area but it ought not to be seen as a cause of social disorder and ill health. Those are affected by poverty, urban management and design but are not fundamentally related to density.

Today, the problems of our settlements (environmental, social and economic) revolve around the struggle to maintain and develop community (Newman and Kenworthy 1999). Health issues are now being related to this loss of community as well (Marmot and Wilkinson 1999). Our research has tried to indicate that there is a link between this loss of community and the density/transport base of a city. When densities reach such low levels that settlements are car dependent, then the notions of community become very difficult to maintain as the opportunities for 'accidental interaction' are reduced, even for children. Low-density planning is not the only cause of loss of community, but it is very difficult to say that density is unimportant to community. The mechanism appears to be through the imposition of a highly privatising device – the automobile – as the key mechanism for linking people. In terms of health the car also has many direct impacts on health due to the lack of physical activity associated with car-based lifestyles. In our studies, a density of around 30 people per hectare seems to be a cut off for an area to have any 'walkability' or viability for public transport. Community occurs of course below this, but it is based on planned trips that are nearly always dependent on motor cars. Most of Australia's inner suburbs are above the critical density of 30 per hectare, but the new suburbs are all below 12 to 15 people per hectare and continue to be planned that way. As shown below, these suburbs are rapidly losing their appeal and are becoming the new poor areas of our cities, thus exacerbating health problems as they are heavily car dependent.

Segregated land use

The traditional city had all kinds of land use mixed in together. This worked well as organic relationships developed between places and their mixture of functions. The links began to break down when industry scaled up during the industrial revolution. Thus, zoning industry into a separate area of the city to prevent pollution was another approach of early health-based town planning. This approach soon led to every function in the city having a zoning and needing a separate area.

Industry was not always required to clean up once spatial dispersion was involved (creating areas of pollution that are often where the poor end up), and the total effect of zoning was an almost complete dismemberment of the city into its parts.

In continental Europe, people were less persuaded by the evils of overcrowding and mixed land use and gave more attention to poverty relief, better housing (still at high density) and direct pollution control. Certainly, they still had their polluted areas but they were less inclined to try and solve their problems by creating zones where people were licensed to pollute.

Lowering density and separating land uses was the town planning solution chosen by the UK and by other Anglo-Celtic cities in the new world. It was rationalised in health terms and so town planners felt they had a scientific basis for sprawling their cities and allowing car dependence to develop. The garden city became the highly spacious garden suburb separated from all the corrupting aspects of city life. The result was increasing travel distances. As these increased further and further in the 20th century the distances became feasible only if the automobile serviced them. The age of automobile dependence emerged directly from these solutions to the 19th century city.

Continental Europe again had a different approach – a more powerful belief in urbanism and the importance of urban design that retained the age-old functions of a pedestrian scale. As Kostoff (1991) says: 'Urbanism . . . is precisely the science of relationships. And these relationships must be determined according to how much a person walking through the city can take in at a glance' (p 83). This element was lost when the adage about 'nothing gained by overcrowding' drove the planning process.

Australian cities however, were driven by this new desire for non-urban space, for the rural village. Thus, the relentless processes of urban sprawl were set in motion with each new spacious suburb being succeeded by another and the rural edge retreating further and further.

The change in the nature of the problems in Australian cities is highlighted by the issue of stormwater in the late 19th century and by smog in the late 20th century. In the 1890s, the filth of the streets was swept away whenever it rained, but due to lack of infrastructure, the garbage, animal wastes and some human wastes all ended up in the streets (and houses) of those who lived down the hill. In the 1890s, the poor lived down the hill. In every Australian city, inner suburbs that have a slum reputation generally are down the hill from the wealthy suburbs. The filth and smell of the poor-crowded slums did not always originate in their 'vice-ridden' lifestyles. The Carlton versus Collingwood football rivalry had its origins in stormwater management.

In the 1990s, we have mostly engineered away the problems of stormwater, though in the sprawling outer suburbs of Sydney and to some extent in Perth, there is a problem with the nutrient loads being washed into water systems. The major problem now is smog. In Sydney, Melbourne and Perth, photochemical smog is a constant reminder of the automobile's impact on our lives. However, it is not widely realised that the major impact of this smog is experienced 'down the hill', by the poor. Smog is generally created in these cities by the intensive use of motor vehicles in the urban areas close to the coast, it is then moved by geographic and climatic factors inland to areas west (in Sydney and Melbourne) and east (in Perth) which are generally where the poor are situated.

Not much has changed. We certainly cannot be complacent about Australia's lovely, spacious cities with their in-built automobile dependence. Professionals must try to understand better this dependence and the many health issues connected with it. The following sections of this chapter attempt to throw some light on costs and patterns of automobile dependence and how new trends in planning are helping us learn to counteract it.

Automobile dependence

When urban land use so constrains choices that there are no options other than to use an automobile to reach most major urban functions, people become automobile dependent. Urban sprawl results from the kind of dispersed urban land use that is planned on the assumption of automobile dependence. Automobile dominance causes or exacerbates such health-related problems as:

- Smog and other air quality problems. Fine particles are now seen as a distinct problem on top of the better-known photochemical smog problem.
- Greenhouse gas emissions. These exacerbate a number of health problems (McMichael 1994).
- Oil vulnerability. This is now one of the great uncertainties facing cities everywhere, but increasingly, those faced with the biggest impact from global oil price rises are the poor who live in car-dependent locations.
- Road accidents. In Australia, they are now costing over $14 billion a year.
- Lack of exercise. Walking is almost non-existent in car dependent suburbs.
- Poverty and inequality. The link to health is now obvious, but increasingly, the divide between rich and poor has become spatially expressed.
- Loss of community. Privatism, consumerism, and alienation from traditional structures of urban life can all be related to the spatial separation inherent in car-dependent parts of cities.

These problems are reaching a series of limits that together mean that cities need a new vision, just as they did one hundred years ago. The industrial cities were able to solve their problems with a combination of vision and engineering. Health professionals were critical then and need to be again. They have insight into the needs of people in cities, as health is so basic to quality of life. And cities are all about quality of life.

If health professionals are to do anything about this, they need to understand more about how automobile dependence is expressed in different cities and how it is being tackled.

Patterns of automobile dependence

The level of automobile dependence varies considerably around the world. Figures 11.1 to 11.4 set out the comparative data on transport, infrastructure and land use from a global survey of 44 cities (Kenworthy et al. 1999; Newman and Kenworthy 1999).

US and Australian cities are considerably more oriented to the automobile. For example, in comparison to European cities, Australian cities have:

- Nearly double the per capita car use while having much lower levels of city wealth (gross regional product per person).
- Less than half the public transport per capita.
- Negligible walking and bicycling for work journeys.
- More than four times the road capacity per person.
- Over 50% more parking in central business districts, and
- Nearly four times less dense urban form.

Figures 11.5, 11.6 and 11.7 show some of the differences in smog, accidents and greenhouse gases associated with these different cities.

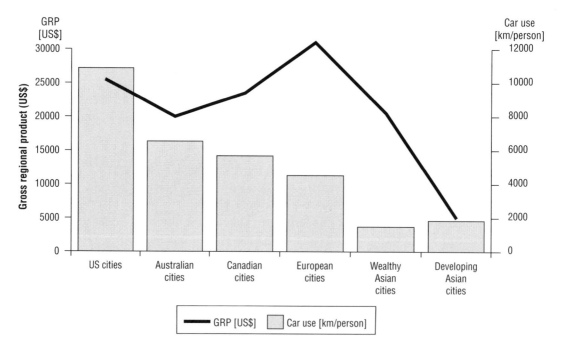

Figure 11.1 Gross regional product and car use per person, 1990

Source: Kenworthy et al. 1999.

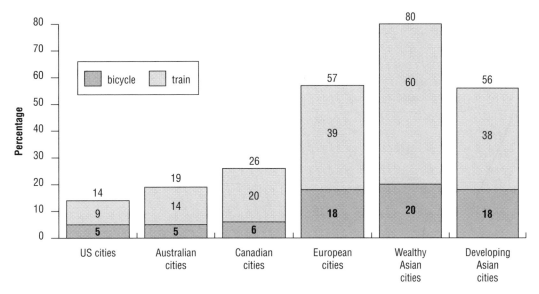

Figure 11.2 Percentage of workers using public or non-motorised transport, 1990

Note: On the side of each column, the lower figure shows non-motorised transport use and the upper figure shows public transport use.

Source: Kenworthy et al. 1999.

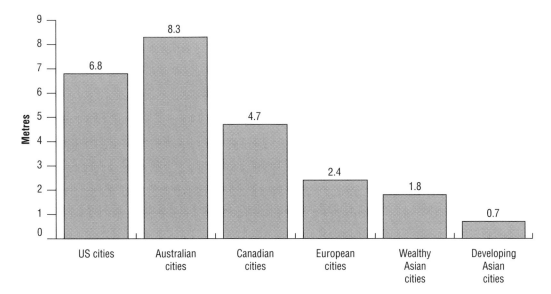

Figure 11.3 Length of road per person, 1990

Source: Kenworthy et al. 1999.

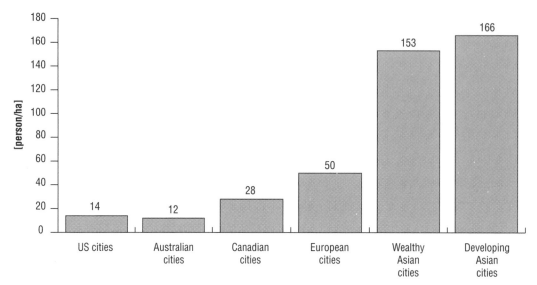

Figure 11.4 Urban density, 1990

Source: Kenworthy et al. 1999.

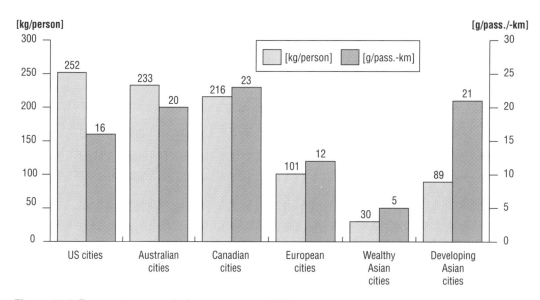

Figure 11.5 Transport smog emissions per person, 1990

Note: For each city group, the left column shows emissions in kilograms per person and the right column shows emissions in grams per passenger kilometer.

Smog emissions include nitrogen oxides (NOx), sulphur dioxide (SO_2), carbon monoxide (CO), volatile hydrocarbons (VHC) and volatile particulates (VP).

Source: Kenworthy et al. 1999.

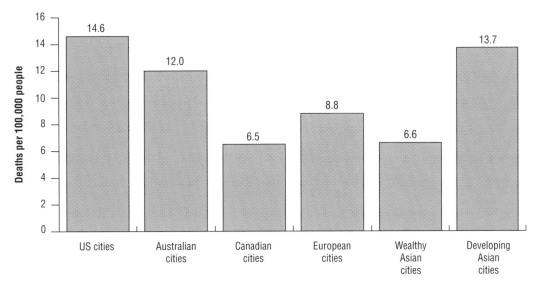

Figure 11.6 Transport deaths per 100,000 people, 1990

Source: Kenworthy et al. 1999.

Solutions to automobile dependence

Not all cities are automobile dependent. The dismal picture of automobile dependence is not inevitable (Rainbow and Tan 1993). There are cities and places that are overcoming automobile dependence (Newman and Kenworthy 1999), and increasingly, the healthy cities movement is seeing these solutions (Foskett 1991).

The rest of this chapter will be oriented to solutions. To each of the identified problems, simple, incremental solutions have been proposed that are increasingly seen to be inadequate and counter-productive. Solutions to one problem can worsen others. For example, solving congestion by increasing road capacity just increases total car use. Switching to non-oil fuels can make greenhouse effects worse and does nothing for traffic problems. The same can be said of electric cars. Even improving fuel efficiency can just lead to greater car use. Solving car use problems by just increasing prices will exacerbate inequity and isolation on the urban fringe.

There is a need to go beyond incremental solutions to more holistic urban system solutions that can make our cities less automobile dependent. This requires several changes in the car-dependent engineering 'mind set,' which is still the dominant paradigm governing our cities. The following five principles are suggested to guide our approach.

1 Accept that the constraints on automobile dependence are real and require new economic approaches

The constraints on automobile dependence are clearly economic and environmental (and increasingly social). There is increasing public awareness of the environmental constraint, but

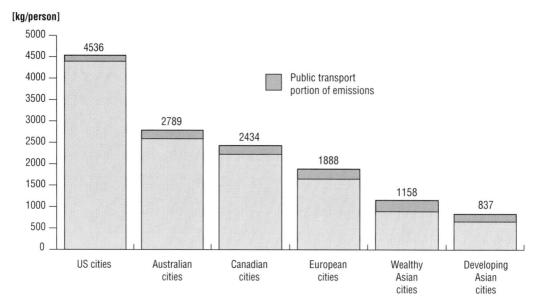

[kg/person]

Figure 11.7 Transport carbon dioxide emissions per person, 1990

Source: Kenworthy et al. 1999.

there is little awareness of the economic constraint. As figure 11.8 shows, transport costs a far greater proportion of city wealth in car-dependent cities.

The automobile is highly subsidised universally. In the US, it is suggested the subsidy is US$4 per gallon or $200 billion a year, provided through roads, parking (eight spaces per car are required), accidents and health. In Australia, Laird (1999) has estimated the subsidy to be at least $8 billion per year. Sprawl is also highly subsidised – around $40,000 per new block of land is fairly well accepted as the kind of figure now at the urban fringe in Australia. These billions of dollars could be redirected into more productive means of supporting human settlement. State and local governments and private investors cannot find the capital for many health services but continue servicing automobile dependence.

The reality of economics is not often seen as impinging on city form and transport but it is fundamental. Lional Frost (1991) has analysed the economics of low-density living and suggests that we cannot continue to sink a large proportion of public and private capital into this kind of fringe development. We are living beyond our means wasting capital and failing to invest in productive means such as value-added jobs. It is not sustainable environmentally or economically to continue to sprawl our suburbs.

The lack of capital for services is also finally hitting home where it counts – road building. This infrastructure is the fundamental building block for urban sprawl both through roads at the fringe and faster roads within the city. We are becoming aware that 'we cannot build our way out of congestion' (Goodwin 1991). This awareness is seeping into transport authorities but is still not institutionalised in Australia. There is much to learn from the US in this regard. They have democratised their transport funding system so that local communities

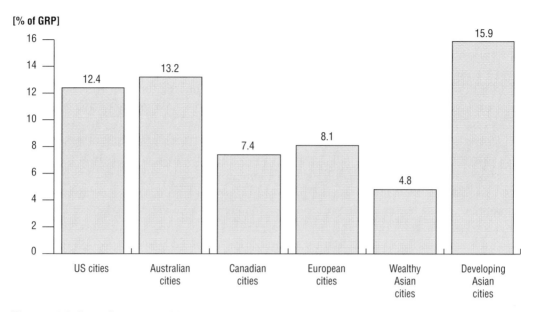

Figure 11.8 Cost of transport, 1990

Note: Figure shows total operating cost of passenger transport, expressed as a percentage of gross regional product.

Source: Kenworthy et al. 1999.

decide their priorities (Newman, 2000). The result has been a major shift away from big road projects to funding for public transport, biking, walking and traffic calming.

Until a similar process is introduced in Australia, we will never turn around the problem of automobile dependence. A survey in Perth showed only 9% of people wanted new roads and 87% supported the conversion of road funds into infrastructure to support other modes of transport. The people are serious about overcoming automobile dependence but the transport planning system is not.

2 Accept demand management as the essential approach to transport and land development

Demand management is well underway in water and electricity agencies. It now needs to be taken seriously (not just talked about) by transport agencies and it needs to be applied for the first time by land development agencies. Statutory planners have seen their job as supplying land to the market, no matter what the market wants. Now, they need to play their role in demand management as well.

Wherever there is a clear link to health problems in food or water or air, there is an immediate move to set up a regulation, and the market is left to adjust. Health professionals have rarely budged when the economic rationalists have applied their simple market analysis and demanded fewer regulations on such obvious health issues. The tightening of regulations on smoking (despite its obvious market) are a good example of the broader view that health professionals have brought to our lives – for the betterment of us all. But, in transport and town planning, we can see so many problems related to automobile dependence and excessive truck use, yet we are in the grip of deregulation and subsidy of these modes.

Will we see a campaign to prevent cities from smoking the fumes of vehicles? Will we ban car advertisements that glorify 4WDs as they tear up fragile mountain slopes or speed effortlessly through empty city streets (as truthful as the Marlboro cowboy in his unspoiled wilderness)? Will we stop land development advertisements that show beautiful 'pristine' bush that can be 'yours' just half an hour from the city? Will we begin to promote healthy modes of transport and the benefits of city lifestyles to community?

Regulations have always been a part of good town planning. But they are not always appropriate, as is often found in proposed development in an older area. Many of the regulations are based on reactions to the great fire of London (preventing a lot of shop-top housing) or on the supposed threat to health from overcrowding or mixed land use (as discussed). These regulations need a total review. They have little relevant basis today and need to be completely revised if we are to overcome automobile dependence. Health professionals need to be critical of existing regulations and assert the need for new regulations to minimise urban car use and to stop the continual spread of our cities.

3 Accept that public transport upgrading and traffic calming are central to the rebuilding of our cities

Better pricing of automobile dependence and better regulations will not guarantee a better city. We still need to plan creatively for public spaces where people can easily meet, and our public transport systems are central to that. Those cities with the least automobile dependence have good, high-profile, electric rail systems and generally slow traffic movement. The two go together and need to be planned into our future.

Light rail is becoming more obviously the solution to public transport, due to its high profile, its ability to move through city streets, and its ability to move at speed on its own right of way. As well, its electric power source appears to be the fuel of the future through dispersed renewable sources linked into the grid.

Traffic calming enables communities to reclaim their streets as well as slowing traffic to allow other modes greater priority.

When cities develop quality public transport, they function better economically, centres and sub-centres become viable, and environments improve. The same can be seen also when urban areas are traffic calmed. People are attracted to areas where cars are managed or removed. These areas are also far better in equity terms. They are better for children and the elderly and are safer for everyone (Engwicht 1992).

4 Accept the need to integrate transport and land use, especially in car-dependent outer suburbs

The great flexibility of cars and buses encouraged cities to scatter and disperse. This meant that no integration of land use was required. If an emphasis on transit and sub-centres guides the city's development, planners will need to work much more closely with transport providers. Transit-oriented development needs to be the goal and assumption of planning from here on.

Urban villages (compact, mixed-use areas near transit services) offer many economic and environmental advantages as the basis of urban development (McGlynn, Newman and Kenworthy 1992). This approach is becoming much more widespread due to considerable market pressure for people to live closer to urban facilities. Our data now show a universal trend to increasing densities after a century of decline, and it seems to be related to the new global 'knowledge economy' jobs, which are all locating in older centres (Newman and Kenworthy 1999). Whilst some of the routine service economy jobs are moving out to the suburbs, the highly paid jobs that are 'knowledge-based' or are part of 'productive services' are going into central areas. The demand for inner-city and central-city housing that is not car dependent defies many of the anti-density pundits in Australia (eg, Troy 1996). The reurbanisation of our inner cities is occurring rapidly but how can we help the outer areas, which are getting so quickly left behind in all Australian cities (see Newman 2000a)?

The solution appears to be an extension of quality public transport and the development around it of real urban centres like the inner city. This means that all suburbs can have access to jobs and services locally and a good transit link to the rest of the city. This can be rationalised in many ways but needs to be seen now in health terms. This is the approach that is becoming described as the New Urbanism in Australian cities.

Mixed land use is the other technique for reducing the need for excessive travel. Modern technology means that industry can be re-mixed into the city along with all other uses to recreate a more urban culture where travel distances are shorter. This should even apply to noxious industries (Newman 1991) where small-scale, hitech animal product processing (biotechnology) can be easily fitted back into our urban areas. At present, noxious industry zones are prevented from being part of a city due to health regulations. The removal of this type of zoning (while insisting on high environmental standards) can lead to a significant reduction in automobile dependence. The use of IT and ET (environmental technology) in rebuilding our industry means that we can build work much more into the fabric of our cities.

5 Accept new institutional approaches to our cities involving health professionals

Planners and transport professionals find it very hard not to think in automobile-dependent ways. They are trained that way, all their manuals say that is how to do it and they are naturally not keen to admit that what they have been doing for the past 50 years or so was altogether wrong. But change is needed and it needs to be reflected in our institutions.

The 'healthy cities' literature advocates a more focused development of urban policies written from a health perspective. Health professionals need to play a more vital role in urban planning. It is rare to have health agencies involved in major decisions across the whole urban region. But this is what we need for well-integrated planning. Greater community input is also needed. The community can often see the broader picture very well, and only by their involvement will NIMBY (not in my backyard) responses to change be avoided.

A holistic approach to problem solving is second nature to health professionals who are oriented to prevention of illness and who appreciate the connection between physical health and mental well-being. This holistic approach is now the kind of approach we need to overcome automobile dependence.

Of course not all aspects of urban health can be reduced to problems of automobile dependence, but its total impact is now quite serious. Good health is threatened by automobile-based planning. The hope is that this threat can be overcome by a combination of technologies, techniques and land use change.

Fundamental to these changes is a change of 'mind set'. We need a mind set that is oriented to the public realm, to public spaces, rather than the privatised world of automobile-dependent suburbs.

Each of the proposed solutions, such as quality public transport, traffic calming and urban villages, requires us to participate more in our city and a little less in our own little private worlds that we create with our house and land and privatised travel patterns. It implies less withdrawal from the city and more of a commitment to our neighbourhoods, our communities, our cities.

For many people, this new mind set is congenial. The new city represents what they want rather than the isolation of suburbia. For many it is a threatening prospect, however, and this fear of change underlies a lot of the NIMBY reaction to increasing densities or to any change planned for an area. These reactions all have to be taken seriously and worked through, but it is my belief that the community can proceed creatively towards a more healthy city as outlined. It is a necessity for our future, but our lifestyle need not be a reduced one as it should indeed be a healthier one.

A healthy city will need to be a more densely populated city. By the same token, rural areas will need to become more rural, eg, with eco-villages based on permaculture (see Newman 1991). However, our basic mind set in urban development should be to 'win back the city'. We should be building the city as a place to delight in, to enjoy in all its urbanity, not to have to escape or withdraw from. This is the source of hope in a city.

Some recent health contributions of potential value to cities

The health profession is obviously seeking to understand health in its broader context. The healthy cities movement has shown that this should involve an understanding of how cities work. Incidental exercise and social anxiety are health concepts that are now being used by health professionals and have considerable potential to be applied more to our cities.

Incidental exercise
The new public health guideline on incidental exercise is that a 10–15-minute walk in the morning and another in the afternoon will significantly reduce cardiovascular disease risks. A problem of urban life in car-dependent cities is a deplorable lack of daily exercise. We go from garage to car park and minimise all unnecessary walking. Incidental exercise fits naturally into any public transport user's routine. But to just state this without looking to structural reasons for the lack of public transport is to be unable to offer much of a solution to the problem of low levels of cardiovascular fitness.

The city has to be addressed at its fundamental level of priorities in transport and land use. If people still believe that high-density housing and mixed land use are to be avoided, it is going to be hard to do much about the level of walking and public transport. To change awareness of how lifestyle affects health, we need to debunk myths about density and mixed use and promote the kind of healthy living principles outlined above.

As well as seeing that incidental exercise will be increased by increases in population density and mixed land use, urban designers are also becoming more aware of the importance of the 'ped shed'. This is the distance from a sub-centre that people can walk to in 10 minutes. This 'ped shed' of about 800 m radius is found to be the critical area for defining a community, for enabling a good public transport link to be available, for ensuring that local services can be provided. Thus the New Urbanist designers suggest a city needs to be planned to this scale, with sufficient residential density and jobs to enable a village centre to be built within a 'ped shed'.

The health profession can now show that a 'ped shed' has a powerful health rationale as well as having the design qualities that are seen to work for other reasons. Walking needs to be facilitated by building 'ped shed' thinking into how we plan and redevelop all our suburbs.

Social anxiety

There is of course an awareness of the social causes of disease, such as inequality-based stress, poor socialisation skills, and the anomie of modern life giving little sense of meaning or hope (Marmot and Wilkinson 1999.) These social problems have been lumped together by some health professionals as 'social anxiety'. This condition and its fundamental causes were seen at a recent Public Health Association conference in Perth to be responsible for maybe two-thirds of health problems (Watson 2000). Such a concept could now be applied to cities to help us begin to face the problems we are building into the urban fabric.

The mechanisms of how 'social anxiety' can cause ill health are being unravelled and the cause of 'social anxiety' is now the subject of much research. It frequently is related to the decline of community and the network of relationships that goes beyond the family and on which we all ultimately depend for our human meaning and purpose. This sense of belonging in a supportive community, the local tribe, the group of people we enjoy being with, are all generally associated with some place. The telephone and internet can help but cannot ultimately replace this. Thus, an element of place is related to social anxiety. So, the concept can legitimately be drawn into urban design debates.

It is essential that health insights into the loss of community also try to identify how community can be facilitated. What can town planning be shown about how to reduce social anxiety? The creativity of personal interactions in our multi communities remains the core source of hope, of the sense that we can expect life to keep opening up rather than shutting down. This needs to be pursued as a part of preventive public health. This sense of hope is the lubricant of community. Yet, the link between finding this more hopeful kind of city environment and overcoming car dependence is not being made.

If a neighbourhood is defined by cars backing out of garages, leaving suburbs with a few odd kids or the unemployed, where is community? If commuting becomes a source of stress where human interactions are reduced to metallic objects flashing past, where is community? If streets are becoming dangerous, where is community? If shopping centres, the only real public spaces apart from the odd sports field and church, become objects designed for consumption and those young, old or non-white who don't seem to be doing that are soon moved on, where is community?

The young in particular have few places to meet and little to do in our new suburbs. The young in Australia are moving rapidly to city locations in search of a lifestyle not provided in these automobile-dependent suburbs. The cafes and pubs and clubs are all in the walkable, tram-based streets of the inner city. Some are even discovering that public transport has its own community – every day, a new set of people full of surprises, and a few friends who make the journey have some extra purpose. But those who have adopted the new urbanity in Australia

Table 11.1 Healthy city strategies for physical health

Healthy city characteristic	Automobile-dependent city characteristic	Anticipated improvements from healthy city development
Clean air	• High smog emissions (and fine particles). • High greenhouse gas emissions. (Possible link between climate change and plague cycles).	• Reduced smog emissions due to reduced car use and more electricity use from renewables. • Reduced greenhouse emissions due to reduced travel, especially car travel.
Clean water	• High stormwater pollution. • High water consumption levels. • Less sewerage (pipes) and treatment, due to costs of sprawl.	• Reduced stormwater, due to reduced sprawl. • Reduced water consumption, due to higher density. • More sewerage and treatment, due to cheaper infrastructure.
Clean food	• Smog impacts on near city market gardens. • Loss of best agricultural land due to sprawl.	• Reduced smog. • Reduced land loss.
Affordable housing (and services)	• Expensive infrastructure, due to low density. • Sprawled low-density housing means increasing proportion of average income goes into house payments.	• Infrastructure costs reduced. • More appropriate housing and less expensive development costs reduces housing costs.
Good, healthy access	• Road accidents. • 'Automobile diseases' related to excess car use. • Lack of exercise.	• Reduced road accidents, due to traffic calming and less car use. • Less car use, less 'automobile diseases'. • More exercise, due to more transit, biking and walking.

Table 11.2 Healthy city strategies for mental well-being

Healthy city characteristic	Automobile-dependent city characteristic	Anticipated improvements from healthy city development
Personal meaning	• Privatism and consumerism dominant values in suburban design.	• Emphasis on 'public realm' in all aspects of city works against privatism and consumerism.
Community	• Community disrupted in older part of city by traffic. • New low density suburbs have little design for community.	• Greater neighbourhood community through traffic calming. • Community design in urban villages and also facilitated by transit and traffic calming.
Financial security	• House ownership an increasing proportion of income. • Transport costs are high and increasing. • High urban costs inherent due to high infrastructure capital drain.	• Housing more affordable. • Transport costs reduced • Capital freed up for more productive purposes.
Lifestyle choice	• Housing choice constrained. • Access limited to cars. • 'Urban' lifestyle not available for more than a few.	• Housing choice increased. • Access available by non-car means. • More 'urban' options available.
'Place' security Historical and natural environment	• Large disruption of historical central business district and inner city by traffic. • Natural environment engulfed and further and further removed from urban life. • Public environmental values surrendered to private, eg, recycling difficult.	• Traffic calming reduces impact on historical areas. • Natural environment made more obvious in city through public spaces and reduced sprawl. • Public environmental values facilitated, eg, recycling easier.
'Future' security	• High vulnerability to global problems like oil and greenhouse; no sense of being able to influence or contribute. • High local environmental costs. • Increased locational inequity and transport disadvantage, increased sense of alienation. • Despair about future.	• Reduced vulnerability to global problems like oil and greenhouse; sense of helping to solve. • Reduced local environmental costs. • Reduced locational inequity and transport disadvantage, increased sense of community. • Hope for future.

are increasingly the wealthy young. The inner areas are now booming as a new urban market pushes densities up. The redevelopment of the Australian inner and central city is reversing the century-long decline in urban densities (Sydney is now back to the density it had in the 1960s).

The inner city is becoming a lively new source of community, but only for those with the financial capital to afford it. Outside this, in the ageing, post-war, car-dependent suburbs, the poor and disadvantaged are increasingly without jobs, services or even the ability to get together. These areas are not ghettos (like the black, inner areas of US cities) as they don't have the places to meet, they are more like unguarded prisons with walls caused by land values closer to the centre. Densities are not rising much here, as the suburbs were not designed to be subdivided, and fringe land continues to be opened up, though the typical Australian demographic family market is vanishing.

The link between social anxiety and poverty is well established. The link between social anxiety and the spatial patterns of our cities is not often seen. It is time that the transport engineers and the town planners were asked to account in health terms for this increasingly divided city. It is possible that it may mean more than the environmental, economic or social analysis which has so easily been cast aside by urban commentators who can see no wrong in car dependence (eg, Gordon and Richardson 1997; Troy 1996).

Conclusion

The involvement of health personnel in the process of creating hope in the city will be crucial, as it is a natural part of their approach to work for a broader common good. Indeed the historical urban precedent is such that the incorporation of broader health goals into urban planning will be a decisive factor in changing the direction of our cities. A central element in this will be a focus on the health aspects of automobile-dependence and the development of viable alternative transport and urban design solutions.

Spiro Kostoff (1991) concludes his monumental study of urban form with:

> If we still believe that cities are the most complicated artifact we have created, if we believe further that they are cumulative, generational artifacts that harbor our values as a community and provide us with the setting where we can learn to live together, then it is our collective responsibility to guide their design.

The collective responsibility must include the health profession.

Further Reading

Newman, P W G & Kenworthy, J R 1999, Sustainability and Cities: Overcoming automobile dependence, Island Press, Washington DC.
   – *A text book on how cities need to respond to the global sustainability agenda, with case studies on the innovative cities showing the way. The book concludes by outlining the changes in professional practice required to adapt to the new agenda and the importance of civil society in providing the values and visions for change.*

UN Habitat 1996, An Urbanising World: UN global review of human settlements, Oxford University Press, Oxford.
   – *Provides a global overview on the status of cities, their populations, health status, infrastructure and other social, economic and environmental data. Policy discussions outline where constructive change is occurring. An update is due in 2001.*

12

Work and health:
the impact of structural workforce changes and the work environment

Anne-Marie Feyer and Dorothy Broom

The centrality of work to health and well-being is unarguable. In industrialised societies, work consumes the greatest active time in adult life, is the most reliable source of continuous access to adequate income, and provides access to a host of key psychosocial dimensions such as identity, self-esteem and social networks. In Australia and New Zealand, as in other developed countries, the relationship between socioeconomic status (SES) and health has been identified: lower socioeconomic status is consistently associated with poorer health outcomes (National Advisory Committee on Health and Disability 1998; Turrell and Mathers 2000). Given that occupation is a key dimension of SES, at least part of the impact of SES on health is likely to be a reflection of differences in working conditions (Marmot, Siegrist et al. 1999). Moreover, the absence of employment is clearly detrimental to both physical and mental health (Bartley, Ferrie et al. 1999). The significant relationship between work and health overall, well beyond traditional occupational health concerns, is therefore widely accepted.

Worldwide, working life is undergoing major changes. Modern established market economies are increasingly characterised by demands for vastly greater labour market flexibility. They have been marked by rising participation by women, as well as increases in long-term unemployment, in temporary employment and in irregular employment contracts. New Zealand and Australia are similar in this regard: rapid and dramatic changes have occurred over recent years in the organisation of labour, of work and of the work environment. The question is what is the impact on health of the sorts of radical changes in working life that are taking place in modern economies? The present paper takes up this issue. Specifically, the aims of the paper are to:

- provide an overview of what we know about the changes that have taken place in working life in New Zealand and Australia;
- consider the mechanisms by which such changes may exert their influence on health; and
- highlight some key areas where gaps in knowledge are critically undermining our ability to identify important adverse health outcomes due to working life and targets for their prevention.

Changes in structure and conditions of employment

It has been observed that the Australian and New Zealand labour markets share many similar characteristics: participation rates, gender distribution, wage structures and unemployment rates are all comparable (Brosnan and Walsh 1998). For both nations, the concept of labour flexibility has become the central issue, and with it, there has been a massive rise in novel work arrangements.

Deregulation

In New Zealand, labour market deregulation is underpinned by the *Employment Contracts Act 1991 (ECA)*, which allowed both the type and content of all employment contracts to be directly negotiated in their entirety by individuals and their employers (Harbridge and Tolich 1992). A principal objective of the ECA was the creation of an efficient labour market by increased flexibility, decentralisation of labour relations decision making and minimisation of monopolistic distortions (unions) (Harbridge and Hince 1994). In Australia, the *Industrial Relations Act 1988*, and the amendments to it, followed by the *Workplace Relations Act 1996*, were designed to encourage a more direct relationship between employers and employees with a reduced role for third party intervention. The general picture in Australia is, therefore, also one of deregulation of the labour market, achieved through 'diminishing the power and scope of the industrial tribunals, limiting the actions of unions and encouraging the development of individual employment contracts between employer and employee' (Richardson 1998).

Hours of work

Changes to hours of work and working time arrangements are among the key adjustment strategies used to achieve labour market flexibility. Analyses in New Zealand indicate that there have been significant changes (invariably reductions) to conditions governing working time arrangements and penal and overtime rates of pay (Harbridge and Hince 1994; Hince and Harbridge 1994) since the introduction of the ECA. Similar patterns have been observed in Australia (ACIRRT 1999).

Disappearance of standard working hours

There has been a trend to extend the Monday–Friday working week to a Monday–Saturday or seven-day working week. Just 39 % of workers in New Zealand are being employed under a contract with ordinary hours stipulated as Monday to Friday (Harbridge, Crawford et al. 1998). Approximately half (56%) of New Zealand employment contracts have been found to stipulate ordinary work on any five days of the week including Saturday and Sunday without premium payment (Harbridge, Crawford et al. 1998). At the same time, the existence of overtime clauses has slowly declined: in 1994/95 85% of employees had contracts that provided for overtime premiums, declining to 72% in 1997/98 (Harbridge, Crawford et al. 1998). In fact, no clock hours were reported in 52% of New Zealand employment contracts, indicating that the majority of contracts no longer have any specified hours of work. The existence of clock hours is a useful indicator of the amount of freedom an employer has to require staff to work irregular hours without the payment of penal or overtime rates (Harbridge, Crawford et al. 1998). Some

15% of employees in the most recent examination of New Zealand employment contracts had no statement in their contract as to the required number of hours to be worked per week with the implication that overtime pay is not available to such employees (Harbridge, Crawford et al. 1998). In general, where they do exist, penal rates are declining, for example double time on Sunday, the previous historical standard, is frequently being replaced by time and a half (Harbridge, Crawford et al. 1998). Women are significantly more likely to be working under contracts where penal and overtime rates were never available or have been removed or reduced; contracts covering 'mainly men' are more likely to have their penal and overtime rates largely preserved (Harbridge and Hince 1994).

In Australia, the disappearance of standard working hours has also been noted (Bittman and Rice 1999). This has been the case in terms of how many hours and when they are worked and the rise of more work at 'unsociable hours' with the expectation of being available at all times (due to mobile phones, telecommuting, for example).

Duration of work hours

There has been an observable trend away from the traditional working week in terms of duration as well, towards both longer and shorter hours in New Zealand (Department of Statistics 1995). The greatest growth has been in numbers who usually work more than 40 hours a week (Department of Statistics 1995).

In Australia, more people in the labour force work more than 44 hours per week, and more people work under 35 hours per week compared to 10 years ago (Australian Bureau of Statistics 1998a). One-quarter of employees participating in The 1995 Australian Workplace Industrial Relations Survey (AWIRS 95) reported that their total weekly working hours had increased in the past 12 months (Morehead, Steele et al. 1997).

Alternatives to full-time work

Over the past decade (1989–1999), part-time work in New Zealand has grown by a massive 42.8% while full-time employment has grown by 7.9% (Statistics New Zealand 2000b). The shift towards part-time employment now sees 23% of the population in 1999 employed in part-time (1–29 hours) employment compared with 17% of the population in 1987. This growth in part-time employment to some extent reflects the increased participation of women in the labour force. Comparisons between 1987 and 1999 show that females have been consistently more likely to be employed in part-time employment than their male counterparts, and that, currently, 38% of the female workforce is employed in part-time positions compared with 11.3% of males (Statistics New Zealand 2000a).

The growth in part-time work is also evident in Australia over the same period. Between the 1990 Australian Workplace Industrial Relations Survey (AWIRS 90) and AWIRS 95, the proportion of part-time workers increased by nearly 40%. One-quarter of the survey population was employed in a part-time capacity in 1995, with the majority of part-time work being performed by women (Morehead, Steele et al. 1997).

Casual employment has also increased in Australia, particularly among women who make up the majority of casual workers (Morehead, Steele et al. 1997). Casual employees increased by around 20% between AWIRS 90 and AWIRS 95, with 70% of workplaces in the survey reporting that they employed casual staff (increased by approximately 10% since 1990). Those employed as contractors increased by around 17% between the two AWIRS survey periods.

A survey-based study suggests similar trends in New Zealand. The number of workplaces in New Zealand employing casual staff rose by around 12% between 1990 and 1995, with contractors/consultants also growing by around 12% (Brosnan and Walsh 1998).

Employment seeking

Increasingly those employed in part-time work are looking for full-time work. In 1991, 5,500 people surveyed for the New Zealand Household Labour Force survey reported looking for full-time work; this had increased to 27,700 in 1999 (Statistics New Zealand 2000a). There has also been a rise in those looking for more hours of work in addition to existing work, with 120,900 seeking more hours of work in 1999 compared with 30,600 in 1991 (Statistics New Zealand 2000a). There are greater numbers of females seeking full-time work or more hours paid employment (Statistics New Zealand 2000a).

In Australia, similar 'polarisation of the workforce into underemployed part-timers who want to work more . . . [and receive] inadequate earnings, and overworked full-timers' has also been noted (Russell and Bowman 2000).

Gender composition of the workforce

In both Australia and New Zealand, the labour force participation rate of women (including women with dependent children) continues to grow. In AWIRS 90, female employees comprised 41% of those working at Australian workplaces with 20 or more employees. By AWIRS 95, this had become 45%. This trend is accompanied however by a persistent occupational segregation and earnings gap (Office of the Status of Women 1999). Similarly, in New Zealand, females comprised 43% of the total workforce in 1989. By 1999, this proportion had risen to 45% (Statistics New Zealand 2000b).

Union density

The trend of placing employees on individual rather than collective contracts, a more general collapse of collective bargaining and the repeal of compulsory unionism provisions, were specific aspects of the new industrial relations environment that have influenced union membership in New Zealand over the last decade (Harbridge and Hince 1994; Henning 1995; Boxall 1997). Union density fell from a high of 73% in 1989 to 46% in 1992, with unions losing 90,000 members in the first seven months after the implementation of the ECA. The decline in union density has continued in the 90s (Statistics New Zealand 2000a), with recent estimates suggesting that 25% of wage and salary earners are union members (Boxall 1997).

In Australia, similar declines in union presence have been observed. According to the Australian Bureau of Statistics, there were more than 3 million financial union members in 1990. By 1995, this had reduced to around 2.5 million financial members. Union density over the same five-year period reduced from 46% to 35%. The results of AWIRS 95 confirmed this change (Morehead, Steele et al. 1997).

Unemployment

Unemployment figures in New Zealand peaked in 1992 at 10.2% to decline to 6.2% in 1996. Currently the unemployment figures are rising, with a rate of 7.5% recorded in 1999 (Statistics New Zealand 2000a). Unemployment rates are greatest in Maori workers with 18.6% unemployed in 1999 compared with 10.8% in 1987 (Statistics New Zealand 2000a). Pacific Islanders have similar growth in unemployment with 14.8% unemployed in 1999 compared with 6.1% in 1987 (Statistics New Zealand 2000a). Unemployment rates for these ethnic groups peaked in 1992 with 25.8% of NZ Maori and 28.8% of Pacific Islanders unemployed. Long-term unemployment (those unemployed for 27 or more consecutive weeks) has increased from 19.1% of unemployed in 1987 to 49.9% in 1993, with a decline to 35.1% in 1999 (Statistics New Zealand 2000a). The number unemployed looking for part-time or full-time work more than doubled between 1987 and 1999 (Statistics New Zealand 2000a).

There is some evidence that a 20-year trend toward rising levels of unemployment in Australia (from post-war lows around 2% to over 10% in the early 1990s) may have stopped and perhaps begun to reverse (Hawke and Woden 1997; see also *Australia Now* www.abs.gov.au). Nevertheless, unemployment remains at 6.7%. Long-term unemployment (more than 52 weeks) is also large as a proportion of overall unemployment in Australia, currently around 29% seasonally adjusted (Australian Bureau of Statistics 2000b).

Changing structure of work and health

In summary, liberalisation of New Zealand's employment laws have allowed employers greater flexibility in work arrangements which has been reflected in significant adjustments to many employment contracts. The result has been increasing numbers of multiple job holders, part-time workers and ordinary hours worked per week, along with changes to the scheduling of the work week, reductions in penal rates and paid overtime hours. Similarly, in Australia, recent years have seen new legislation, and conditions of employment such as hours worked, security of tenure, flexibility of hours, benefits and remuneration have been changing rapidly (ACIRRT 1999). All of these rapid changes in both nations have occurred against a background of intractable high unemployment and increased participation by women.

The changes in the way labour is organised, the way work is organised and the consequent changes to work environment could all be expected to have an impact on the health of workers and their families. There are at least four broad dimensions that are likely to be significantly affected.

Direct effects of work organisation on occupational health and safety

There is a growing body of evidence that those working on contingent arrangements are at elevated risk of work-related injury due to economic pressures, inadequate occupational health and safety information and regulation, and reduction in working conditions such as sick leave and annual leave (Quinlan, Mayhew et al. 2001). Higher occupational health and safety risks have long been associated with contract labour. Diminished employer incentives to provide temporary workers with on-the-job training and socialisation necessary for skill development mean that contingent workers are liable to be less integrated into the organisation and less familiar with standard safe operating procedures (Sverke, Gallagher et al. 2000). Where sub-contracted and casual workers perform the jobs traditionally undertaken by permanent employees, this can result in part of the workforce being less stringently supervised and trained in workplace safety than permanent employees (Kochan, Smith et al. 1994; Rousseau and Libuser 1997). In settings where such arrangements have traditionally been common, construction for example, the hazards associated with the workforce being largely temporary, mobile and often self-employed have been clearly associated with increased risk of injury (Ringen, Englund et al. 1995). The influence of piece-rate arrangements is also clear. Among New Zealand forestry workers for example, those employed on a quota system were more likely to report having had an injury than those working on an hourly wage (Lilley, Feyer et al. 2001).

There are, however, few systematic examinations of the impact of employment arrangements on injury rates. In part, this reflects that injury patterns are reported from routine data collection (eg, national morbidity registers, workers' compensation databases). These data sources have not been established with distinguishing key aspects of work arrangements in mind. Even quite coarse indicators are difficult to obtain regarding the influence of structural changes on injury occurrence. Recent data from New Zealand for example indicates that self-employed workers are at much greater risk of work-related fatal injury than employees (Feyer, Langley et al. 2001). For comparable Australian data, it was not possible to make even this most gross distinction reliably with respect to employment arrangements (National Occupational Health and Safety Commission 1998). Reliance on special studies is always likely to be problematic because they lack timeliness and tend to be flawed proxies for national data on injury patterns associated with different employment arrangements.

The changing patterns in work hours are also likely to have an impact on occupational health and safety. The problems associated with working longer non-standard hours are among the best-documented hazards in occupational health (Spurgeon, Harrington et al. 1997). Night work per se has been shown to be hazardous to health and safety, as have long work hours (Folkard 1997; Akerstedt 1998). Chronic sleep disturbance (and its sequelae), reduced alertness and performance capacity, and reduced quality of social and family life are well documented consequences of poorly designed working hours regimes (Spurgeon, Harrington et al. 1997). The relationship between work hour regimes and adverse outcomes is not an entirely linear one however. Recent evidence suggests that self-selection of work hours has strong positive effects which to greater and lesser degrees may offset the negative impact of working longer and working at non-standard times such as evenings and overnight (Barton 1994; Akerstedt, Kecklund et al. 2000).

On the other hand, little is known about the impact of the sort of irregular work hours that are becoming increasingly evident with flexibilisation, where work hours are stretched to meet operational demands. Existing data largely relate to circumstances where working hours are very long, exceeding 50 hours per week, and the effects of traditional shift arrangements. There is little information about hours below this level, about *ad hoc* hours arrangements and, in particular, about the effect of overtime and overtime arrangements where compensation is forfeited in exchange of time much later, say as an additional week of annual leave (Harrington 1994; Spurgeon, Harrington et al. 1997; Aronsson 1999).

Job insecurity

It has been argued that the other side of flexibility is job insecurity (Marmot 1999). The over-simplified distinction between having a job and being unemployed has been replaced by the understanding that there are degrees of insecurity in the work conditions that people experience and that insecurity itself may be a health hazard (Bartley, Ferrie et al. 1999). There is ample evidence that health begins to be affected when people anticipate unemployment but are still at work (Bartley, Ferrie et al. 1999). For instance, investigation of privatisation in the public sector in the UK showed that deterioration in health status occurred during the period of anticipation of the changed organisation, and that significant increases in cardiovascular risk factors occurred before the finalisation of the change (Ferrie, Shipley et al. 1995; Ferrie, Shipley et al. 1998). Similarly, during 'downsizing' in the private sector, psychological distress symptoms were evident during the period of change, with one of the most important predictors of distress found to be perceived job insecurity (Isaksson, Hellgren et al. 2000).

Job insecurity has a number of dimensions. It can be that the job itself ceases. Alternatively, the job may continue but not with the same incumbent. Some forms of employment are by their nature more secure than others. At one end of the spectrum lies a contract of permanent on-going employment which offers a great deal of security so long as the job itself continues, so that at times of low unemployment, such jobs are particularly secure. At the other end of the spectrum, casual employment provides almost no security for the individual worker (irrespective of whether or not the job continues). Between these two, there are a host of time-restricted employment arrangements. Flexibility in the new labour market has been achieved by increasing the proportion of workers employed on less secure forms of employment. Time-restricted or contingent employment arrangements have been used to assure organisations' flexibility in response to troughs and peaks in production through variation in the number of employees, work hours and skill mix (Aronsson 1999).

The growth of arrangements based on short-term or fixed-term contracts has been the hallmark of the new labour market in Australia and New Zealand. Between 1990 and 1995, the largest net increases for both full-time and part-time employment were the categories offering the least secure employment (Brosnan and Walsh 1998). Such arrangements reflect multiple employer objectives: lower labour costs, increased temporal flexibility with employment reflecting demand and reduced responsibilities for management and supervision of employees.

Little is known about the impact on health of such labour differentiation or the impact on health of the contingencies that operate for the various forms of insecure employment. It has been argued that contingent work can offer control to the worker, for example access to variable working hours can provide opportunities to balance home and work responsibilities (Reilly 1998). On the other hand, high unemployment reduces the options that workers might otherwise have to exercise such control, both with regard to work tasks and job form. That the proportion of part-time workers seeking more employment is growing in both Australia and New Zealand, for instance, suggests that current arrangements may not necessarily reflect choice or the exercise of control.

The implications of lack of job control, both related to task/environment conditions and also related to more macro work environment conditions, have been extensively considered and their health effects are well documented. There is abundant evidence that job strain due to an imbalance between demands placed on a worker and the extent of decision latitude or control available to the worker to meet those demands is related to adverse health outcomes. Work environments characterised by high demand and low control are positively associated with, for instance, coronary heart disease (Bosma, Marmot et al. 1997; Hallqvist, Diderichsen et al. 1998). Control in relation to job insecurity is more likely to reflect a related conceptualisation, the imbalance between work effort and reward. Occupational rewards include such dimensions as money, security/career opportunities, and psychosocial benefits such as self-esteem and membership of a social network (ie, work colleagues). Effort by the worker is exchanged in return for these rewards, as part of a social contract based on reciprocity and fairness (Aronsson 1999; Marmot, Siegrist et al. 1999). Job strain results where effort and reward are not balanced, or are perceived as not balanced. Job contracts or agreements that do not reward work efforts will be viewed as unfair, and have been shown to lead to emotional distress and physical health problems. Adverse health outcomes, coronary heart disease for example, have been shown to be positively associated with high effort/low reward conditions of work in a number of studies (Bosma, Peter et al. 1998; Marmot, Siegrist et al. 1999).

There is growing evidence for the association between dimensions of job control and adverse health outcomes. It has been argued that under conditions characteristic of the new labour market, with its flexibilisation, increased job insecurity and structural unemployment, the imbalance between effort and reward, that is high cost/low gain conditions (and presumably the associated health consequences), becomes more marked (Marmot, Siegrist et al. 1999). There is inadequate evidence, however, documenting changes along these dimensions as a consequence of the structural changes in the labour market evident in Australia and New Zealand, or indeed the health consequence due to exposure to the new working environment.

Skill change and work intensification required under flexibility

It is widely believed that skill requirements have increased in market economies due to changes in technology and in managerial philosophies which accompany flexibilisation (Gallie 2000). Between 1986 and 1992 in Great Britain, jobs requiring no or low-level qualifications decreased while those with higher prerequisite qualifications increased, and the rise in skill levels was positively associated with a marked increase in intensification of work effort and with greater job strain (Gallie 2000). Overall, the new labour market is thought to impose greater demands for adaptability, partly reflected as changes in skill level and work intensity.

Little research has examined national trends in skill requirements or work intensification in New Zealand or Australia. However, trends along similar lines are suggested. Approximately half of respondents to the third New Zealand National Survey of Labour Market Adjustment under the Employment Contracts Act reported that their skills had increased over the previous 12 months (Industrial Relations Service 1997). In Australia, about half of workers in a recent national survey reported that, over the year prior to the survey, effort required by their jobs had increased (59%), stress had increased (50%), work pace had increased (46%), and close to one-third of workers had a high work intensification index based on pattern of responses to the effort, stress and pace questions (Morehead, Steele et al. 1997). The empirical evidence for the relationship between these trends in skill change and work intensification on the one hand, and structural changes in the labour market on the other, is lacking, as is information about health impact of the trends.

Wider health implications

Flow-on effects from changes in working life to family and social life are also likely to be significant. While there is general acceptance that work does not occur in isolation from family life, little is known about the impact of the sorts of radical changes in working life that have occurred in recent decades for health of the workers' family members. The full impact of paid work may not be evident unless workers' domestic workloads are also considered (Aneshensel and Pearlin 1987), but health is rarely considered in research on how changes in employment and work conditions affect family life (Wolcott and Glezer 1995; Russell and Bowman 2000). The strain and time pressures of the 'second shift' (Broom 1986) may compromise time and energy available for childcare and maintaining family relationships. When work hours are irregular, work/non-work conflict may be intensified, and these conflicts are especially acute for parents (and other workers with domestic caring responsibilities). Some aspects of work arrangements may enhance parental resources such as time, income and care, while other aspects are likely to constrain them. It would seem logical that those workers whose households are entirely dependent on income from their job will be more vulnerable to deleterious effects, particularly when there are fewer options for change of employment. When employment is insecure, a straightforward relationship with fluctuations in income is also likely. Through their effects on parental resources therefore, work conditions may well have flow-on effects for children's health.

There has been considerable attention paid to the impact of traditional shift work arrangements on non-work life in terms of satisfaction with the interface (Barton 1994). There has been little research examining the impact of the sorts of changes to work that have occurred with flexiblisation or examining the health outcomes of family members. Yet, the interaction of insecure employment with domestic workload, parental resources and the impact of fluctuations of income are all likely to be important in terms of health outcomes.

Variation in the impact of the new labour market

The effects of work on health are likely to be shaped by such dimensions as age, ethnicity, socioeconomic status and gender. Thus, while there may be population trends in health impact, there are also likely to be key gradients of effect also. For example, it is likely that the nature and impact of structural changes in the labour market will differ across the socioeconomic gradient. It seems likely that vulnerability to poor health outcomes due to insecure employment will be intensified among those on low incomes and those with the least control over their work circumstances. There has been little examination of the differential impact that recent changes in working life might have on different groups within a society.

Conclusions and future directions

It could be expected that the trends towards a greater proportion of the work force being employed on less permanent arrangements and working longer/more irregular hours might be accompanied by an increase in adverse occupational health and safety outcomes. There has been little systematic investigation of changes in the distribution of such health outcomes in relation to structural changes in the workforce.

Besides more traditional occupational health outcomes, there are a number of new potential issues associated with increasingly widespread job insecurity, the flip side of flexibilisation, against a background of intractable unemployment. The impact of insecurity itself, work intensification and other related issues is not well understood. From international research, these dimensions are likely to have an important impact on health. However, it is also likely that social and cultural systems have a substantial modifying influence on the impact of insecure employment. This is certainly the case with the impact of unemployment. While unemployment has strong negative psychosocial and health consequences in all European countries, the severity of the impact varies (Gallie 2000). The relative deprivation of the unemployed in Denmark, for example, has been found to be less marked than in Britain (Gallie 2000). The nature of welfare institutions and the extent to which social support networks and social organisation provide a buffer are thought to modify the risk that unemployment will result in its most dire consequences (Gallie 2000). Direct transfer of experience with insecure employment from, for instance, Scandinavian countries, to Australia and New Zealand is, therefore likely to be limited. This suggests that it will be imperative to build up knowledge of how the same general structural changes operate against the background of different societal environments.

While the structural changes in the labour market are increasingly well described, there have not been parallel advances in either understanding the impact on population health or the mechanisms by which quite radical changes in working life might have their impact in Australia and New Zealand. At present, it is not even possible to make connections between information collected nationally about health and information collected about work arrangements. A range of research activities would be appropriate to fill these gaps in knowledge. At the broadest level, one avenue might be linkage of national census data with national morbidity and mortality data. This could provide some general information about relationships between relevant broad dimensions of work arrangements and health outcomes. However, national census collections are not designed for obtaining detailed information about working life. National surveys that are designed to obtain information about relevant parameters of both working life and health status would provide a better starting point for understanding the broad picture. If repeated regularly, such surveys could provide important benchmarking information against which the impact of changing trends in working life might be assessed. Purpose-specific surveys might be used, or there might be adjuncts to existing national surveys already undertaken in both countries. Ideally, the surveys would be designed to allow comparison between Australia and New Zealand, as well as with other surveys undertaken internationally. While providing an important starting point, national surveys will necessarily always be broad-brush tools. In-depth studies will also be needed to investigate the mechanisms by which aspects of working life may have their impact in the Australian and New Zealand context. As a case in point, very little is known about the extent, nature or mechanisms of flow-on effects of changed working environments for family life, or of any consequent effects for the health and well-being of workers' family members. Examination of such issues would require detailed purpose specific studies.

The extent and pace of change in working life here, as elsewhere in the world, has been striking. Knowledge about the key health outcomes due to these changes in working life and their determinants are urgently needed. Without such knowledge, it is impossible to identify priorities for intervention, or the nature of potentially effective interventions, in order to maintain and improve population health in Australia and New Zealand.

Acknowledgements

We would like to express our thanks to Rebbecca Lilley, Melissa Purnell and Anna Wilkinson for their assistance with obtaining data required to produce this paper.

Further Reading

Isakson, K, Hogstedt, C, Eriksson, C & Theorell, T (Eds) 2000, Health Effects of the New Labour Market, Kluwer Academic/Plenum Publishers, New York.
  – *Provides a good overview of the issues for the restructuring of traditional labour organisation to fulfil the modern demands for ultimate flexibility from an international perspective.*
Sennett, Richard & Sennett, Bob 1999, The Corrosion of Character: The personal consequences of work in the new capitalism, WW Norton, New York.
  – *Disturbing essay on the health, social and individual impacts of new working arrangements.*
Macintyre, S 1997, The Black Report and Beyond: What are the issues?, Social Science & Medicine 44, 6: 723–47.
  – *Succinct summary of two decades of research linking health to socioeconomic inequalities including employment.*
Turrell, G, Oldenburg, B, McGuffog, I & Dent, R 1999, Socioeconomic Status and Health: Towards a national research program and a policy and intervention agenda, Commonwealth Department of Health and Aged Care, Canberra.
  – *A detailed review of Australian research.*

13

Health, inequities, community and social capital

Robert Bush and Fran Baum

Introduction

The health status and life opportunities of those in poorer communities are less than those elsewhere (Australian Institute of Health and Welfare 1998). Responding to this situation is internationally recognised as requiring a multifaceted national as well as community approach that includes both social and economic initiatives (World Health Organization 1986a). This chapter explores the potential for social capital to provide a framework for developing communities in such a way that the health and life opportunities of poorer communities are improved.

We address the relationship between social capital and the health and life opportunities of people in communities. This includes not only the individual health of those in communities, as often measured by mortality, morbidity, and quality of life instruments, but also the idea that there are 'healthy communities' in and of themselves – communities in which there is a good stock of social capital and other forms of resource. 'Life opportunities' refers to the equality of opportunity that comes about through the local availability of many types of resources – for example, access to local childcare to encourage early child development that is so important to later achievements at school and beyond. Indeed, where access to and availability of social, economic and cultural resources are limited, so the life opportunities are also limited and this eventually becomes reflected in health statistics.

The breadth of views about social capital necessitates a brief investigation of its historical origins and the way different disciplines have conceptualised the links to health and life opportunities. We begin with the theoretical underpinnings, address some of the key empirical findings and them describe the Adelaide study of health development and social capital. This is a study that pays attention to levels and types of local participation in community life, the role of organisations and groups in the generation of social capital in communities, and the predictive value of social capital on health status.

Historical and theoretical underpinnings

The 1960s saw the adoption of ideas about social capital as the source for social action in a range of community studies. Concern over the decline of the city neighbourhood in the US (eg, Jacobs 1965) and the old inner-city areas of Britain (eg, Frankenberg 1966; Young and Wilmot 1962) led to studies that sought to understand people and the places where they live through the lens of cross-cutting networks that had developed over long periods of time. These networks were the source of trust and local cooperation that benefited individuals, families and the communities as a whole. Networks were shown to be particularly strong among women. Urban redevelopment, rapid changes to industry leading to limited local employment opportunities and the necessity to be more mobile led to the breakdown of these networks as the bedrock of community life.

The eventual demise of these studies was due to a failure to adequately link the social dynamics of social capital to changes in economic conditions. New forms of collective action were needed that could take into account these larger structural changes. Many attempts to link such larger structural adjustments to changes in the lives of people and their communities have occurred since. Three of these are closely linked to ideas of social capital, as this is understood forty years on.

Cox (1995) introduced the term 'social capital' into the lexicon of contemporary Australian public debate in her 1995 Boyer Lecturers. She drew heavily on the work of the American Robert Putnam (1993, 1996) in which norms such as trust and reciprocity embedded in social networks became the substance of civil society. It is through these networks that wealth and public goods are created. Cox differed from Putnam by acknowledging the significance of informal local networks in peoples' lives while Putnam stressed the significance of formal group membership. Putnam's work is aligned with the Weberian traditions of US political science. In this tradition, face-to-face local relations rather than hierarchical structures generate the capacity for civic engagement. It is these relations that health advocates wish to study and use in the production of better health and well-being.

Critics of this popular view of social capital stress the neglect of any analysis of power and the unequal distribution of resources between individuals and across different communities. They argue that without such analysis an important dynamic in the causes of inequality is missing. There is no analysis of the impact of wider global economic pressures to advance competitiveness for example. Nor is there an analysis of the limitations of market-driven public policy to address civic concerns beyond economic issues.

A second source underpinning concepts of social capital lies in the original work of the American sociologist James Coleman (1988, 1993). Coleman's description of social capital is firmly entrenched in the functionalism of Durkheim and Parsons and has two basic components. First, social structures consist of networks that surround individuals and second, these provide the resources through social relationships for a variety of needs. He is influenced by Granovettor's (1985) empirical analysis of the function of different types of networks, each providing a list of potential benefits such as access to information and employment. The benefits are accrued to the individuals under conditions of compliance with obligations enforced through group norms. Coleman, like Putnam, does not address power and resource distribution. The emphasis appears more concerned with satisfying self-interest as a motivating force for network membership.

A third approach to social capital has received much less attention in Australia to date. Bourdieu's (1977) ideas about social capital have been described as combining both a structuralist and a constructionist position (Bedharz 1994). The value of his work lies in the attempt to discover the socio-cultural processes that lie behind the problem of inequalities. Bourdieu's social capital combines with other forms of capital (economic, cultural and symbolic) to explain the dynamics of difference in societies. It is differential access to these various forms of capital that explains the difference between individuals and also communities. Bourdieu's thought derives from Marx but he moves well beyond the traditions of economic class struggle to describe how structured cultural differences come about through the way social relationships are endlessly formed and transformed. Thus, economic capital (money and material objects that can be used to produce goods and services), social capital (positions and relationships in social networks), cultural capital (habits, lifestyles, linguistic styles, educational credentials) and symbolic capital (use of symbols to legitimate possession over other forms of capital) combine in the creation of inequalities of various kinds.

Bourdieu's analysis of various forms of capital permits us to approach communities in terms of the economic and social processes that lead to various forms of access to and denial of resources and opportunities that make a difference to people's lives and their health. Some social networks are rich in these resources and others are not. Those in relative poverty with little access to social networks that include decision-makers, for example, suffer poorer health and premature death (Wilkinson and Marmot 1998). Bourdieu's ideas have been applied in Europe to improve community well-being by working with local networks, not only on the creation of cohesion and trust but by linking communities to resources and decision-makers.

From ideas to actions

This brief outline of theoretical work on social capital from wider afield serves to provide a set of ideas that informs empirical investigation, policy and practical action. These are:
- Reconstructing social capital as a public good over and above private benefit.
- Reconstructing social networks beyond those that surround the individual or family unit to those that include the formal and informal structures that link people to other forms of capital.
- Reconstructing participation to include a wider range of actions encompassing individual and collective action, social and self-interested participation, and collective civic activity for the public good.

We used these starting points to develop the study of social capital in the Adelaide Health Development and Social Capital study, described later in this chapter.

Social capital and the public good
Recognition of the limits and the recent failure of the market and neoliberal economics as a model for government have lead to experiments with new social and economic strategies in

public policy (Blair and Schroder 1999; Giddens 1998). One rationale for such new experiments is the belief that public institutions such as large government departments are now inadequate for the provision of public goods, equitable social protection and civic order that lie at the root of community concerns. Central to this recognition are debates about re-establishing local governance over many local affairs and resources (Stewart-Weeks 2000). Local governance over local affairs is about building new institutional arrangements that protect public goods. Such arrangements are more about structural reforms than about adopting market or quasi-market forms of government (Giddens 1999).

Such new arrangements are central to the health and well-being of communities. These are concerned with the non-monetary values of community life such as justice and protection against injustice, the possibilities for friendship, addressing the local causes of crime and ill health, and the moral resources of a community such as volunteering, being a good neighbour and willingness to help strangers (Sampson 1997). It also concerns other more tangible public goods such as the provision of public space and facilities that are associated with health gains for all in a locality (MacIntyre et al. 1993).

The important aspect of such public goods is that their creation and consumption do not diminish the quality or value of these goods for other local people as other forms of private capital may do. The involvement of a diverse range of people, groups and organisations in deciding what public goods to invest in becomes a central purpose of social capital building in local communities.

Social capital and network structures

There is enough research evidence to assert the benefits of personal support networks for health. An overview of the findings of several prospective studies on social support indicate that it is an independent risk factor for mortality (House et al. 1988, pp 540–5); House et al. 1982; Berkman and Syme 1979, pp 186–204; Schoenbach et al. 1985, p 585).

Community networks stretch beyond the idea of the personal network to include the many groups and organisations, both formal and informal, to which locals may belong. These structures have been described as health development or mediating structures (Baum and Kahssay 1999, Couto and Guthrie 1999) and are seen to serve several functions. For Couto and Guthrie (1999), these are a moral resource that counters the alienation of individualism implicit in market relations. For Giddens (1999), mediating structures allow for identity formation in a diversified society. It is the availability of many groups and organisations that allows for the expression of both unity and difference in a vibrant community. For Baum et al. (1999), health development structures provide for the well-being of both the community as a whole and the individual through opportunities to participate in decisions that effect our well-being.

Salamon (1993) cited in Couto and Guthrie (1999) presents a less certain view of mediating structures, suggesting several possibilities. The first is that mediating structures are essential to the democratic state. Mediating structures are the conduits between the individual and government. These mediating structures may serve to temper the excesses of the government and for that matter the markets through their collective action. The second possibility is that mediating structures essentially impede proper democratic process. Many groups and organisations are undemocratic and concerned with self-interest rather than the interests of the community as a whole. The third possibility is that mediating structures are essentially dis-engaged from the political process. It would seem the extent and quality of networked mediating structures within communities can provide the possibilities for creating health and improving life opportunities, but the existence of mediating structures is not in itself a guarantee of such an eventuality.

Social capital and participation

Participation has been central to primary health care and health promotion strategies since the WHO *Health for All 2000* strategy was launched in 1978. This direction was reinforced by the Ottawa Charter for Health Promotion (WHO 1986b), which placed considerable emphasis on strengthening community action as a mechanism to achieve health-promoting changes in physical and social environments. These participation-oriented strategies urge citizens to become involved in planning for and achieving better health through active involvement with non-government and government agencies.

The health promotion literature of the last decade has seen participation in social and civic life as a central factor in empowerment. Empowerment is also emphasised in a number of other disciplines relevant to public health including: radical social and community work (McKnight 1985; Freire 1972; Ife 1995), health promotion and education (Wallerstein 1992; Labonte 1990, 1997; Tones 1992; Israel Checkoway and Schulz 1994) and community psychology (Rissel 1994; Zimmerman 1990; Hawe 1994). Israel et al. (1994, p 153), based on a review of literature from a range of disciplines and professions, offer the following definition of empowerment:

> Empowerment, in its most general sense, refers to the ability of people to gain understanding and control over personal, social, economic and political forces in order to take action to improve their life situations. In contrast to reactive approaches that derive from a treatment or illness mode, the concept of empowerment is positive and proactive.

This sense of empowerment is determined in part by the extent to which people participate in activities outside their immediate home and work lives. It is here that the reason for the recent interest in social capital from health promoters becomes apparent. The strength of participation in social and civic life becomes one of the indicators of how healthy a community is. Despite this considerable interest in participation and its impact on health, there have been few empirical studies of participation in communities, and this was one reason for undertaking the Adelaide Health Development and Social Capital study.

Empirical investigations of social capital

There are four basic ways in which researchers have approached studies on social capital. First, there are studies of different levels of social structure, ranging from large-scale concerns over social capital and the well-being of the state, the role of social capital in the region and local community and studies of the individual and social capital. Second, there are studies that seek to identify what makes up the components of the stock of social capital. Third, there are those studies that seek to identify the benefits that are derived form the presence or absence of stocks of social capital. Fourth, there are studies that tend to limit the identification of social capital to attitudes and norms, while others have focused on the structural properties of networks and the benefits of these. Use of these approaches tends to be differentiated according to the discipline guiding the research.

Social capital across levels of society

If we consider communities as some middle level between the individual and family on one side and the state on the other, then our interest can be in how the stock of social capital is both used and invested at the community level from both sides. It is the linkages across levels of society that is the research focus.

At the individual level, for example, it has been found that children that live in families where there is an investment in intergenerational communication have access to a wealth of information and resources linked to their parents' community and work networks (Boisjoly, Duncan Hofferth 1995; Frustenbergen and Huges 1995). Majoribanks (1991) showed that young Australians coming from families that invested time and energy in community groups and organisations increased knowledge and skill development through these linkages. At a wider level, Coleman (1988) cites several studies that demonstrate how tight matrices of relationships with characteristics of trust and mutual obligations across larger regions are conducive to aiding a wide range of local and individual benefits.

An important indicator of links between the state and the community is the proportion of gross domestic product (GDP) assigned to social investment by governments to build and support social structures. This is an under investigated area that is of interest to a number of western governments.

The make-up of social capital

This research direction seeks to identify the characteristics of communities and public policies that either enhance or diminish the stock of social capital as a public good in its own right. Types of community organisations such as self-help organisations that produce local social opportunities beyond state provision have been consistently investigated (Banks 1997; Stolle and Rochon 1998). Volunteers are more prone to engage in a wide range of community activities beyond their specific volunteer activity that seems to increase the stock of local social capital (Baum et al. 1999). Linkages between schools and youth programs and the availability of programs for youth at risk appear to increase the stock of social capital among younger people (Donald and Dower 2000; Youniss et al. 1997).

Recent studies on the production of social capital reveal just how widely the concept has been applied. Its application crosses local and national issues, the structural aspects of networks and spatial design and the effects of attitudes such as trust in government.

What social capital produces

Commonly, studies seek to establish whether or not the presence of social capital helps to produce a range of other benefits. In such studies, social capital is the independent variable affecting a range of outcomes (Foley and Edwards 1999). Knack and Keefer (1997), using the

World Values Survey to capture indicators of trust, civic norms and group membership, found social capital does matter to economic performance but not in a straightforward way. Trust and civic norms are higher in countries where there are higher and more equal incomes, for example. Better economic performance was also associated with the presence of civic institutions that restrained the predatory actions of chief executives and where populations are better educated but also more homogeneous.

Various aspects of social capital have now been linked to reduced levels of crime in local areas (Sampson 1997; Saegert and Winkel 1998) greater availability of volunteers (Baum et al. 1999), neighbourhood stability (Temkin and Rohe 1998), the growth of intellectual capital and local economic opportunities (Nahapiet and Goshal 1998; Burt 1997), levels of juvenile crime (Rubio 1997) and mortality rates (Kawachi et al. 1997b). The tendency thus far to measure social capital at one point in time and to use predictive modelling leaves us with a wide range of associations between indicators of social capital and several community outcomes but we are short on understanding the causal pathways.

Attitudes and norms versus networks and structures

Two broadly-based approaches have been used to operationalise social capital regardless of whether the research purpose has been to identify what makes up its substance or to examine how it contributes to other outcomes. Economists and community psychologists in general have operationalised social capital as survey items about social trust in other people, in local communities and in larger institutions such as government. Often included in the montage of trust questions are items about reciprocity norms. Measures of civic engagement such as extent of voting, contact with political leaders and public officials, group activism, local council attendance and so forth are also commonly included in survey research. These are seen to arise as a consequence of the attitude/normative measures rather than the other way around. These items of civic engagement are in turn seen to produce improved economic performance or health and well-being in a population. The empirical foundations for this order of connectedness is a matter for research validation.

Several interrelated concepts about community norms that represent aspects of social capital have also been operationalised in survey instruments. One of the earliest of these concerned psychological sense of community or community mindedness (Sarason 1974). This idea was later refined by MacMillan and Chavis (1986) into a four-dimensional scale that includes items to represent 'sense of feeling part of a community', 'influence in a community', 'integration' in terms of needs being met and a shared sense of history and 'attachment'. Sampson (1997) developed a small range of questions to represent 'collective efficacy' to measure the extent of support for a common set of local values such as willingness to help a stranger in the neighborhood. Eng and Parker (1994) constructed an eight-dimensional set of questions to measure 'community competence' made up of a combination of the concepts previously described. Measures like these are potentially useful because the focus is on perceived community attributes rather than individual attributes. However, the efficiency and predictive validity of these measures remains largely untested (Lochner et al. 1999).

A different approach, favoured more by social scientists, operationalises social capital through identification of the qualities of social structures such as networks. Key items measured include the availability of local groups and organisations and the linkages between these and individuals, other groups and organisations and wider institutions. Common measures include size, reach, density and interconnectedness of mediating structures. This approach often defines how access to resources may be sought and the extent of availability of resources within existing network structures. Studies of health development structures (Baum et al. 2000) and other mediating structures (Couto and Guthrie 1999) that take this approach pay attention to the way non-economic community resources are identified, maintained and used to produce other forms of capital.

The first approach (that which collects information about attitudes and norms) is common in large-scale population studies and in trans-national comparative studies because it has been relatively easy to aggregate individual survey responses into population or national mean scores. The loss of contextual information about social capital in this approach has adverse consequences for understanding social capital formation and function. It has not been possible to describe differences across communities in large-scale studies using aggregation methods based on attitudes/norms in a convincingly reliable way. On the other hand, the second approach (that which emphasises social structures) does not easily lend itself to large-scale population studies and rests mainly within the realm of local community investigations.

Newton (1999), in commenting on attempts to demonstrate the predictive value of attitudes and norms of social capital, concludes that, 'those who are satisfied with life are trusting, and they are satisfied with life because their income, education and skill [as well as] . . . social position that gives them good cause to be so'. In other words, social capital is a product of structural advantage. Smith (1997) found 'negative trust' for example was associated with lower education, income, recent financial misfortune, marginalisation and poorer health. This is not to suggest attitudes and norms representing trust are not important, but rather that these appear secondary to the availability of networks that provide life opportunities.

Social capital and health status

Health inequalities are primarily produced by differences in socioeconomic status (Wilkinson 1992). It also appears that health inequalities worsen as the wealth gap widens, even when economic growth is strong. In other words, public policies that seek to consider resource distribution across communities may be necessary to address health inequalities rather than encouraging economic growth alone. This has lead to the search for evidence about the effects of not just material deprivation but also social circumstances to explain health inequalities across communities (Kawachi et al. 1997b; Marmot 1998).

Kawachi and Kennedy (1997) suggest two possible reasons why income inequality and health (measured by mortality rates) are linked together. The first reason is that the link simply reflects a linear relationship between poverty and health. However, accumulating evidence suggests that the relationship exists even when absolute poverty is accounted for (Marmot 1988). The second reason may be that as the income gap widens both within and between communities, investment in the social capital of communities begins to decline. The lower socioeconomic strata disinvest because of very limited resources and the upper strata disinvest by increasingly isolating themselves through use of private means – the move to walled communities and the use of private education are examples.

It appears reasonable to assert that one reason why economic growth alone does not translate into equitable health gains is that disinvestment in social and community infrastructure leads to a lack of networks, groups and organisations that can translate economic capital into public goods (Kawachi et al. 1997b). Tentative evidence for this assertion comes from a cross-sectional community study between the US states showing the relationship between income distribution, investments in social capital (measured by group membership and levels of trust) and mortality rates (Kawachi et. al. 1997b). States with lower investments in social and community infrastructure had greater income inequalities and strongly associated mortality rates.

There is, then, tentative evidence for the potential and vital role of social capital in its various forms in communities as a mechanism for ensuring access to resources that make a difference to health status. The suggestion is that a widening gap between richer and poorer communities diminishes social capital investment in the very mediating structures and network relationships that make up the glue that binds us together for good health.

The Adelaide Health Development and Social Capital study

Our study commenced because of a desire to look beyond what were often rhetorical statements about the role of participation and social capital in contributing to health. The study was designed to enable a picture of the patterns of participation and component parts of social capital to be documented, measured and understood.

The Adelaide Health Development and Social Capital study[1] has considered the levels of participation in social and civic activities of a random sample of the population in the western suburbs of Adelaide who responded to a mailed questionnaire survey (2,542 people responded out of an initial sample of 4,000). The study also explored reasons for these participation patterns through detailed in-depth interviews. Community groups and organisations were surveyed to determine the role they played and had the potential to play in promoting health at a local level. Twenty-five case studies of these groups were also developed to explore their health development role as mediating community structures in more detail.

Measuring Participation

Participation was conceptualised as being broadly either social or civic. Civic participation is divided into two types: individual and collective. A detailed epidemiology of participation using this Index is reported elsewhere (Baum, Bush et al. 2000). The study found that people are most likely to participate in informal social activity and least likely to participate in collective civic activity. In fact participation in this later activity was rare with only 3–5 % of the sample regularly undertaking civic activities. Most significantly, we found that individual household income and educational level structured rates of participation in each form of social activity. People living in households with comparatively higher incomes are significantly more likely to participate in civic activities whether these are individual or collective activities. They are also more likely to take part in social activities outside their home. A similar but more significant pattern emerges for people with higher education attainment.

These are data based on correlations so they do not tell us much about patterns of causality. For instance, do people have higher household incomes because they are have good networks, or does their higher income level enable them to gain access to networks?. The most significant factor is that the determinants of health advantage are also those associated with higher social and civic participation.

We have also conducted some analysis of our data by postcode and found that the average scores for participation differ according to the average household income. There are, however, a few pointers that civic participation (even though low overall) was significantly higher in some areas than others even though the areas had a lower average household income. It may be that the characteristics of a neighbourhood could be related to participation and health patterns. Indeed, if it can be shown after controlling for socioeconomic status of individuals that such a pattern persists, then this points to the value of investments aimed at reducing health inequities through direct local area strategies rather than individualised services exclusively.

In general, we found that age and gender shapes people's experiences of participation. Younger people were the least likely to be involved in civic activity but the most likely to be involved in social activity in public spaces. Older people and women were most likely to be involved in community groups. The overall conclusion from our measures of participation is that, just like health, its distribution is socially and economically structured.

Explaining patterns of participation

Twenty-nine percent of our sample reported that they would like to be more involved in groups aiming to improve conditions, facilities or services in their area. This suggests that policies to encourage greater social and civic inclusiveness could make sense. The barriers to participation are, however, complex. On the mail questionnaire, people indicated that barriers to participation included transport difficulties, childcare problems and lack of time. Our qualitative data suggest that participation is influenced by a complex set of forces, both psychological and sociological. There is, of course, also an interaction between these forces which are very hard to untangle.

Low-income and older people were the most likely to report interaction with their neighbours. The qualitative interview data suggested that the costs associated with more formal types of participation such as joining a sporting or a social club often excluded those in a lower income bracket. Those on low incomes tend to become involved in a host of informal social activities that rely on neighbourly trust, reciprocity and minimal amounts of disposable income. Typical examples were chatting over the garden fence, offering support to neighbours and swapping produce from the garden. The picture that emerged from the in-depth interviews was that patterns of social interaction of some of the people living in working class suburbs were similar in feel to the accounts from the British community studies conducted in the 1950s and 1960s. Some reported intense local networks that involved a fair degree of reciprocity.

Table 13.1 Social and civic participation

Activities contained in each index of participation from the survey

Activities contained in each index of participation from the survey

Indices of participation were measured by counting the number of items in each measure that individuals answered 'yes' to. The higher the number, the higher the level of civic or social participation.

1 Social participation – informal (3 items)

If the respondent had done any of the following activities monthly or more often in the past twelve months:

Visited family or had family visit; visited friends or had friends visit; visited neighbours or had neighbours visit.

2 Social participation – activities in public spaces (4 items)

If the respondent had done any of the following activities monthly or more often in the past twelve months:

Been to a cafe or restaurant; been to a social club; been to the cinema or theatre; been to a party or dance.

3 Social participation – group activities (6 items)

If the respondent had done any of the following activities monthly or more often in the past twelve months:

Played sport; been to the gym or exercise class; been to a class; been involved in a hobby group; singing/acting/musician in a group; been involved in a self-help or support group.

4 Civic participation – individual activities (7 items)

If the respondent had done any of the following activities at all in the past twelve months:

Signed a petition; contacted a local MP; written to the council; contacted a local councillor; attended a protest meeting; written a letter to the editor of a newspaper; attended a council meeting.

5 Civic participation – group activities (4 items)

If the respondent had been involved in any of the following groups at all in the past twelve months:

Resident or community action group; political party, trade union or political campaign; campaign or action to improve social or environmental conditions; local government.

6 Community Group Participation – mix of civic and social (5 items)

If the respondent had been involved in any of the following groups at all in the past twelve months:

Volunteer organisation or group; school-related group; ethnic group; service club.

If the respondent had done the following activity monthly or more often in the past twelve months:

Attended church.

But alongside these stories of community cohesiveness, we also had neighbourhood conflict reported and a sense of distrust and ill-ease. Such feelings were often expressed in racist terms against particular groups such as Aboriginal or Asian people and often reflected a strong nostalgia for the past when communities were perceived to be more trusting and friendly by some. Amongst some of the people who recorded low participation rates, a strong distrust of others was evident. They were also more likely to perceive their communities to be unsafe and to be less safe than they had been in the past. Certainly, our qualitative data suggests that not trusting can lead to a reluctance to participate both in social and civic activity.

Amongst some of our sample, we found a profound lack of trust in formal institutions and politicians. Typical of such views was the 66-year-old man who said in response to the question, 'So you don't have much faith in the government?': 'Not really . . . They're all a pack of liars. They promise you the bloody world but when they get in they knock it out from underneath you. Labor or Liberal – they're all the bloody same.' Such attitudes were prevalent among low participators and certainly suggest a feeling of lack of control.

People's self-image also affects their willingness to participate in activities with others. People with low self-esteem appear likely to be low participators. The qualitative interviews suggest a language of low self-esteem, with people referring to themselves as 'loners', 'losers' and 'nobodies' to account for their lack of participation. This is illustrated by this account from 'Rob', 56 years old, who was a low participator and housebound with a host of physical and social problems:

> I've always been a loner and I don't make friends easy because I don't trust people . . . I've always been hard to make friends with because I've always been a loner and this is it. When I was working I never mixed with anybody. Always stuck to meself. Maybe I don't trust people, I don't know.

Physical surroundings may affect the ways they participate. For instance, street-level shopping strips were seen as friendlier and more conducive to a sense of community than large undercover shopping centres. Others mourned the loss of local shops that had given them a local destination on the way to which they often experience a sense of connectedness and links with other locals. Here, they were expressing the importance of weak social links, which were seen as part of what makes a community tick.

Some of the respondents reported that their physical health status was a barrier to their participation. Often this was a barrier to participation in sport but, for older people, ill health acted as a more general barrier. We also noticed that men who had worked in manual occupations reported their occupational-related diseases as a barrier to participation and women that children could restrict their participation outside child-related activities.

Our study suggests a complex picture of why people do and don't participate in social and civic activities. While it is hard to derive firm lessons from it, it is clear that people's extent of participation reflects a mixture of their economic and educational position, their life experiences and their feelings of control and self-esteem.

Path model showing the relationship between social and civic participation and two health outcomes, individual health status and sense of control in community.

Participation, self-reported health status and sense of control over community affairs

We have used the findings from the population survey to construct several path models to test the relationship between types of participation, demographic characteristics and measures of health status. Figure 13.1 describes the relationship between a set of participation activities clustered into social or civic participation and outcomes of self-reported health status, measured by responses to the SF12 (a self-report physical and mental health questionnaire), and a measure of sense of control over community affairs. In the model presented here, the influence of demographic characteristics are not accounted for. In other models, however, it is clear that these do have moderating effects in line with the description outlined earlier.

The path model shows that informal social participation, like doing something for a neighbour, social activities like visiting friends and family, and group activities like going to the gym or a hobby group are strongly associated with the construct 'social participation'. Collective civic participation, such as attending a residents' action group, and individual civic participation, such as contacting a public official or politician about a local issue, are both strongly associated with the construct 'civic participation'.

As we would expect, following extensive research on the benefits of support networks (House et al. 1988), social participation predicts health status but it is a much weaker predictor of sense of control over community affairs. It is engagement in civic participation that predicts sense of control. However, engaging in civic matters is not a predictor of individual health status. It would seem that different types of participation in communities lead to different benefits. In the case of this path model, outward-looking civic actions may well give a sense of control and perhaps assist in the collective 'well-being', whereas more social activities seem good for your individual health overall. What appears clear from this model is that a

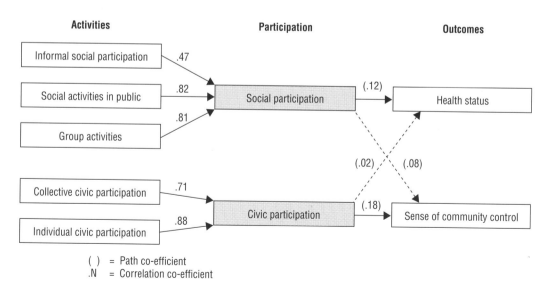

Figure 13.1 Outcomes of social and civic participation

vibrant community is one where there are many opportunities to engage in connectedness in both simple ways and in terms of encouraging control over local affairs.

Mediating structures

Our study of health development and social capital was designed to allow for both a consideration of individuals' attitudes and behaviours and of the structures within communities that might encourage participation. These structures were studied through the compilation of an inventory and a series of case studies. Of the 240 groups and local organisations upon which data was collected, 75% stated their activities were health-promoting activities and 40% reported that they had worked with a health service in the past two years. Social contact and social support were reported to be the most central functions of these groups.

The ways in which they may assist health promotion are[2]:

- Their activities may in and of themselves be health promoting (eg, sporting clubs).
- They bring people together and contribute to building networks and trust, the components of social capital (Country Women's Association, service clubs such as the Lions and Probus).
- They may support health services functions (Red Cross volunteers, rural chronic illness peer support groups for young people with chronic illness).
- They may advocate and lobby on issues that will improve health (eg, Local Consumer Advisory Group which advocates on behalf of people with mental illness, or a Friends of the Coroong group, and a local progress association that saw its health role as representing the community on health services).

From these descriptions it is clear that the groups have a mix of social and civic functions. Our suggestion is that they strengthen communities by increasing trust and networks among people. Some of these groups also act to create spaces between community members and government services or mechanisms of governance (such as local government). Our case studies illustrate the ways in which these health-promoting roles of the groups are played out in everyday life. Individually, none of the workings of the groups appear significant. Yet, when viewed as a whole their potential for strengthening communities becomes less elusive. However, we are unclear whether the groups play much of a role in linking people across different social classes. We also found that most of the groups are ethnic specific and so do not currently play much of a role in forming 'alliances across difference' (Reid 1997).

Conclusions

We began this chapter by asking a question about whether or not social capital can improve the health of communities and the life opportunities of those within them, given the evidence that there is a widening gap between those with wealth and those in relative poverty. This is a significant community question because of the concentration of those with wealth and those in relative poverty in separate communities. Moreover, the health and life opportunities differ across these different communities.

The concept of capital seems a useful one for understanding how investing in social infrastructure and connectiveness helps in the production of other forms of capital. Equally, the idea that there exists a stock of social capital, which individuals, communities and governments can all draw on and replenish, takes us well beyond the restrictions of economic concerns to address a wider range of issues that are central to the very life of the democratic state, namely the health of civil society. But we have been hampered so far in the health field by the uncritical adoption of theory about social capital, principally through the lack of attention to the power relationships that are expressed through the ownership of forms of capital. Bourdieu's analysis shows promise because it not only allows us to consider community relationships but also access to resources through social relationships that shape our thinking, our actions and our access to other forms of capital.

There is also considerable value in now reshaping some core ideas about social capital and its distinctive properties. Its importance to the creation of public goods is the first and most fundamental of these. If the origins of health and life opportunity are to be taken seriously, then how public goods are stimulated by public policies, and how health researchers measure the stock and the value of these goods for health, is one place to begin. One way forward here is to generate a renewed interest in mediating or health development structures in communities. The way these link people to resources that create opportunities for difference and diversity is essential in contemporary heterogeneous communities – a type of community different to the old romantic view of the 1960s and 1970s community. This was a view that in the end failed because of a limited vision devoid of the interconnectedness between various forms of capital. It will also be beneficial to accept that participation takes many forms and helps to produce many outcomes, some of immediate personal gain and others for collective benefits.

A wide field of research across several disciplines demonstrates an untidy but emerging evidence base that will help us not only to define the social determinants of health, but also to address these through population health measures in communities and through large scale public policy. Policies that encourage local involvement in limiting exclusion of specific groups from resources and life opportunities, that encourage use and a sense of ownership of public space, that enable stability in basic shelter and housing are among several public policies that are immediately amenable to empirical research. There is room for a much more vigorous research agenda at the cross-over points between levels of society and how social capital can be generated and passed on across generations – as within the family and community studies – as well as passed on by government policies that stimulate social investments – as in an investigation of returns on investment in social infrastructure as a portion of GDP.

There is at least some evidence that social infrastructure in the form of networks, and mediating groups and organisations are a prerequisite for a 'healthy' community. While trust and reciprocity oil the relationships around these structures, their importance to the issue of redressing inequities in health status lies primarily in the role these can play in redistributing resources among groups in society. The view of social capital we have taken accepts that material deprivation is one of the key factors underlying health inequities (notwithstanding the importance of more psychological factors which contribute to the existence of health gradients among different groups). Social capital's role is in serving to improve the access individuals within communities have to resources that provide access to material and intellectual benefits such as employment and education. Some of these resources operate invisibly so that a community in which a rich fabric of community organisation and physical features encourage the formation of trust and thin and thick networks leads to communities in which economic success may be more likely.

The data we have presented from the Adelaide Health Development and Social Capital study indicate that those who are most likely to participate in society are also those who are better off economically and who have higher educational levels. While the direction of causality is not clear there is enough evidence to suggest that policies should aim to encourage an environment in which the features of social capital flourish. Social attributes such as trusting networks are to be valued in and for themselves. But, they also appear to play an important function in encouraging participation in both civic and economic life in a community. The aim of public policy should be to assist communities that are relatively poor in these social capital resources to become less so.

Acknowledgements

The Adelaide Health Development and Social Capital study was funded by an NH&MRC grant.

Notes

1   The Adelaide Health Development and Social Capital team comprises Fran Baum, Robert Bush, Eva Cox, Kathy Alexander, Carolyn Modra, Charlie Murray, Robert Potter, Catherine Palmer, Samantha Miller.
2   These examples were compiled by Rosie King, Project Officer, Hills Mallee Southern Health Development Structures study being conducted jointly by SACHRU, Department of Public Health at Flinders University and the Hills Mallee Southern Regional Health Service.

Further Reading

Ian Winters (Ed.) 2000, Social Capital and Public Policy in Australia, Australian Institute of Family Studies, Melbourne.
   – A stimulating collection of Australian perspectives on the implication of the current social capital debates for public policy. The chapters are a mix of theoretical perspectives and reports based on empirical data, and include an excellent overview of the major themes and debates in the social capital literature. Topics covered include citizenship, business and social capital, non-profit organisations, trust, family health and social capital, politics and policy.
Woolcock, Michael & Narayan, Deepa 2000, Social capital: implications for development theory, research and policy, World Bank Research Observer 15: 1.
   – An extended essay from the active group within the World Bank. It is written through the lens of the needs of developing countries, but contains many useful perspectives on the conceptualisation and theoretical approaches to social capital that are more generally applicable.

Part D
Developmental and biological perspectives

14

Health inequalities:
the seeds are sown in childhood, what about the remedies?

Graham Vimpani

There is growing evidence from fields as diverse as education, criminology, child health, public health and mental health that early childhood is a more critical period in the life cycle than has been previously recognised. For example, the recent Acheson report (1998) concluded that:

> While remediable risk factors affecting health occur throughout the life course, childhood is a critical and vulnerable stage where poor socioeconomic circumstances have lasting effects. Follow up through life of successive samples of births has pointed to the crucial influence of early life on subsequent mental and physical health and development. The fact that the adverse outcomes, for example, mental illness, short stature, obesity, delinquency and unemployment, cover a wide range, carries an important message. It suggests that policies which reduce such early adverse influences may result in multiple benefits, not only throughout the life course of that child but to the next generation.

Socioeconomic gradients in outcomes vary between countries

In each of these areas, there are data to suggest that there are gradients in a variety of health and education outcomes across the socioeconomic spectrum. Countries with social policies that invest more in social assistance for workless and low-paid parents have lower child poverty rates, which in turn are associated with shallower gradient slopes and better mean outcomes for the whole population (UNICEF 2000; Keating and Hertzman 1999; McCain and Mustard 1999). The Scandinavian countries, for example, have lower rates of both relative and absolute child poverty at least in part because of taxes and transfers. These countries achieve higher overall literacy standards and shallower socioeconomic gradients than many other OECD countries, despite having relatively high rates of single parent families, which, in most other industrialised countries, is highly correlated with child poverty. The extent to which this outcome is a consequence of more generous parental leave provisions and high quality child care for young children is worth pondering. Mean outcomes and gradient slopes in Cuba are also much more impressive than those in many South American countries.

Poverty, inequality or both?

While there is no doubt that poverty on the scale experienced in many third world countries is a major determinant of poor health status within their populations, in industrialised countries there is considerable evidence that health is related to relative rather than absolute income. Indeed, in more egalitarian societies, such as the Scandinavian countries where differences in income and social status are smaller, not only are there shallower gradients in health and other outcomes in childhood, but there are also signs of greater social cohesiveness (Wilkinson 1999). Poverty itself can undoubtedly have a major impact on the way life is experienced by children in poor families. For example, Brooks Gunn, Duncan and Maritato (1996) discuss the extent to which poverty constrains the ability of families to purchase goods for their children, affects their emotional well-being which in turn impacts upon their parenting style and limits access to high quality child care. But for those lower in a steep social hierarchy, Wilkinson (1999) contends that it is the experience of 'shame, inferiority, subordination, being put down and not respected' that is an extremely important, if largely unrecognised, source of recurrent anxiety. Low social status is known in animal and human studies to have a significant impact on raised basal cortisol levels, the effects of which appear 'to be so far-reaching that they have been likened to the process of rapid ageing' (Sapolsky, 1998). It is important to note that professional home visitation models which are based on theoretical models that directly address the impact of this experience, through the promotion of self-efficacy and empowerment of mothers are amongst the most powerful early intervention strategies that have been demonstrated for poor, single, young mothers (Karoly et al. 1998; Davis 1993).

Timing of exposure to adversity is important

The timing of exposure to low income in childhood is important. For example, the correlation coefficients for family income–developmental outcome links are smaller for high school completion than for earlier school achievement. A longitudinal study in Baltimore found that welfare receipt in the preschool years was more highly associated with adolescent outcomes such as literacy, high school completion and school failure than was family welfare receipt during the mid-childhood or early adolescent years (Brooks-Gunn, Guo and Furstenberg 1993) a finding comparable to that found in the US Panel Study of Income Dynamics (Axinn et al. 1997). Brooks-Gunn et al. (1999) attribute this to the impact that low income has on preschool readiness and verbal scores; low readiness test scores are associated with subsequent grade failure, school disengagement and school dropout.

Biological embedding

There is a growing body of evidence that suggests that the origins of socioeconomic differences in a range of life-course outcomes are established in foetal life and early childhood by a process of biological embedding of environmental experience that particularly affects neuropsychological development and its impact on the function of other biologic systems. 'Variations in social status are associated with important differences in the quality of the social and physical environments that are encountered by young children, and these differences in turn produce variability in the specific experiences that contribute to neural sculpting and thus to potentially enduring differences in health, coping and competence' (Keating and Hertzman 1999).

Latent versus Cumulative effects

There is debate about whether the influence of adverse childhood circumstances affects later adult health and well-being through latent or cumulative effects. That is, are adverse circumstances early in life part of a continuing and cumulative pattern of disadvantage, the so-called *'pathways'* model, whereby socioeconomic and psychosocial adversity in childhood is followed and reinforced by an ongoing sense of powerlessness and alienation allied to a social support network made up of others who have been similarly disadvantaged and socially excluded, with those affected at increased risk of participating in a vicious cycle of educational failure, criminality, substance misuse, teenage pregnancy with subsequent poor employment opportunities, and risks for chronic disease and early onset of degenerative disease (Keating and Hertzman 1999)? Or are adverse circumstances very early in life likely to impact on health and well-being later in life regardless of intervening circumstances, except for perhaps being triggered by proximate re-exposure to a related risk – the so-called *latency model* – for example, adult-onset obesity triggering emergence of raised blood pressure in those who had experienced poor nutrition prenatally (Barker 1994), or where the risks of adult depression following divorce are greater in individuals who had experienced divorce of their own parents during childhood (Rodgers 1994).

Experiential and environmental impacts on early brain development

The role that the impact of adverse environmental influences on early brain development may be contributing to these differences is receiving increased attention, particularly in North America and Australia. Whilst genetic influences are important in laying down the broad framework for brain development, the mammalian limbic and neocortical brain relies on exposure to high probability environmental circumstances likely to be encountered at a critical time in the normal life of the species for the fine-tuning and organisation of its synaptic networks. For example, the development of binocular vision in humans is dependent upon images from both eyes being transduced to the visual cortex within the first six or eight months of life – there is no inbuilt genetic code that ensures normal vision. In ducks and other avian species that are mobile and self-feeding shortly after birth, there is a critical age for imprinting the behaviour that usually ensures mutual bonding between parent and offspring, a behaviour that forms the foundation for later learning of survival skills (Cynander and Frost 1999).

The importance of good enough parenting and attachment

The assertion that parenting is probably the most important public health issue facing many industrialised countries (Hoghughi 1998) is increasingly recognised as having validity in the light of evidence demonstrating the long-term risks to health and well-being of poor attachment between young children and their primary caregivers, and of the impact of maternal depression on developmental health outcomes. Attachment is a special type of social relationship, most notably between an infant and caregiver, involving an affective bond which provides the context in which the infant learns to regulate emotion (Sroufe 1995). Not only is this 'affective interchange paramount for the development of emotion, but also the maturation and development of the child' (Spitz 1965) in all aspects of personality and social development. There are clear links between early attachment experiences and later adaptation, with infancy assessments of attachment predicting self-regulation, self-reliance, self-efficacy and the development of autonomy in four-year-old to eight-year-old children in longitudinal studies. Children who had experienced a secure relationship with their parents as infants were more likely to be rated by their teachers as competent, socially oriented, empathic and able to form deeper relationships with others; these differences persist into middle childhood and early adolescence (Fonagy 1995). Patterns of attachment in infancy are strongly correlated with subsequent adult patterns with between 68% and 75% correspondence found between the two age groups (Fonagy 1995).

There is clear evidence of a strong association between the determinants of poor attachment, parenting difficulties and socioeconomic status. For example, poor parenting skills and maltreatment of children are more commonly found in families suffering socioeconomic hardship (Belsky 1993; Garbarino 1992). Social advantage on the other hand is more often associated with secure attachment. Broussard (1995) found that only 24% of infants in an inner-city sample were securely attached whilst 32% were found to be insecure/disorganised. In contrast, around 65% of middle-class children are normally securely attached with only 10% having a disorganised pattern (van Ijzendoorn et al. 1992). Moreover, while there is a strong correlation between multiple forms of deprivation in childhood and later adult criminal behaviour, 'good parenting' can protect against the acquisition of a criminal record in children from deprived backgrounds (Kolvin et al. 1990). These findings are consistent with those of Constantino (1996) who showed that insecure attachment is associated with abnormal levels of aggression in preschoolers and Tremblay et al. (1995, 1999) who found that whilst many children show signs of aggressive behaviour at age two ('the terrible twos'), in most children this pattern has been inhibited by age five years, in large part through good limit setting and the development of brain functions that inhibit this kind of behaviour. However, those children who at school entry were still exhibiting oppositional behaviour, physical aggression and hyperactivity were more likely to become violent and nonviolent delinquent teenagers; about 28% of those who were demonstrating antisocial behaviour at school entry were delinquent by age 13 years, and around 70% of crime is committed by those who had difficult behaviour from an early age (Tremblay et al. 1994).

Some writers go so far as to argue that attachment theory is probably the most useful organising framework for understanding the impact of socioeconomic inequality on health and well-being outcomes (Fonagy 1995), since adverse attachment experiences in the early years impact upon an individual's educational achievement, sense of self-esteem, quality of interpersonal relationships, social support systems and sense of self-control throughout life.

Attachment and early brain development

Evidence is now starting to accumulate from animal and human imaging studies that attachment behaviour affects early brain development (Schore 1994). For example, a recent study has shown a 12% reduction in the volume of the hippocampal region – part of the limbic brain system, which is associated with memory and cognitive function – in children with a history of early childhood abuse and neglect who have ongoing symptoms consistent with post-traumatic stress disorder (Bremner et al. 1997). The extent to which this may be due to excessive activation of the HPA axis and excess cortisol production, known to produce neuronal death and a loss of dendritic branching in animal studies (Uno et al. 1989; Sapolsky et al. 1990) is intriguing. The degree and quality of caregiving may thus be critical for the long-term biological organisation of the child as the regulatory experiences between infant and caregiver strengthen or eliminate synapses which are overproduced in the infant's brain (Fonagy 1995).

Environmental and experiential impact on neuroendocrine and neuroimmunological responses

The quality of sensory stimulation in early life thus helps shape the brain's endocrine and immune pathways (McCain and Mustard 1999). Studies of newborn rat pups have shown that early modest exposure to handling (Meaney et al. 1988), that in turn results in more frequent licking and grooming by their mothers, results in better regulation of their response to subsequent stressful events than in rats who are not handled, or handled for longer periods (Francis et al. 1996; Francis and Meaney 1999). The pups who were more frequently groomed and licked had lower cortisol levels in response to acute stress as adults (Liu et al. 1997). There thus appears to be a critical period for gaining effective neural control over the stress response (Cynander and Frost 1999). Sustained or chronic stress has the opposite effect and reduces the capacity to process new sensory stimulation, influences behaviour and has a negative impact on memory (McCain and Mustard 1999). Indeed, Perry (1996) asserts that deprivation of optimal stimulation or disruptive experiences in infancy may lead to abnormal behaviour and cognitive disabilities through their impact on the development of the midbrain and limbic areas; because of the dysfunctional development of these parts of the brain many of these children spend most of the time in a low level of fear or abnormal arousal, appearing inattentive, learning disabled and reacting aggressively to perceived threats from their peers.

Goldstein et al. (1999) have suggested that individual differences in children's cardiovascular reactions to stress may mediate the association between socioeconomic status (SES) and health. Preschool children who were of low SES, identified by observation to be nondominant with their peers and highly reactive in measures of cardiovascular reactivity (high mean heart rate during tasks and high heart rate recovery difference score) had the poorest measures of global physical health.

Stress and immune function

McEwen (1998) has shown that chronic stress can suppress the immune system. Meyer and Haggerty (1962) showed that poor family functioning influenced the incidence of streptococcal infection and the likelihood of a positive throat culture and symptomatic expression over a period of one year. Boyce et al. (1977) also found that environmental and family stability influenced the severity and duration of upper respiratory illness in children. Boyce et al. (1995a) observed that evidence of the pathophysiological changes that accompany emotional stress had led to speculation that it may account for the uneven distribution of illness in childhood populations wherein 15–20% of children incur the majority of illness visits in primary care settings and sustain over 50% of overall paediatric morbidity. He and his colleagues examined adrenocortical and behavioural predictors of immune responses to starting kindergarten and pneumococcal vaccine immunisation in 39 mainly upper middle-class five-year-old children. They found that school entry evoked elevations in cortisol and behaviour problems accompanied by shifts in functional and enumerative measures of immune status. Children with greater markers of stress had less effective B-cell mediated antibody production. Coe (1999) notes that, even in monkeys, the magnitude of the immune suppression that occurs after separation from their mother can be modulated and largely ameliorated by a more benevolent separation environment.

Lower plasticity of stress-regulating systems

One of the reasons why experiences of adversity in the early years may be so critical throughout the life cycle is that once the regulatory systems concerned with emotional regulation and arousal that are sited in the limbic and midbrain areas are organised early in life, it may be difficult to modify them, whereas other more plastic parts of the brain, such as the neocortex continue to undergo use-dependent modification throughout life. Once the critical periods for these aspects of brain development have passed it may be difficult, despite the provision of nurturing environments to achieve the brain's full potential. Evidence from UK studies of the outcomes of institutionalised Romanian orphans shows that those who were adopted in the UK under the age of six months had markedly higher cognitive performance at age four years than those adopted between six months and two years; the former group had scores that were no different from UK born adoptees (Rutter et al. 2000a). Moreover, there was a close association between the duration of deprivation and the severity of attachment disorder behaviours which in turn were correlated with attentional and conduct problems and cognitive level (O'Connor and Rutter 2000).

Early intervention is a cost-effective investment

Longitudinal follow-up of rigorously planned and executed interventions that aim to support families with very young children in North America suggests that investment in such strategies is a cost-effective means of improving a diverse range of educational, health and well-being outcomes. A recent review by the Rand Corporation (Karoly et al. 1998) provides evidence that long-term returns over fifteen years on investment during the early childhood window of opportunity may be as high as 5:1. Follow-up into young adulthood shows additional cost–benefits (Schweinhart et al. 1993). These strategies aim to minimise risk of adverse outcomes and create the conditions that are likely to promote resilience. Evidence suggests that strategies such as extended home visitation, group work with parents and early preschool, that offer a broad range of support that addresses unmet emotional, developmental and relationship needs of the primary caregivers as well as their young children's needs for developmentally enriching environments are most effective (Olds et al. 1997, 1998a; Cox et al. 1991; Schweinhart et al. 1993). Programs that seek to facilitate attunement between mothers and infants and other programs designed to enhance emotional literacy (Steiner 1997; Gordon, 1975, Gottman and Declaire 1997) offer particular promise (van den Boom 1994).

Need for longitudinal data

Good policy development in Australia has been hampered by the absence of longitudinal datasets that, depending upon the design, would enable us to trace the impact of social change and socioeconomic disadvantage on health and well-being outcomes as well as providing a framework whereby the benefits of early intervention strategies could be evaluated in our own social context. The recent policy decision to establish a national childhood longitudinal study as part of the Stronger Families and Communities strategy is welcomed although it needs to be recognised that without additional funding, its aims will need to be kept relatively modest. For example, the budget for a single year of the Canadian National Longitudinal Survey of Children and Young People (which is following-up a sample of children intially aged 0–11 years every two years, as well as adding a new birth cohort at that time, will also be able to examine community-level, or social capital, effects on outcomes) is greater than that proposed for the initial nine years of the Australian study (Zeesman 2000).

The need for national investment in early childhood

The wide-ranging nature of the research outcome data challenge the prevailing view that the promotion of developmental health and well-being in early childhood should be primarily a private responsibility, especially in the context of building a knowledge-based society able to play an effective role in the emerging Information Age. Current social investment in the support of families with young children, especially in the context of the additional demands placed on families as a result of increased workforce participation of women, fails to reflect the crucial lifelong influence of this developmental period. The largely unacknowledged but uneven access that exists across different regions in Australia to various early childhood services – such as free preschool for four-year-olds – institutionalises disadvantage.

In Canada, the Vanier Institute of the Family recently issued this challenge in 1998:

> For Canada and Canadians to prosper in the 21st century, we must find ways to harmonise the demands of paid work and the responsibilities of family life. Achieving a balance between employment and family is a key strategy for increased productivity, enhanced creativity, global competitiveness, family security and civic vitality. So pervasive is the issue in our everyday lives that such a balance also holds the promise of improving the healthy development of our children and the well-being of our individual lives as men and women . . . The Work and Family Challenge, as it has been called, is the pivotal issue that confronts Canada and other industrialised nations as we enter the new millennium.

Duncan and Brooks-Gunn (1996) conclude that 'programs that raise the incomes of poor families will enhance the cognitive development of children and may improve their chances of success in the labour market during adulthood. Most important appears to be the elimination of deep and persistent poverty during a child's early years'.

In Australia, despite the promise of new investment in strategies such as Families First (NSW), Stronger Families and Communities (Commonwealth), and the Good Beginnings National Parenting Project, it needs to be recognised that these are miniscule responses in comparison both to the resources that are consumed in downstream responses to managing problems of developmental health and well-being, and to the extent of unmet family needs for support and the potential offered by the plasticity of the young human brain. In a globalised economy, we need social goals as well as economic ones if we are to remain competitive. A national debate on the importance of the early childhood years for the rest of the life-cycle and the role of government and the private sector in providing support to families in their task of promoting developmental health and well-being of young children, similar to that which preceded the introduction of universal school education, is needed to enhance our capacity to create a learning society. Accepting the status quo would be a prescription for disadvantaging ourselves in a global market and amount to setting a course for declining competitiveness and status on the world stage.

Further Reading

Brooks-Gunn, J, Duncan, G J & Maritato, J 1996, Poor families, poor outcomes: the wellbeing of children and youth, in Duncan, G J & Brooks-Gunn, J (Eds) Consequences of Growing Up Poor, New York: Russell Sage Foundation, pp 1–17.
– A very comprehensive recent review from a North American perspective.
Evans, R G, Barer, M L & Marmor, T R (Eds) 1994, Why are Some People Healthy and Others Not? The determinants of health of populations, Aldine de Gruyter, New York.
– A good summary of the current thinking about mechanisms by which disadvantage gets translated into health inequalities.

Shonkoff, J P & Meisels, S J (Eds) 2000, Handbook of Early Childhood Intervention (2nd edition), Cambridge University Press, UK.
  – *One of the best overviews of different models of early intervention for children who are disadvantaged.*

15
Family, early development and the life course:
common risk and protective factors in pathways to prevention

Judy Cashmore

Developmental outcomes and pathways

The current and generally accepted model of development views children's development as the result of the ongoing interaction and transactions between the children and the environment they grow up in. Those interactions have effects on both the child and the environment, and include transactions between the child's family, the neighbourhood and the wider community. All are variously affected as well by the policies and the structures of the government and the broader society in which they exist (Bronfenbrenner 1979; Shonkoff and Phillips 2000).

Throughout their development, children follow various pathways to particular physical, social, emotional and cognitive developmental outcomes. There is no single straight pathway from early to later development but a number of 'straight and devious' pathways to various developmental outcomes (Robins and Rutter 1990). Children may reach the same outcome or 'point' in different areas of development by a number of different pathways, but the research evidence suggests that certain adverse outcomes in adolescence and adulthood such as criminal behaviour and substance abuse are continuations of anti-social behaviour and mental health problems in childhood (Farrington 1994; Nagin and Tremblay 1999; National Crime Prevention 1999; Robins and Rutter 1990; Werner 1987).

At various points along the pathway, there are a number of points of change or *transitions* which involve major re-orientations in how a child relates to his or her environment (Shonkoff and Phillips, 2000). These are important because they tend to be periods when individuals and/or others around them are looking for information and are likely to be more open to some assistance or intervention. Transitions may occur as particular aspects of the child's development (for example, when children are acquiring language or trying to increase their independence from their parents, either as toddlers or as adolescents) and they may also be a result of changes imposed by the child's environment or stage of life. Such life-stage transitions include entering child-care or school, changing from primary to secondary school, and getting a job and leaving home. In addition, certain life events such as moving to a new area, changing schools, and changes in family structure as a result of divorce, the birth of a sibling or the death of a family member also bring with them changes in various aspects of a child's life. How well children manage these changes is likely to be affected by the level and type of support they receive, the choice they have about making that transition, and the timing and spacing of those transitions and life events.

Risk, protection, vulnerability and resilience

One of the central questions in relation to developmental outcomes is how and why some individuals do well despite adversity and why others do poorly. Increasing attention is now focusing on the various risk and protective processes that children are exposed to, both in terms of their own characteristics and the features of their environment. At each level, various factors as well as significant life events and transitions can either increase vulnerability and the probability of an adverse outcome (*risk factors*) or reduce the risk or promote resilience and increase the probability of positive developmental outcomes (*protective factors*).

There is, however, no evidence that single risk factors by themselves lead to a negative outcome; rather, risk factors seem to interact, with a combined effect that is not simply additive but multiplicative. For example, Rutter's (1979) early study of children's adjustment difficulties found that an increase from *no* risk factors to *one* risk factor resulted in no increase in the incidence of these problems, but an increase from no risk factors to four to six risk factors resulted in a 20-fold increase. Bebbington and Miles (1989) provide a good example of the cumulative effect of risk in relation to the probability of children entering care in the UK. A combination of five factors – family structure (single parent), family size (four or more children), income level (low or welfare dependency), housing conditions (fewer rooms than people in the family) and ethnicity (white Anglo) – multiplied the risk of entering care from a 1 in 7000 chance for the most favourable combination to a 1 in 10 chance for the least favourable combination.

Furthermore, it may not be just the number and combined effect of various factors but their timing, both in terms of when they occur in the child's life and how closely they are spaced. While it may be possible to cope with one or two risk factors or adverse life events over a relatively long period, another 'event' or less spacing between them may provide the 'tipping point'. This may apply to transitions and other life events. A good example of an accumulation of risk, together with a number of transitions over a short period of time is evident in the circumstances of young people leaving out-of-home care. For many of these young people, their time in care is characterised by multiple placements and living arrangements, minimal security and stability, irregular contact with their family, and compromised educational achievement. They often face leaving 'care', leaving school, and having to learn to live independently with little, if any, financial or emotional support. Within a year or so of leaving care, many have seriously considered or attempted suicide and many of the young women have had one or more pregnancies. Those who do better tend to be those who have had greater stability in care, have continuing support from a member of their extended or foster family or have a supportive network at work or in a religious organisation and see some hope for their future (Cashmore and Paxman 1996).

Risk and protective mechanisms

The mechanisms by which risk factors and risky situations function to increase the probability of adverse outcomes is not yet clear. What is clear, however, is that negative outcomes are often not directly *caused* by the obvious risk factors. Some factors, for example, that appear to be associated with or predict later outcomes may operate as markers for or as proxies for other factors. For example, while a number of studies have found an association between family structure (single parents *versus* two-parent intact families) and children's academic performance and mental health problems, it appears that single parenthood *per se* does not 'cause' these poor outcomes. The underlying mechanism is likely to have more to do with the emotional distress, financial stress, residential mobility and reduced resources that are often associated with single parenthood and the effects of those factors on the parent and the parent–child relationship (Fergusson 1998; Silburn et al. 1996). There is, for example, considerable evidence that parents' warmth, consistency and responsiveness to their children often suffer as a result of the emotional and financial stress following separation (Dodge, Pettit and Bates 1994; Fergusson 1998; Sampson and Laub 1994). A more punitive and inconsistent approach to discipline is in turn a risk factor for children's behavioural and mental health problems. Thus, it is not necessarily single parenthood but the circumstances and the associated difficulties that may affect children's outcomes.

Adding to the complexity is the effect of further interactions involving protective factors and mechanisms. Indeed, Rutter (1990) argues that the effects of protective processes are 'apparent only by virtue of their interactions with the risk variable' (p 188). He outlined a number of ways in which protective processes may bolster children's resilience – by reducing the impact of the risk either by changing children's exposure to it or its meaning for them; by interrupting a negative chain reaction; by opening up positive opportunities, and by promoting the child's self-esteem and self-efficacy. Rutter suggested, for example, that the protective value of a child having a positive relationship with at least one parent may function in several ways. It may be that this positive relationship promotes the child's self-esteem and confidence in dealing with difficulties or that the presence of one positive relationship means that the overall level of discord within the family is less than it would otherwise be. Alternatively, it may mean that this parent actively works to protect the child from exposure to the discord and other difficulties within the family.

In summary, it seems that the 'children showing resilience are generally those who have been exposed to fewer risk factors for a shorter period of time' and/or protected by positive experiences or exposure to buffers or compensatory mechanisms (Rutter 2000b, p 670). What is clear then is that resilience – doing well against the odds – is not an individual characteristic but reflects a range of processes and the complex interplay of factors across a number of different levels (child, family, school, community and societal). While there is still much to learn about the way these processes work, the current understanding of development does provide some directions for policy and preventive interventions.

Table 15.1 Risk and protective factors for adverse outcomes for children

Child factors	Family factors	Community & social factors
Risk	**Risk**	**Risk**
• Prematurity • Low birth weight • Difficult temperament • Aggressiveness • Insecure attachment • Poor attention and impulsivity • Behaviour problems • Low self-esteem and self-efficacy • Poor problem-solving skills • Chronic illness • Disability	**Parental characteristics** • Teenage mothers • Substance abuse • Mental illness **Family environment** • Family structure • Low income/unemployment • Social isolation • Family violence • Intergenerational abuse • Criminality • Conflict **Parenting style** • Harsh, inconsistent discipline • Abuse or neglect • Lack of warmth • Lack of involvement • Inadequate supervision	• Socio-economic disadvantage • Long-term high unemployment • Poor social networks • Poorly serviced area • Income inequality – predicts violence • Ineffective public policies re children • No coherent focus on promoting well-being of children and young people
Protective • Easy temperament • Secure attachment • Intelligence • Social skills	**Protective** • Family coherence • Warm supportive relationship with child • Secure, stable care • Strong family norms	**Protective** • Strong social networks and community support • Access to support services • Cultural norms against violence

What does a developmental approach propose in relation to preventive intervention?

Despite the limits of current developmental research and knowledge, there are a number of promising strategies which may guide interventions to divert children from pathways leading to adverse outcomes to pathways that lead to more positive outcomes:

• Intervene early in life and early in the pathway.
• Aim at reducing the accumulation of risk at multiple levels (child, family, community, society).
• Use a coordinated approach that takes into account common risk and protective factors.

- Make any interventions acceptable and accessible to the participants, including the children and the young people themselves.
- Target transitions and prepare and support children and their families through transitions.
- Evaluate preventive interventions to learn what makes a difference and why.

Intervene early in life and early in the pathway

The first suggestion to intervene early – both early in life and early in the pathway – is based on the idea that it is easier to produce positive change before any negative effects are well-established and before the child progresses far down the path to one or more adverse outcomes, which may in turn cut off other options (Coie et al. 1993).

An emphasis on intervening *early in life* arises from concern about the impact of early experience on brain development and the 'biologically embedding' of behaviour and developmental health (Keating and Hertzman 1999). This is linked to notions of critical and sensitive periods in early development and suggests that particular experiences are crucial during these periods and have an impact on later development *'independent of intervening experience'* (Keating and Hertzman 1999, p 7). While there is evidence for critical early experiences for particular areas of development such as visual development, other areas show more plasticity and appear to be open to influence from various sources of vulnerability and resilience throughout childhood and even into adulthood. As Shonkoff et al. (2000) point out, however, there has as yet been no systematic testing of the 'earlier is better' hypothesis, and the 'best' times to intervene during the early years are likely to depend on the nature of the parent or child risk.

A focus on intervening *early in the pathway* and at particular transition points arises from concern about the cumulative effect of various life events and risk and protective factors on later development. The key here is to interrupt the chain of negative events and to divert the child from a pathway leading to an adverse outcome. For example, young children who have been subjected to physically abusive parenting are more likely than other children to misinterpret and react aggressively to the benign behaviour of others (Haskett and Kistner 1991). This means that they often provoke negative reactions from other adults and children, thereby setting up a chain of negative experience. Similarly, children's disruptive and aggressive behaviour may make it difficult for them to concentrate at school and to get along with their peers. This in turn may lead them to seek support in a deviant peer group and become involved in delinquent behaviour (Loeber et al. 1999). Intervention before such behaviour and ways of relating with others become established therefore has the potential to shift the odds and move the child from a deviant to a more positive pathway.

Aim at reducing the accumulation of risk at different levels

The evidence for the combined effect of risk factors being much greater than their individual effects indicates the need to prevent risk factors accumulating – both across levels (concurrently) and over time (Coie et al. 1993; Rutter 2000). While it may not be possible or desirable to intervene to modify some risk factors (eg, socio-economic status, parental intelligence), it may be possible to reduce the negative impact of these and other factors by enhancing the appropriate protective factors and promoting alternative pathways. One way of doing this is to build on the strengths of families rather than simply focusing on their weaknesses and problems. This is usually more effective when families are involved in making decisions about the intervention process and their part in it.

Reducing the accumulation of risk also means that early intervention or prevention programs need to focus on the risk and protective factors at more than one level. Working with children only is likely to be much less successful than a multi-level approach which also involves working with parents and families, and with the school and community. Indeed, Durlak's (1998) review of 1200 prevention studies found that the risk and protective factors associated with eight major adverse outcome areas (including school failure, teenage pregnancy and drug use) were not restricted to any one level but were spread across *all* levels of the ecological model (individual child, family, peer group, school and community). Furthermore, several comprehensive reviews have found that the more promising and successful prevention programs dealing with children's anti-social and difficult behaviour have offered a range of elements in multiple settings (home, child care centre, school) focusing on multiple levels (Durlak 1998; Yoshikawa 1994).

Use a coordinated approach that takes into account common risk and protective factors

There is increasing evidence that a number of risk and protective factors are common to a range of adverse developmental outcomes and social problems across fields that often deal with these problems separately (Coie et al. 1993). These include poor school performance, mental health problems in children and adolescents (including anxiety, depression and suicidality), juvenile crime, substance abuse, domestic violence, and teenage pregnancy. In particular, Durlak's (1998) review found that a number of risk factors were common to a range of maladaptive outcomes (such as school failure, teenage pregnancy, drug use and physical health), leading him to argue that:

> Categorical approaches to prevention that focuses [*sic*] on single domains of functioning should be expanded to more comprehensive programs with multiple goals. Future prevention programs, therefore, will need to be more multidisciplinary and collaborative ... Restricted funding for prevention creates artificial boundaries and turf battles among investigators who could otherwise be working cooperatively to achieve common goals. Prevention funding ... should permit researchers to combine interventions for different areas in innovative ways (eg, melding components that target drug use, physical and mental health, and academic performance) (Durlak 1998, p 518).

Interventions that are acceptable and accessible to the participants

Interventions that are not easily accessible to those they are trying to benefit or not able to keep participants engaged are unlikely to have a demonstrable effect. Families are unlikely, for example, to participate in a program or service which is labelled as 'crime prevention' or 'child abuse prevention' or which is seen to be overly intrusive and without direct benefit to them. They are also less likely to be willing to participate in a program which is imposed on them and where they have little say in the way it is run.

Because of the difficulty of predicting which children will go on to experience adverse outcomes, and the problem of labelling particular children as 'high risk', one approach is to use naturally occurring and non-stigmatising ecological niches such as child care centres and schools within high risk communities.

Another useful approach, where problems have already been identified, is to encourage families to participate in finding their own workable solutions using processes such as family group conferences and family decision-making. The efficacy of such approaches is now evident in a number of jurisdictions (Burford and Hudson 2000).

Target transitions

Transitions, as points of change, usually involve some uncertainty about the change and what is likely to happen, so they tend also to be times of openness to new information and assistance. Perhaps the most widely known and successful intervention programs focusing on one of the key transitions in family life, the birth of the first child, are the Elmira and Memphis home-visiting programs targeting first-time mothers (Olds, Henderson et al. 1998a; Olds, O'Brien et al. 1998b). The inclusion of these programs in Durlak and Wells (1997) meta-analysis of a range of prevention programs led them to conclude that transition programs targeting first-time mothers were 'among the most effective of all interventions' (p 142).

Evaluate preventive interventions to learn what makes a difference

Quality evaluation and research in relation to intervention programs is essential for several reasons. First, it is important in order to understand developmental processes and to learn what works for different children. It is not sufficient just to know whether an intervention works; it is also important to know how and why it works. This includes knowing how the intervention was implemented and what features of that process affected outcomes for particular groups of children. Ideally, research and rigorous evaluation studies should advance our understanding of the mechanisms and 'causal links' between the features of an intervention and the outcomes for children (Shonkoff and Phillips 2000, p 407). If it were possible to identify the key factors that influence child outcomes and those that are amenable to intervention, this would provide a very useful underpinning for good policy development and effective practice.

Second, good evaluations are needed to determine the most cost-effective means of intervening. This means translating research results into measures and findings that are useful to policy makers. It also means examining the efficacy of a program under optimal conditions (for example, good funding, skilled and trained staff) as well as its effectiveness under more typical conditions. Well-funded model demonstration projects that are found to be effective may not accurately reflect the way the program works when it is widely replicated with less adequate funding and less skilled personnel.

Rather than simply being used to determine whether particular projects and programs should receive on-going funding, a more constructive process might focus on 'what specific *actions* should be implemented to effectively utilise the available resources' (Scott, Mason, and Chapman 1999, p 1263). Research findings that are reported in terms of means and correlation coefficients do not, however, 'easily translate into indices of a reduction in the prevalence of a disorder, reduction in risk to an individual, or specific cost savings that policymakers desire'

(Scott, Mason and Chapman 1999, pp 1263–4). For example, a small and statistically insignificant change in group means may result in significant changes in the *proportion* of extreme cases where there are maladaptive or adverse outcomes for children. Conversely, while factors may be found to be highly significant statistically, they may explain only a small proportion of the variance; this may be partly because they include only the relatively easily measured proximal factors at the individual and family level rather than the more distal and less quantifiable factors at the community and societal levels.

Similarly, person-oriented analyses in which the *person* is the main focus are also needed to complement developmental psychology's usual *variable*-oriented analyses in order to provide a means of examining typical and atypical relationships between childhood factors and later patterns and clusters of outcomes (Magnusson and Bergman 1990). As Cichetti (1996, p 34) points out, a focus on group means and modal pathways is likely to 'overlook or obscure' important findings by missing the *patterns* that lead to similar-looking outcomes for children who have had different experiences (equifinality) and those that lead to different outcomes (vulnerability and resilience) despite apparently similar experiences (multifinality). By analysing the various clusters of outcomes, Magnusson and Bergman (1990) were, for example, able to show that aggression at age 13 did not predict officially recorded criminal offences and problems with alcohol in adulthood unless aggression was part of a syndrome of severe behaviour problems at the earlier age.

Ideally, evaluations should involve measures that are both qualitative and quantitative, that assess both the process and the outcomes, and that are both short-term and long-term across a range of outcome areas. One of the lessons from the long-term follow-up studies of Headstart and the Perry Pre-school Project is that there were benefits across a broad range of outcomes (greater stability in relationships, increased likelihood of completing secondary school, getting a better paid job, and reduced criminality) and after periods in which the benefits appeared to have faded. If the follow-up studies do not continue for long enough or measure a wide enough range of outcomes, then they will not be able to provide any evidence of long-term or broadly-based benefits as a result of the intervention. If process measures are not included, it will not be possible to assess whether the program was implemented as planned, and what aspects of the implementation made a difference (Tomison 2000).

In summary, the developmental approach to prevention is applicable to a range of 'social problem' areas. Indeed an important aspect of this approach is that it encourages a more coordinated approach to prevention, early intervention and to evaluation – what the Blair Government has called 'joined up solutions' to 'joined up problems'. The focus on pathways, on risk and protective factors as sources of vulnerability and resilience that are common to a number of adverse developmental outcomes and social problems provide some promising directions in the development of guidelines for preventive intervention.

Further Reading

Shonkoff, J P & Meisels, S J (Eds), Handbook of Early Childhood Intervention (2nd edition), Cambridge University Press, New York.

– A thorough and excellent overview of the theoretical and conceptual underpinnings of approaches to early intervention and an analysis of service delivery models and evaluation, with an excellent final chapter on resilience.

Shonkoff, J & Phillips, D (Eds) 2000, Committee on Integrating the Science of Early Childhood Development, Board on Children, Youth, and Families. 2000. From Neurons to Neighbourhoods: The science of early development. National Academy Press, Washington DC.

– An excellent summary of the core concepts of development, including an analysis of the recent neurological research on early brain development and the environmental influences and contexts of early development.

16

Health inequalities:
is the foundation for these laid before the time of birth?

Terry Dwyer, Ruth Morley and Leigh Blizzard

Introduction

Barker's original idea of the 'foetal origins' of cardiovascular disease (CVD) and chronic lung disease in adulthood relates to foetal under-nutrition in a malnourished mother. There is evidence suggesting that when the foetus receives an inadequate supply of nutrients, its growth is slowed and blood flow is redistributed preferentially towards the brain. It is hypothesised that these adaptions result in reduced weight at birth, and structural or metabolic adaptations that predispose the foetus to disease in adult life (Barker 1991).

Lower socio-economic status (SES) is associated with lower birth weight (Pattenden et al. 1999), and it has been suggested that the harmful effects of low SES on adult health may be mediated via a pathway involving foetal under-nutrition and low birth weight (Barker and Martin 1992). The implication is that preventive efforts aimed at reducing diseases of adults need to embrace measures to alleviate social inequalities in women of reproductive age

In this paper, we discuss the findings of our own research that suggest the link between social status and adult disease can be explained largely by differences in foetal development.

Health effects of low birth weight

There are now a very large number of studies that have shown that babies who are small at birth have a higher risk of adult cardiovascular disease (Leon et al. 1998) and diabetes (Hales 1997). The following data (table 16.1) from the Nurses Health Study in the United States (Rich-Edwards et al. 1997) demonstrate just how strong an effect this might be.

Risk factors for these diseases such as higher blood pressure and impaired glucose tolerance are also found more commonly among children and adults who were small at birth.

Table 16.1 Relative risk of non-fatal coronary heart disease to 1992 for 70,297 nurses who were full-term singleton births and who were recruited into the Nurses' Health Study in 1976 when aged 30–55 years

Relative risk, adjusted for	Birth weight (grams)					
	<2268	2268–2495	2496–3175	3176–3856	3857–4536	>4536
Age	1.36	1.22	0.99	1.00	0.97	0.75
Other risk factors	1.32	1.15	1.02	1.00	0.92	0.68

Note: Other risk factors = body mass index, cigarette smoking, reported hypertension, reported raised cholesterol, parental history of myocardial infarction to age 60, diabetes, menopausal status, use of postmenopausal hormones.

The association between low birth weight and SES

Could this apparent effect of low birth weight explain the known associations of SES with CVD and diabetes, and possibly with other diseases? The available evidence does show that low birth weight is more common in lower SES families.

For example, we have found that 30% of the occurrence of low birth weight (defined as less than 2500g) in a sample of British children can be attributed to the effects of social inequality. These subjects were 921 children recruited into two large infant nutrition studies (Lucas et al. 1999; Lucas and Morley personal communication) and randomised to bottle-feeding or to the breast-feeding 'control' arm. Whilst not representative of their source population, extensive social and demographic data on these children were collected by maternal self-report, including information on maternal education, social class and maternal smoking during pregnancy. Birth weight was significantly related to both maternal education and social class, and to maternal smoking during pregnancy (table 16.2).

Smoking, which was strongly associated with lower birth weight, was also more prevalent in mothers with less educational attainment and with lower social class (table 16.3).

There are two main possibilities here. The first is that low birth weight occurs more frequently as an effect of exposures, in particular to smoking, that are more common in some social environments. The second is that smoking explains part but not all of the effect, and there are other – not so easily defined – effects of social deprivation that also lead to lower birth weight.

To investigate whether maternal education and social class affect birth weight independently of maternal smoking, each of these factors was included in the same linear regression model using the UK data. The results are shown in table 16.4. The significant association between social class and birth weight remained after adjustment for smoking. Women from lower social class families were more likely to have smaller babies than women from higher social class families, even if they did not smoke.

When data for non-smoking women were analysed separately, we found that birth weight of their offspring fell by 37 {95%CI 6, 67} grams with each decrease in social class category after adjusting for sex and gestation.

Table 16.2 The effect of a unit change in maternal education, social class and maternal smoking on birth weight of 921 children in two studies of infant nutrition in the United Kingdom

Factor	Change in birth weight (g)
	Change {95% CL}
Maternal educational attainment (per category)	38 {11, 66}
Social class (per category)	−42 {−63, −21}
Mother smoked during pregnancy	−220 {−298, −143}

Notes: Change {95% CL} = regression coefficient adjusted for sex and gestational age {95% confidence limits}. Maternal educational attainment = 5-point scale where 5 = university degree or higher and otherwise based on results in nationally standardised examinations up to age 18 (1 = no examinations passed), with n = 915. Social class = Registrar General's classification of the 'breadwinner's' occupation where social class 1 includes all professionals and social class 5 unskilled manual workers, with n = 899. Mother smoked during pregnancy = (0/1) binary variable based on maternal self-report of prenatal smoking.

Table 16.3 The association between maternal education, social class and maternal smoking in pregnancy for the mothers of UK children

Maternal education	N	Percentage of smokers	Social class	N	Percentage of smokers
1 (Low)	144	50%	1 (High)	101	4%
2	71	40%	2	173	10%
3	434	23%	3N	87	15%
4	89	9%	3M	325	34%
5 (High)	177	6%	4	118	38%
			5 (Low)	38	47%
			Unclassified	57	51%
Chi-squared test of proportions		P<0.001	X test of proportions		P<0.001

Notes: Maternal educational attainment = 5-point scale where 5 = university degree or higher and otherwise based on results in nationally standardised examinations up to age 18 (1 = no examinations passed). Social class = Registrar General's classification of the 'breadwinner's' occupation. Social class 1 includes all professionals and social class 5 unskilled manual workers (3N = non-manual, 3M = manual). The category of unclassified included unemployed persons, students and others not included in the workforce.

Evidently there are modifiable risk factors for low birth weight in poorer families, such as smoking, but other factors must be at work as well. These other factors may include maternal nutrition, availability of financial support to enable the mother to stop paid work and even home duties during pregnancy, and access to antenatal care.

We used some Australian data to further explore the possibility of an independent effect

Table 16.4 The effect of female sex, gestation, maternal education, social class and maternal smoking on birth weight of children in two large infant nutrition studies in the UK after adjustment for each of the other factors

Factor	Change in birth weight (g)
	Change {95% CL}
Female sex	−95 {−164, −26}
Gestation (per week)	238 {214, 263}
Maternal educational attainment (per category)	−6 {−39, 27}
Social class (per category)	−28 {−53, −3}
Mother smoked during pregnancy	−187 {−271, −103}

Notes: Change {95% CL} = regression coefficient adjusted for all other factors {95% confidence limits}. Maternal educational attainment = 5-point scale where 5 = university degree or higher and otherwise based on results in nationally standardised examinations up to age 18 (1 = no examinations passed), with n = 915. Social class = Registrar General's classification of the 'breadwinner's' occupation where social class 1 includes all professionals and social class 5 unskilled manual workers, with n = 899. Mother smoked during pregnancy = (0/1) binary variable based on maternal self-report of prenatal smoking.

of SES (see table 16.5). The subjects were children in the Tasmanian Infant Health Survey. Included in that survey were all infants born of multiple pregnancies, and approximately one in every five infants born of singleton pregnancies, in Tasmania during 1988–95. The singleton born infants were selected using a scoring system (D'Espaignet et al. 1990) based on six risk factors for sudden infant death syndrome (young maternal age, male sex, low birth weight, autumn or winter season of birth, maternal intention to bottle-feed, and duration of second stage labour). Those with a composite score over a cut-off point were eligible for inclusion. Infant data on the children were obtained on three occasions (a hospital interview at day four of life, a home visit during the fifth postnatal week, and at telephone interview at 10 weeks of age), but only the at-birth data are used here. The analysis was restricted to the children born in 1988 or 1989 and living in southern Tasmania in 1996 or 1997 because they have been followed up to 8 years by us in a recent study of blood pressure (Dwyer et al. 1999).

The UK data on social class were based on occupation, and we used the reports by the Tasmanian mothers of the usual occupation of herself and of the current occupation of the baby's father at the time of birth to obtain roughly comparable information. The data for occupation were coded using the Australian Standard Classification of Occupations (Australian Bureau of Statistics 1986). Using the first digit of these classifications gave an 8-point scale from 1 (managers and administrators) to 8 (labourers and related workers), to which we added a ninth category for unemployed persons, pensioners and students. The linear regression results were adjusted for gestational age and for the selection factors that determined eligibility for inclusion in the survey. As noted above, those selection factors included maternal age and the mothers' stated intention at the time of the birth to bottle-feed rather than breast-feed.

Table 16.5 shows that birth weight was estimated to be higher in the offspring of more highly educated mothers and parents in skilled occupations. Mothers who smoked during

Table 16.5 The effect of maternal education, parental occupation and maternal smoking on birth weight of children in two year-of-birth cohorts of the Tasmanian Infant Health Survey

Factor	Change in birth weight (g)	
	Adjusted	**Adjusted also for prenatal smoking**
	Change {95% CL}	**Change {95% CL}**
Maternal education (per category)	80 {30, 131}	59 {9, 109}
Maternal occupation (per category)	−36 {−58, −14}	−29 {−51, −7}
Paternal occupation (per category)	−19 {−32, −6}	−14 {−27, −2}
Mother smoked during pregnancy	−235 {−302, −168}	

Notes: Change {95% CL} = regression coefficient {95% confidence limits}. Adjusted = adjusted for gestational age (weeks) and cohort selection factors (maternal age, sex, month of birth, intention to breast-feed, duration of second stage labour). Maternal education = primary to year 6 (1), some secondary (2), completed secondary to year 12 (3), attended university of other tertiary institution (4), with n = 865. Occupation = managerial (1), professional (2), paraprofessional (3), trades (4), clerical (5), sales and service (6), plant and machinery operators (7), labourers (8), unemployed, pensioners and students (9), with n = 543 (maternal occupation) or n = 851 (paternal occupation). Househusbands (n = 3) and housewives (n = 325) were excluded. Mother smoked during pregnancy = (0/1) binary variable based on maternal self-report of prenatal smoking, with n = 868.

pregnancy had smaller babies, and the result of adjusting for maternal smoking was to diminish but not eliminate the associations of birth weight with maternal education and parental occupation.

Adjusting the measured association between birth weight and maternal prenatal smoking for maternal education reduced the estimated difference in birth weight of children whose mothers smoked during pregnancy to −219 {−287, −152} grams.

Is low birth weight a cause of disease or a marker of low SES?

Is it possible that there is no true causal link between low birth weight and disease, but there appears to be because low SES causes disease and low SES families are more likely to have low birth weight infants?

We addressed this question in a relatively novel way using data collected on twins (Dwyer et al. 1999) in the Tasmanian Infant Health Survey. The analyses made use of a unique feature of twins – that they shared the same uterus – to test hypotheses about maternally related causes of the inverse association between birth weight and blood pressure. This was done by calculating the differences in birth weight and in blood pressure for each twin pair, and testing whether the within-pair differences were associated. Twins have most commonly been used as subjects to separate environmental from genetic causes, and we took the opportunity to examine this as well.

When the observations on our 55 pairs of eight-year-olds were treated as if they were unpaired, we observed a strong inverse association between birth weight and blood pressure (a 7mm Hg fall in systolic blood pressure for each 1kg increase in birth weight). This should have been reduced on within-pair analysis for both dizygotic and monozygotic pairs if maternal factors were confounding the relationship, and in monozygotic pairs if genes were responsible. In fact, the estimated association was little changed on pairing. Our study lacked power to rule out chance, but another twin study (Poulter et al. 1999) published in the same edition of the British Medical Journal on 492 pairs of adult female twins obtained the same result.

We concluded from this that factors associated with each individual twin itself – located somewhere in the foetoplacental unit – were responsible for the association between blood pressure and birth weight.

Supporting our conclusions is the analysis of the US Nurses Study (Rich-Edwards et al. 1997) referred to at the beginning of this paper. The authors had shown that birth weight predicted coronary heart disease in adults (see table 16.1). They found that adjusting for socio-economic factors made little difference to the association, again suggesting that it is something connected to birth weight that was causing the disease. The association of coronary heart disease with birth weight appears not to have arisen merely because birth weight is associated with low SES.

Further Reading

Kramer, M S 2000, Invited commentary: association between restricted fetal growth and adult chronic disease: is it causal? Is it important? American Journal of Epidemiology 152: 605–8.
  – *Discusses confounding by socio-economic status in the context of questioning whether the association between size at birth and adult disease is causal.*
Kuh, D, Ben-Shlomo, Y (Eds) 1997, A Life Course Approach to Chronic Disease Epidemiology, Oxford University Press, Oxford.
  – *Another perspective about how exposures relevant to adult disease differ in each stage of life.*
Vågerö, D, Koupilová, I, Leon, DA, Lithell, U-B 1999, Social determinants of birthweight, ponderal index and gestational age in Sweden in the 1920s and 1980s, Acta Paediatrica 88: 445–53.
  – *Explores the socio-economic factors associated with low birth weight.*

17
How social factors affect health:
neuroendocrine interactions

Kerin O'Dea and Mark Daniel

Introduction

Hierarchy is associated with health. Resolving what it is about hierarchy that influences health has important implications for health and social policy. Large gradients in health status and life expectancy by income level, education and occupation were repeatedly observed in various parts of the developed world in the 20th century (Antonovsky 1967; Cassel 1976; Marmot and McDowell 1986; van der Meer and Mackenbach 1998). Income, education, and occupation indicators are interrelated and, individually and in various combinations, have been used to measure socioeconomic status (SES). That associations between SES and morbidity and mortality are found for *each* indicator suggests some underlying primary causal process, correlated with relative social position, which expresses itself through pathways of health and disease.

Much research has targeted a better understanding of health disparities. Disease incidence, mental illness, morbidity and mortality have been shown to vary between groups rated, in terms of SES, as more or less 'advantaged' or 'disadvantaged.' Multiple studies have generated strikingly similar conclusions about the reduced life expectancy, greater frequency of chronic disease, and greater prevalence of behavioural and affective disorders for disadvantaged versus advantaged groups (Bennett 1995; Fiscella and Franks 1997; Lantz et al. 1998; Shouls et al. 1996).

That low-SES groups are characterised by obesity, poor diet and physical inactivity, and are deprived of adequate medical care and exposed to environmental pollutants, crowding, sub-standard housing, violence, and infection does not fully explain the relationship between SES and health. *Risk factors* (eg, poor diet, physical inactivity, or obesity) and *risk conditions* (eg, social, or living, conditions) differ by level of SES in their distribution and relationship to health. An underlying causal determinant of the relationship between SES and health appears to operate across the entire range of SES. It has become clear that the impact of SES on health is *not* a threshold effect due to poverty, but is a graded effect across the social hierarchy (hence the term 'social gradient') (Adler et al. 1994).

The Whitehall study (which takes advantage of the ranked grades of employment in the

British civil service) is probably the most telling of the studies examining the social gradient in health outcome. Compared to the top administrators, the relative risk of mortality over 10 years was 1.6 for the professional–executive grades, 2.2 for the clerical grades, and 2.7 for the unskilled workers (Marmot et al. 1984). A 25-year follow up of civil servants from the first Whitehall study indicated that differentials in mortality persist at older ages for almost all causes of death (van Rossum et al. 2000). Other studies indicate that there is a social gradient in infant mortality, which parallels that of total mortality (Martuzzi et al. 1998).

In the remainder of this paper we focus on the possible mechanisms of the social gradient in health, beginning with a discussion of behavioural factors, before moving on to a discussion of the psychosocial factors and the possible biological pathways that could plausibly mediate their impacts on health.

Behaviours affecting health

Coronary heart disease (CHD) is a major cause of death in western societies and its aetiology has been the subject of intensive study for over 50 years. Yet the three major risk factors for CHD (smoking, elevated plasma cholesterol levels, and hypertension) explain less than half of the variance in mortality associated with CHD. Cohort studies have found that SES differentials in health status persist despite improvements in health behaviour among low SES groups (Bennett 1995; Lantz et al. 1998). Overall, known risk factors account for just part of the morbidity (Brunner et al. 1997; Lynch et al. 1996) and mortality (Davey Smith et al. 1990; Lantz et al. 1998) associated with SES. Statistical adjustments that 'control' for common behavioural risk factors do not significantly attenuate or otherwise 'explain' the SES-health gradient (Lundberg 1991; North et al. 1993; Stronks et al. 1997).

While behaviours such as cigarette smoking, physical inactivity, poor diet, and substance abuse cannot fully explain the SES–health relationship, they are not irrelevant, being closely linked both to SES and health outcome. Further, they are the most proximal influences on health outcome, amenable to public health and medical intervention at the individual level, and important in their own right.

Cigarette smoking is strongly linked to SES. For example, in the Whitehall II study smoking rates for men in the lowest employment grades were four times higher than those for men in the highest grade (33.6% versus 8.3%). The gradient in smoking was not as steep or as consistent among the women civil servants, with those in the highest grade smoking more than those in the grade immediately below them (Marmot et al. 1991).

Physical inactivity is one of the major determinants of obesity, and both are linked inversely to SES. Results from the Whitehall II study (Martikainen and Marmot 1998) indicate not only differences in body mass index (BMI) across employment grade, but increasing differentials over time (ie, those in the lower employment grades were more overweight at baseline and then gained weight more rapidly over time). Furthermore, in addition to being more overweight, those in the lower employment grades had a more central distribution of body fat, which is a well-established independent risk factor for a cluster of chronic diseases (most notably Type 2 diabetes and cardiovascular disease). The possible role of psychosocial factors in mediating the deposition of intra-abdominal fat via stimulation of the hypothalamic-pituitary-adrenal axis is discussed in more detail below.

Poor quality diet may also contribute to the social gradient in health. Using a seven-day diet diary to assess dietary intake in a stratified random sub-sample of the Whitehall II study, Stallone et al. (1997) concluded that type and amount of dietary fat did not appear to be protective. However, intakes of vitamin C and potassium (surrogates for vegetable and fruit intakes) were strongly linked to employment grade. Consistent with this hypothesis that diets low in fresh vegetables and fruit could contribute to the poorer health outcomes for those in the lower employment grades, Bobák et al. (1998) concluded that low intakes of dietary antioxidants could play a role in the high rates of CHD in the Czech Republic. The low standardised mortality rates in people who have migrated to Australia from southern Europe are also consistent with a protective role of diets rich in vegetables and fruit (Mediterranean diets are rich sources of antioxidants from high intakes of plants foods and olive oil) (O'Dea and Walker 1995).

Alcohol shows an opposite pattern, with higher intakes in those of higher SES. Interpretation of these data is more complex, as alcohol abuse has adverse health outcomes, but moderate alcohol consumption may have health benefits (McCarty 2000).

Psychosocial factors

In seeking to explain the primary basis of the social gradient in health, attention is now focusing on the role of social position in relation to psychosocial characteristics such as depression, hostility and perceived psychological stress, all of which are clearly linked to various measures of SES and health outcomes (Ickovics et al. 1997). We use the term 'psychosocial' broadly, in keeping with the social gradient having to do with hierarchy as affecting health through relative rather than absolute deprivation. This is a psychosocial conceptualisation that implies the circumstances in which people live and work could affect health via psychological pathways according to where individuals are situated in terms of their social position. This emotionally-oriented perspective preferences subjective feelings over objective instrumental supports (eg, the number of friends or social supports one may have). While we have separated our discussion of behavioural from psychosocial factors, this distinction is for the benefit of exposition only. Health-related behaviours and psychosocial factors are intimately connected, and capable of influencing health status both independently and together through their interaction (Marmot et al. 1998).

Depression
Depression, both as a pathological state (major, or clinical depression) and as general depressive symptoms, is inversely related to SES. A classic study in a Canadian community-based sample found a more than six-fold higher prevalence of major depression in the low versus high SES groups, and over the subsequent 16 years, the incidence of new cases showed the same marked SES differential (Murphy et al. 1991). Further, the Whitehall II study documented the existence of an inverse gradient between depression and employment grade

(Stansfeld et al. 1998). In community-residing men and women aged 62 and older, depression predicted declines in self-efficacy perceptions of domains of living, including family relationships, relationships with friends, living arrangements, and financial, safety and transportation domains (McAvay et al. 1996). In this study, while demographic factors were predictive of decline for some domains of living, the most constant predictor of decline was depression.

Depression is related to multiple adverse health outcomes, particularly increasing the risk of CHD as well as suicide (Barefoot and Schroll 1996). A systemic review of controlled studies assessing depressive symptoms and disorders in relation to death rates between 1966 and 1996 found that suicide accounted for less than 20% of deaths in psychiatric samples, and less than 1% in medical and community samples (Wulsin et al. 1999). The same study also found that, besides increasing risk of death by unnatural causes, depression substantially increases risk of death by CHD but not cancer (for reasons unknown). In persons surviving an acute myocardial infarction (MI), depression in hospital after MI is a significant predictor of one-year cardiac mortality in women (odds ratio (OR) = 3.3, 95% confidence interval (CI): 1.0–10.6) and well as for men (OR = 3.1, 95% CI: 1.3–7.2), and its impact is largely independent of other post-MI risks (Fraser-Smith et al. 1999).

In persons hospitalised for CHD, social support assessed during hospitalisation is negatively associated with depressive symptoms one month after discharge, while hostility is an indirect predictor of post-discharge depressive symptomology by way of its negative relation with social support (Brummett et al. 1998). Such findings point to the interaction of depression with other affective states and more contextual factors.

Hostility

Defined as angry, antagonistic, cynical, distrusting behaviours and attitudes, hostility is strongly inversely related to SES measured by level of education, occupation or income (Barefoot et al. 1991; Caroll et al. 1997; Kubzansky et al. 1999). Numerous prospective studies have demonstrated strong links between hostility and risk of CHD (Barefoot et al. 1995; Miller et al. 1996). Situational (Porter et al. 1999) and contextual (Gump et al. 1999) factors play an important role in anger expression. On-going exposure to challenging life experiences associated with low SES can lead to the development of a hostile response pattern (Kivimaki et al. 1998), and it has been suggested that the association between SES and health might be partially mediated by hostility (Pincus and Callahan 1995; Seeman and McEwen 1996).

An analysis of data from a 22-year mortality follow-up of 750 men (from the Western Collaborative Group Study) showed that, both in interaction with and separately from hostility, social dominance (defined in terms of verbal competition, immediateness of response, and fast speaking rate) was positively related to mortality (Houston et al. 1997). These relations held after controlling for diastolic blood pressure, total cholesterol, and smoking status. A pattern of characteristics of individuals neither hostile nor socially dominant was significantly negatively related to mortality. These results are important, because characteristics of social dominance are more highly correlated with self-reported dominance than outwardly directed, expressive, hostility.

Psychological stress

Both exposure to, and experience of, stressful events and circumstances may contribute importantly to the social gradient in health outcome. Exposure to major life events requiring substantial adaptation (death of a loved one, job loss, etc.) is well recognised as increasing the risk of a range of adverse health outcomes, including CHD. It is the perception of stress to the individual, however, which is increasingly recognised as a critical factor in linking psychological stress to ill health: the subjective perception that demands exceed one's capacity to cope (Stansfeld et al. 1995). It is in this key area of coping skills and cognition where the differential impact of SES and social hierarchies is most pronounced (Taylor et al. 1997). There are wide individual as well as gender and cultural differences in personal characteristics that influence one's response to life events (one person's insuperable barrier is another's exciting challenge) (Kaplan 1992; Muecke 1994). There is little doubt, though, that those lower down the SES scale are less likely to have acquired the coping skills and social support networks (through family example, educational or occupation experience) to buttress them through stressful times. As a result of fewer material and personal resources, those individuals at lower levels of SES can experience greater vulnerability to stressful exposures, which can itself both contribute to and exacerbate further stressful events (Gump et al. 1999).

Social position

Social position, through social hierarchy, is associated with health (Evans et al. 1994). This has obvious implications for health in terms of the absolute impact of income and material comforts, as well as more complex, relative effects. One of the more intriguing observations to emerge from the Whitehall study is that position in the social hierarchy, *independent of income or educational disadvantage*, is a major determinant of health outcome (Marmot et al. 1984; van Rossum et al. 2000). British civil servants employed at professional–executive levels (well-remunerated and highly educated, often in high-status professions such as law or medicine) had a higher mortality than their immediate superiors the top administrators, and so it went on down the line. The Whitehall study demonstrated evidence of the effect of employment grade on health at each level of the social hierarchy, where individuals with the highest grade had better health than those just below them, who, in turn, had better health than those below them did.

What is it about hierarchy that has such a profound impact on health? That relations between SES and morbidity and mortality have been found for each indicator of SES (education, occupation and income) suggests some underlying primary causal process which expresses itself through pathways of disease. The particular diseases to which illness and death are attributed may then be alternative pathways to, rather than the 'causes' of, outcomes determined by the underlying causal mechanism. This position is supported by the persistence of the gradient between social class and mortality in Great Britain over most of the 20th century (Black et al. 1988; Office of Population Censuses and Surveys 1978). The gradient changed little over time, despite major changes in the causes of death from infectious diseases to heart disease and cancer.

Insights about the effect of hierarchy on health can be gained from studies in experimental animals. In studies of wild baboons, Sapolsky and Mott (1987) reported lower levels of high-density lipid (HDL) cholesterol, a marker of CHD risk, in subordinate relative to dominant male animals living in a socially stable group. This changed under conditions of social instability (threat to dominance). More recent work with baboons points, however, to the dynamic relationship between behaviour and hierarchy, where particular behavioural styles may attenuate the endocrine indices of stress among low-ranking animals (Virgin and Sapolsky 1997). Related work with rats also supports the need for a detailed behavioural analysis to undertake meaningful biological evaluation of stress-induced immune changes, because different coping strategies result in different immunological consequences (Stefanski 1998).

An example of the effect of social instability in humans is provided by gay men who are particularly sensitive to social rejection, where accelerated HIV progression is not observed in men who conceal homosexual identity, suggesting that concealment as a way to maintain social position may protect such individuals from negative health effects (Cole et al. 1997). Lack of social integration in gay and bisexual men is associated with more rapid decline in immune function relative to those more socially integrated (Miller et al. 1997). There is no consistent evidence in humans, however, that integration in the social hierarchy affects the incidence of disease, although social isolation and unstable social interactions can result in lower immune function and accelerated neuroendocrine and cardiovascular activity associated with disease outcomes (Seeman 1996).

Studies with female macaques who, like women, are resistant to atherosclerosis, have found that this resistance is modified by social dominance, whereby subordinate females resemble males in the size of atherosclerotic lesion that develops, and are characterised by hypercortisolaemia, behavioural dysfunction, and impaired ovarian function (Kaplan JR et al. 1996). Similar results have been reported in other primate studies (Cameron 1997). Manuck and co-workers (1988) observed decreased coronary atherosclerosis in socially dominant cynomolgus macaques, but only under socially stable conditions. Under conditions of unpredictable but recurrent threats to their dominance, dominant animals had more atherosclerosis than submissive ones. This adverse effect of unstable social conditions on the development of atherosclerosis in dominant macaques was reversed by the administration of propanolol – a beta-adrenergic antagonist, a response that is discussed below. These data provide clues to the biological pathways mediating the health impacts of social hierarchies, but also indicate that the adverse health outcomes are a consequence, rather than a cause, of social status.

Neuroendocrine aspects of the social gradient

All illnesses have a biopsychosocial component to their causes and effects. We take for granted that stressors and 'stress', a state of threatened homeostasis, reestablished by a complex repertoire of *physiologic* and *behavioural* adaptive *responses* of the organism (Chrousos 1998), can make you sick. So, too, that social injustices, racial inequities, and status disparities contribute to stress, and hence stress-related illnesses, and are present in disease outcomes. But how does stress 'make you sick'? And how do social and status inequalities or disparities make you stressed (Taylor and Repetti 1997), and hence 'sicker' (Brunner 1997)?

There are varying approaches to an understanding of stress and its consequences, but in all approaches there is agreement on the central role of discomforting life situations, sociocultural background and rapid environmental change (including social, cultural and economic shifts) in the occurrence of stress-related outcomes. The body of research on stress and health dates back more than 70 years. Pioneers studying the biopsychosocial pathways of stress responses include both Cannon (1929) and Selye (1956) who linked stress with sympathetic and pituitary adrenocortical stimulation respectively. More recent work, targeting understanding of the interrelations between stress, health and contextual or social environments, owes its development to these earlier contributions.

The biological pathways mediating psychosocial influences on health emanate from the central nervous system (CNS), the source of the organism's perceptions of, and responses to, the external world. In considering such biopsychosocial pathways, it is useful to introduce the concept of allostasis: the altered response of the organism to challenge that enables it to function in the face of increased demand (Sterling and Eyer 1988). The basis of this concept is that the body does *not* conserve the same metabolic status and regulate strict homeostasis. Rather, the autonomic nervous system, the hypothalamic-pituitary-adrenocortical (HPA) axis and the metabolic, cardiovascular and immune systems attempt to achieve homeostasis by establishing a new metabolic equilibrium at an entirely different series of set points. Allostatic load is the cumulative 'cost' of accommodating stress through allostasis (McEwen 1998) whereby prolonged, on-going activation of the HPA axis by environmental challenges leads to maladaptive changes in regulatory systems (Chrousos and Gold 1992, McEwen and Stellar 1993, Seeman et al. 1997).

The empirical relationship between SES, psychosocial factors and allostatic load has been established only recently (Checkley 1996; Kubzansky et al. 1999; Seeman et al. 1996; Stansfeld et al. 1998). It draws, however, upon a solid foundation of research by another pioneer in research on the physiology of stress, James Henry, who conducted creative and perceptive work in this field until his death in 1996. Together with others in the field, Henry and co-workers developed an integrated hypothesis to explain how a range of psychosocial influences affect health and disease risk (Henry and Wang 1998).

Their thesis is that the right brain controls the positive 'species preservative' behaviours of animals living in social groups, including humans. Oxytocin has been identified as the primary hormone stimulating affiliative behaviour (maternal, social, sexual) between parents and offspring and between individuals within groups. A number of stages of the neuroendocrine response to stress are described using a classic inverse 'U' shaped relation between challenge and performance. All forms of response to effort show the same flattening of the curve as the limits of response are reached. Beyond a point, despite continuing increase in effort, further demand is met by falling performance ('burnout'). The slope of the curve varies, however, between individuals. Those with the healthiest response to stress – due to genetic inheritance and/or differences in early life experiences – have a steeper curve than those with an impaired response to stress (flatter, and with limit to performance reached earlier).

A set of predictable hormonal changes accompanies this 'challenge–performance' relationship. Early in the process, the individual responds to a stimulus that may be perceived as a threat to control by stimulating the sympathetic-adrenal-medullary system. Norepinephrine (the 'fight' hormone) rises during this phase, as does testosterone. At this early stage, there is no loss of activity of the oxytocinergic system, and positive immune system responses may be observed. It is therefore the classic 'species-preservative' activity, also referred to as 'healthy stress'.

If the stress stimulus persists, it may be accompanied by uncertainty over control. As status and control are increasingly challenged, there is a falling off of the 'species-preservative' activity, with falls in the gonadotrophins and oxytocin, and an increase in the 'self-preservative' activity. With the perception that loss of control is possible, and as the threat develops, that it is probable, *anxiety* becomes the predominant emotion associated with increasing production of the 'flight' hormone epinephrine, and cortisol concentrations increase. Self-esteem may, however, modulate (buffer) patterns of neuroendocrine response to cognitive challenges in daily life (Seeman et al. 1995).

Further along the 'challenge–performance' continuum, there is an increasing sense of helplessness and loss of control as fatigue and exhaustion are approached. This is associated with activation of the hypothalamic-pituitary-adrenal (HPA) axis, and the oxytocin-gonadotrophic 'species-preservative' system shuts down. By this stage there has been a shift from active defence to a passive non-aggressive coping style, with the emphasis on 'self-preservation'. For example, in rhesus monkeys experimentally inoculated with the simian immunodeficiency virus, changes in housing, particularly those involving social separations, are associated with shorter survival times, with housing disruptions occurring earlier after inoculation associated with the shortest survival times (Capitanio and Lerche 1998).

Henry and Wang (1998) suggest that self-preservation is associated with left hemispheric brain function and that species-preservation is associated with right hemispheric function. They speculate that extreme stress during infancy and early life may create insecure attachment (suppression of the oxytocinergic system), and result in a permanent bias towards self-preservative behaviour (poor social interaction). This manifests as a hostile personality, quick to anger, suspicious of the motives of others. Children who demonstrate psychobiological reactivity experience greater rates of respiratory illness (Boyce et al. 1995c) and school absence due to illness (Johnston-Brooks et al. 1998) than less reactive children given adverse conditions and exposure to stressors. Such individuals can demonstrate impaired corticoid responses as adults (Boyce et al. 1995c; Carlson and Earls 1997). Further, it is proposed that the coronary Type A behaviour pattern may be related to such a deficit (Henry and Wang 1998).

Environmental influences on foetal and neonatal development are thought to effect long-term alterations in the function of the sympathodrenal system that may contribute to the development in adulthood of the constellation of disorders variously referred to as 'the insulin resistance syndrome', 'syndrome X', or the 'metabolic syndrome' (Young and Morrison 1998). Numerous studies have indicated a relationship between low birth weight (LBW) and increased risk of chronic lifestyle-related conditions including Type 2 diabetes and cardiovascular disease in later life (Barker 1994). LBW has also been associated with centralised distribution of body fat and insulin resistance in adult life. These associations are consistent with a relationship between reduced foetal growth and the insulin resistance syndrome in later life. Whilst the mechanism is not yet fully understood, studies in both humans and experimental animals indicate that elevated activity of the HPA axis may mediate these associations. Phillips et al. (1998) have recently reported an inverse relation between birth weight and plasma cortisol concentrations in adult life for men born between 1920 and 1930 in Hertfordshire, UK. This is consistent with data from much more rigorous studies in rats showing that foetal growth retardation induced by dexamethasone leads to permanently greater activity of the HPA axis, with elevated circulating levels of corticosterone and hypertension in the adult animals (Benediktsson et al. 1993).

Hormones are key regulators of gene expression throughout the body, and the actions of hormones on the brain are instrumental in shaping sex differences and in determining the effects of stress on brain function. Key brain areas, such as the hippocampus, are essential to the processing of information that affects how an individual adapts to and responds to potential stressful life events, including social stress (Schulkin et al. 1994; Tidey and Miczek 1996). The response of the brain to chronic stress through control of endocrine, autonomic, and immunologic function (Cirulli et al. 1998; Flugge et al. 1997) determines the degree of allostatic load an organism will experience. Allostatic load, in turn, interacts with genetic susceptibility to influence health outcomes (McEwen 1997). This is thought to be how CNS-mediated effects influence the positive graded relation between breadth of exposure to abuse or household dysfunction during childhood and the presence in adults of multiple health risk factors (alcoholism, depression, smoking, drug abuse, physical inactivity, and obesity) and disease (CHD, cancer, lung disease, and liver disease) (Felitti et al. 1998).

Health consequences of excessive stimulation of the HPA axis

Per Björntorp has argued for many years that central obesity and other manifestations of the insulin resistance syndrome such as Type 2 diabetes and cardiovascular disease have a neuroendocrine basis (cf. Björntorp 1999). Low SES is linked to high waist/hip ratio (WHR) (Rosmond et al. 1996), and the Whitehall II study showed unequivocally that for both men and women there is a strong inverse social gradient in the prevalence of the insulin resistance syndrome, as well as in WHR (Brunner et al. 1997). These findings of the Whitehall II study, and the fact that health-related behaviours accounted for little of the social patterning of the prevalence of the insulin resistance syndrome, suggest that the insulin resistance syndrome itself may contribute to the biological explanation of the social gradient in CHD risk.

There is abundant evidence that insulin resistance and its associated abnormalities are major risk factors for CHD, and insulin resistance is likely to be an important component of the greatly elevated risk of cardiovascular disease associated with Type 2 diabetes (Reavan 1988). Most research on this topic has focused on the pathogenesis of insulin resistance, searching for a genetic basis. Particular metabolic defects have been shown in muscle and liver tissues (cf. Björntorp 1999): poor insulin activation of glycogen synthase in skeletal muscle; elevated mobilisation of free fatty acids (FFA); muscle fibre types and/or capillarisation; and resistance to insulin suppression of hepatic glucose production. Despite intensive research, however, functional genetic defects have not been established for any of these candidate pathways. Acquired determinants of insulin resistance are age, abdominal obesity, physical inactivity, smoking and hypertension.

Only recently, and due in large part to the persistence of the highly respected Björntorp and co-workers, have increasing numbers of researchers in the diabetes/CVD fields begun to take seriously the possibility that the insulin resistance syndrome and its adverse sequelae may be related to over activity of the HPA axis, secondary to psychosocial stress. This possibility has strong biological plausibility.

Early work by Björntorp and others on a neuroendocrine role in the insulin resistance syndrome built on similarities observed between the clinical features (anthropometric, metabolic and endocrine) of visceral adiposity and mild–moderate Cushing's syndrome. For example, hypercortisolism in Cushing's syndrome is associated with enlargement of the abdominal but not gluteofemoral fat depots in women (Rebuffé-Scrive et al. 1988). Persons with Cushing's syndrome have higher levels of subcutaneous abdominal fat by a factor of two and greater levels of intra-abdominal fat by a factor of five in comparison to matched controls (Mayo-Smith et al. 1989). Further, administration of glucocorticoid antagonists (acting at the receptor level) ameliorates the central adiposity of Cushing's syndrome (Nieman et al. 1985). Such data support the possibility that visceral obesity may be a function of elevated cortisol levels, secondary to abnormal regulation of the HPA axis in response to chronic psychosocial stress. The impact of increased cortisol secretion on visceral fat deposition, insulin sensitivity, and the associated changes in hormonal and metabolic profiles is consistent with this possibility.

High doses of cortisol, when given for therapeutic usage, increase abdominal adiposity independently of the degree of obesity in persons ranging from non-obese to more than twice their ideal body weight (Vague et al. 1969). Patients on extended glucocorticoid therapy also have larger mediastinal fat areas relative to controls (Horber et al. 1986). High concentrations of cortisol have been found in abdominal adipose tissue (Newton et al. 1986), and mid-morning plasma cortisol levels (0900 hours) correlate weakly ($r = 0.29$) with WHR in obese women (Hauner et al. 1988). Glucocorticoid receptor density is higher in intra-abdominal relative to subcutaneous abdominal tissue, but there are no differences in receptor affinities between these two sites (Rebuffé-Scrive et al. 1985).

Cortisol opposes insulin action at many levels, resulting in compensatory increases in basal and glucose-stimulated insulin secretion. The effects of cortisol excess on the glucoregulatory actions of insulin (reduced glucose transport and glycogen synthesis in muscle, enhanced hepatic glucose production) may be mediated by enhanced release of FFA from adipose tissue.

The apparent link between perturbations of the HPA axis and weight gain is intriguing in itself (aside of its effects on patterns of body fat deposition). Björntorp et al. (1999) have speculated that increased food intake may be secondary to glucocorticoid-induced resistance to leptin. This is consistent with data from animal studies indicating that adrenalectomised rats have high sensitivity to leptin in association with low food intake and leanness, whereas corticosterone administration is associated with resistance to leptin, increased food intake and weight gain.

Whilst there is biological plausibility in the notion that general neuroendocrine reactions to stress are associated with the development of disease, it is unclear whether the effect of stress is mediated through abdominal obesity (Björntorp 1988) or directly on glucose and insulin concentrations (Landsberg 1986). Standardised stress, however, can invoke neuroendocrine dysregulation at the hypothalamic level in mice, primates and humans (Jeanrenaud 1994, Mårin and Björntorp 1993). As postulated by Björntorp (1988), it is possible that hypothalamic dysregulation in response to environmental stress could induce engagement of: (a) the sympatho-adrenal axis (causing hypertension and increased concentrations of free fatty acids); (b) the pituitary-adrenal axis (causing increased secretion of adrenal steroids); and (c) the pituitary-ovarian or gonadal axis (causing altered sex steroid concentrations, anovulation in women, and abdominal obesity). Stress-induced engagement of these central nervous system and autonomic-neuroendocrine system axes could thereby contribute to the development of most risk factors for stroke, cardiovascular disease, Type 2 diabetes and some cancers.

The foregoing discussion has particular relevance for the interpretation of the results of a study published many years ago on the impact of a temporary reversion to traditional hunter-gatherer lifestyle on carbohydrate and lipid metabolism in diabetic Australian Aborigines (O'Dea 1984). This seven-week lifestyle change intervention resulted in marked improvements in all of the metabolic abnormalities of diabetes, as well as reduction in a number of risk markers for cardiovascular disease (blood pressure, dyslipidemia, and bleeding time). The cluster of metabolic characteristics which make up the 'insulin resistance syndrome' were all ameliorated. These beneficial changes were interpreted as being due to a combination of weight loss secondary to increased physical activity and a low fat, bulky diet which altered energy balance. In a brief review paper published elsewhere (O'Dea 1983), the following quotation implies, however, that the explanation was likely to be considerably more complex:

> The Aborigines in this study were very impressed with the possibility of understanding why they had diabetes and how they could treat it themselves. They could see that this was an area of their health that they could potentially control themselves – that they did not need drugs or doctors.
>
> We discussed the problems they would have in continuing their treatment once they were back in Derby. Many expressed the desire to go back to their traditional country and live there permanently – partly living off the land and partly having 'good' Western food. They saw this as their only chance of controlling their own lives again, and they realised that it was only by regaining power over their own lives that they could come to grips with many of their health problems – diabetes and heart disease being only two amongst many. Alcohol was seen as a much more damaging problem.
>
> When the people in this study went back to their own land – even for only a few weeks – they changed greatly. Not only did their health improve, but also, so it seemed to me, did their self-respect. In this sense there is a direct relationship between health, the outstation movement and land rights.

Markers of the stress pathways

Neural and endocrine changes associated with the acute stress response include release of norepinephrine and epinephrine, which remain elevated for one to two hours. Endocrine systems are stimulated to increase cortisol and glucagon concentrations, and perpetuate a response over the longer term if stressors are perceived still to be present.

Perturbations in the activity of the HPA axis are reflected by deviation in the circadian rhythm as well as in the concentrations of adrenal hormones. Salivary cortisol is a measure of the activity of the hypothalamo-pituitary-adrenocortical (HPA) system. Increases in cortisol concentrations are reflected in saliva (Akanji et al. 1990; Lo et al. 1992). Salivary cortisol is a better measure of HPA activity than total plasma cortisol concentration, since it is highly correlated with bioavailable unbound plasma cortisol and corticotrophic hormone concentrations (Aardal-Eriksson et al. 1998). The assessment of cortisol in saliva has proven a valid and reliable reflection of the relative amount of the unbound hormone in blood (Kirschbaum and Hellhammer 1994). It is also an excellent tool for assessing variation in diurnal secretion patterns (Shinkai et al. 1993).

Salivary cortisol assessment is non-invasive, easy to collect, and requires only that the subject chew on a cotton swab. Salivette samples are stable frozen or unfrozen for up to 30 days after use, and thus can be self-administered by the subject and in some cases mailed to researchers for analysis (Clements and Parker 1998). Salivary cortisol also has advantages over blood cortisol analysis, such as non-reactive sampling, low cost and laboratory independence. As circulating cortisol fluctuates both diurnally and in response to acute stressors, researchers can focus on distinguishing either elevated reactivity of cortisol (eg, response to an acute, standardised stressor) or blunting of the diurnal variation in circulating cortisol (requiring several measures over at least one 24-hour cycle). Both states are a function of exposure to chronic stress (Brunner and Marmot 1999).

Salivary cortisol concentration is correlated, and cortisol reactivity or altered diurnal cortisol secretion pattern associated, with both perceived (van Eck et al. 1996) and anticipatory (Lupien et al. 1997) stress, stressful daily events (Samuels et al. 1997), general psychological affect (Smyth et al. 1998) and measures of depression (Galard et al. 1991, Odber et al. 1998, Strickland, P et al. 1998) mastery (Grossi et al. 1998), and anxiety (Rosmond and Björntorp 1998b). These relationships, and links to somatic arousal and chronic burnout (emotional exhaustion, physical fatigue and cognitive weariness) (Melamed et al. 1999) as well as high blood pressure and elevated insulin concentration, themselves related to abdominal adiposity and obesity (Rosmond and Björntorp 1998a), are thought to be part of the mechanism underlying associations among stress, diabetes and cardiovascular disease.

Environmental factors affecting salivary cortisol concentration in humans include social hierarchy (Hellhammer et al. 1997), psychosocial (Earle et al. 1999) and physical (Miki et al. 1998) environmental characteristics, and financial strain (Genco et al. 1998), all of which are associated with elevated morbidity and premature mortality in disadvantaged populations subject to a high allostatic load (McEwen 1998).

Besides salivary cortisol, an alternate, more stable measure of stress with utility under the less controlled conditions of field surveys is glycosylated haemoglobin (GHb), concentrations of which are elevated by stress-related catecholamine-mediated increases in blood glucose (Netterstrom et al. 1998). The population distribution of GHb is well understood (Simon et al. 1989, Yudkin et al. 1990) and it has utility as a practical biomarker of stress for population health surveys (Kelly et al. 1997). Associations between GHb and psychogenic stress have been reported for non-diabetic persons (Arnetz 1984, Netterstrom and Sjol 1991, Theorell et al. 1988) as well as for people with Type 1 (Auslander et al. 1993, Goldston et al. 1995) and Type 2 (Demers et al. 1989, Okada et al. 1995) diabetes. GHb concentration is proportional to the time-averaged concentration of blood glucose over the two to three months preceding its measurement (Folling 1990).

Notwithstanding that GHb is closely related to glucose tolerance and that its distribution is a function of similar determinants, it is not necessarily the case that the population distribution of GHb can be predicted entirely from fasting or 2-h glucose. Factors other than degree of glucose tolerance or ambient blood glucose influence GHb concentration (Davidson et al. 1999, Gould et al. 1997). Social environmental stress could be one such determinant (Daniel et al. 1999b). Correlation coefficients for the relationship between GHb and 2-h glucose concentrations in normoglycaemic individuals are but moderate, ranging from 0.43 and 0.64 (Yudkin et al. 1990).

The potential impact of environmental stress on GHb was recently illustrated in a contrast of populations genetically and culturally distinct within and between indigenous and non-indigenous groupings. The analysis, which included Torres Strait Islanders, Australian Aborigines, Native Canadians, Greek migrants to Australia, and Australians of Anglo-Celtic descent, accounted for more than 72% of the variance in GHb, and controlled by stratification glycaemic status (by oral glucose tolerance test) and adjusted for age, gender and 2-h glucose (Daniel et al. 1999a). Mean GHb was greater for each indigenous group than for either non-indigenous group. Differences specific to glycaemic classifications were significant for *normoglycaemic* persons as well as for those with diabetes. Mean GHb did not differ between the three indigenous groups or between the two non-indigenous groups. Despite differences between indigenous populations in the prevalence of diabetes, GHb did not differ at any level of glycemic status. Native Canadians with the lowest prevalence of diabetes of *any* group still had mean GHb no different from Torres Strait Islanders and Australian Aborigines. The study populations differ in geographic area, culture and genetic composition. The primary commonality among such disparate peoples is exposure to Westernisation, that is marginalisation, social disadvantage and inferior status relative to Greek migrants to Australia and Australians of Anglo-Celtic origin. Such stress, systemic with its origins in the very fabric and structure of society, was proposed as allostatic load exemplified, in part, by consistently elevated GHb not accounted for by other influences for which the study controlled.

Concluding comments

There is abundant evidence that psychosocial factors have a profound impact on health. Nonetheless, little research to date has targeted the possible biopsychosocial pathways by which social environmental and contextual conditions of living affect health. There are few published reports of empirical studies linking SES, psychosocial factors, and stress responses or allostatic load, and none that attempt to move beyond the empirical basis of these relationships through examination of the underlying theory, methodology and politics of the work. There is a significant need for testing and refining of social theory to supplant the primarily atheoretical work conducted thus far and to serve as a guide for further studies. The reasons for this stymied development of the field, at least beyond investigation of individual-level relationships, are complex: difficulties in measurement, challenging analytical issues, conservatism of the research establishment and funding bodies, the dominant molecular paradigm, and the relative paucity of multidisciplinary research. Understanding how social factors affect health is increasingly recognised, however, as one of the great future challenges in health and social research. The implications are immense. As the biological pathways of the social gradient in health become better understood it should be possible to develop properly theorised and well-targeted interventions to attenuate its impact. For example, identification of the critical intervention points in early life should, in theory, provide the opportunity to 'reprogram' infants and young children for resilience. In terms of public health significance this is arguably the most important and challenging future field of research.

Further Reading

Brunner, E, Marmot, M 1999, Social organization, stress, and health, in Marmot, M, & Wilkinson, R G (Eds) Social Determinants of Health, Oxford University Press, New York, pp 17–43.
  – *Reviews biopsychosocial pathways by which the social environment influences biology.*
Brunner, E J 2000, Toward a new social biology, in Berkman, LF, Kawachi, I (Eds) Social Epidemiology, Oxford University Press, New York, pp306–31.
  – *Applies a life course perspective in examining the biological impact of social and psychological factors in health inequalities.*
McEwen, BS, Seeman, T 1999, Protective and damaging effect of mediators of stress: Elaborating and testing the concepts of allostasis and allostatic load, in Adler, NE, Marmot, M, McEwen, BS, Stewart, J (Eds) Annals of the New York Academy of Sciences, Volume 896, Socioeconomic status and health in industrial nations, New York Academy of Sciences, New York, pp 30–47.
  – *Examines the concepts of allostasis and allostatic load in relation to factors mediating the impact on health of psychosocial stress.*

Part E
Implications for policy, interventions and health research

18

Aboriginal health, policy and modelling in social epidemiology

Ian Anderson

Aboriginal health and social disadvantage

In Aboriginal health it is generally assumed that the determinants of mortality and morbidity are complex and multidimensional. The parameters of Aboriginal health disadvantage have been well documented. For example, Aboriginal and Torres Strait Islander life expectancy at birth for the period 1991–6 was estimated to be 56.9 years for males and 61.7 years for females. Life expectancy for nonAboriginal people during the same period was 75.2 years for males and 81.1 years for females. (AIHW 1999, p 134). Death rates, according to available data, are elevated in all age groups of Aboriginal and Torres Strait Islanders relative to nonAboriginal Australians (AIHW 1999, p 131). Aboriginal disadvantage is also well documented with respect to a range of other social indicators. For instance, according to the 1996 census:

- Forty-one percent of Aboriginal and Torres Strait Islanders aged 15–64 years were employed (including employment the Community Development Employment Projects (CDEP) scheme jobs); 12% were not employed but seeking work and 47% were not in the labour force. The unemployment rate is calculated as a percentage of those in the labour force, so that at this time, the Aboriginal and Torres Strait unemployment rate was 23%, compared with 9% for nonAboriginal Australians (AIHW 1999, p 19).
- The median weekly income for Aboriginal and Torres Strait Islander males over the age of 15 was $189 in 1996, compared with $415 for nonAboriginal males. At the same time, the median weekly income for Aboriginal females was $190, compared with $224 for non-indigenous females (AIHW 1999, p 22).
- Forty percent of Aboriginal and Torres Strait Islander people left school before the age of 16 years, compared with 34% of nonindigenous Australians. Two percent of Aboriginal and Torres Strait Islander adults aged 15 years and over had completed a bachelors degree or higher, compared with 11% of nonindigenous Australians (AIHW 1999, p 19).

Even a superficial investigation of Aboriginal health disadvantage underscores the need for a complex multi-layered response by Australian governments. A growing body of evidence from social epidemiology that points to the role played by social factors such as relative economic status, educational attainment or social capital in the production of health inequalities. Despite this evidence, there has been limited success in achieving effective co-ordination of governmental interventions in the social determinants of Aboriginal health in sectors other than health. Current Aboriginal health strategy has a significant focus on promoting access to health care and co-ordinating the development of appropriate housing and environmental health infrastructure (Anderson 1997; DHFS 1994; DHFS 1997, DHAC 1999). However, strategies that align health policy with the policy and program development in potentially relevant policy sectors have yet to be consolidated. This possibly reflects the significant institutional barriers to effective cross-sectoral action in health. Certainly, cross-sectoral policy development can too easily become a frustrating exercise in bureaucratic process. A more systematic and evidence-based approach to the development of policy that effectively addresses the social determinants of Aboriginal health would guide action in what is a complex area of health policy. This is the context in which I want to explore the potential contribution of modelling in social epidemiology to Aboriginal health policy development.

There have been several recent attempts to develop multi-level explanatory models that organise the evidence from social epidemiology along with data from fields as diverse as behavioural psychology, risk factor analysis, physiology, pathology and biochemistry (eg, Marmot and Wilkinson 1999; Marmot 2000). The development of these explanatory frameworks reflects a growing recognition that the 'multiple cause, black box paradigm of the current risk factor era in epidemiology' has significant limitations in a health policy environment that is increasingly focused on addressing complex health inequalities (Susser 1998, p 612; see also Krieger 1994). Susser argues that this problem requires a multi-level eco-epidemiology that has the potential to bind together the strands of an increasingly diversified epidemiology – from the molecular to the global. The implication of this to Aboriginal health is that a strategy for health gain requires more than a series of interventions designed to reduce individual risk (for example, in terms of diet or the consumption of tobacco or alcohol). Such interventions need to be embedded in a broader, whole of government strategy that also coordinates action to address known social determinants of health.

There has not been, to date, any work on the development of explanatory models in social epidemiology that are particular to the social and historical context of Aboriginal health in Australia. Nevertheless, it is hoped that such models can be applied to the context of Aboriginal policy development, as they have been used for mainstream health policy (Oldenburg 2000). However, I will argue in this chapter that the value of such explanatory models in Aboriginal health policy would be enhanced with some further theoretical and methodological development (see also, Anderson 2000b). A greater conceptual clarity in the use of social constructs such as 'race' or 'Aboriginality' in social epidemiology would assist this. To be an effective tool in policy, these models need to draw out the relationship between governmental interventions, social determinants of health and health outcomes. It is also important to consider the way in which these models frame the relationship between social phenomena and individuals in whom disease is expressed.

This chapter will largely focus on Aboriginal health issues, reflecting my own experience and identity. Torres Strait Islanders are the other culturally significant indigenous people in Australia. Although I do not directly address issues relevant to Torres Strait Islanders, the arguments developed are broadly applicable to this context.

In the following sections, I describe what is meant by explanatory models in social epidemiology, and clarify concepts such as 'Aboriginality' or 'race'. I then explore the potential value of modelling in social epidemiology in Aboriginal health by examining in more detail the application of one such model to current policy practice. In the concluding section, I consider some of the theoretical and methodological challenges such analysis presents.

Explanatory models and social epidemiology

Brunner and Marmot (1999) developed a social model of health that 'links social structure to health and disease via material, psychosocial and behavioural pathways. Genetic, early life, and cultural factors are further important influences on population health' (pp 19–21; see also figure 4.1, Eckersley, this volume, p 53). In this explanatory model, social categories such as 'work' and 'social environment' are interposed between categories representing the 'social structure' and 'psychological domains' as 'they are among the upstream factors now reemerging in thinking about public-health policy' (p 21). Turrell and Mathers (2000), in another explanatory model (see figure 6.2 Turrell, this volume, p 98), alternatively proposed a multi-level framework that draws together:

- upstream (macro) factors that include 'global forces', government polices, and the social, physical, economic and environmental determinants of health, with
- midstream (intermediate) factors such as psychosocial factors, health care system characteristics, health behaviours, with
- downstream (micro) factors such as physiological systems and biological reactions.

These multi-level explanatory models organise sets of empirical observations by mapping the relationships between them. Such models encompass a number of analytical realms (such as the social, individual and biological). The models are necessarily complex, and their validation requires a form of inductive argument that can synthesise empirical claims established by a range of methodologies from studies based in diverse disciplines. The organising assumptions (or theoretical bases) that underpin the approach taken to achieving such a synthesis are not always made explicit in social epidemiological analysis. In fact, there is sometimes a tendency to represent epidemiology as a discipline that is a-theoretical and methods driven. However, whether or not such theoretical principles are declared, modelling in social epidemiology is not possible without a coherent set of ideas about abstract concepts such as 'society'. Such theoretical assumptions are necessary in order to interpret and represent the relationship between discrete data. As Krieger (2000, p 891) observed in relation to epidemiological modelling:

> Models do no exist independently of theories . . . Theories attempt to explain why phenomena exist and are interrelated. By contrast, models attempt to portray how these connections occur and are always constructed with elements and relationships specified by particular theories.

In this way, modelling in social epidemiology is both a methodological and theoretical challenge. It requires evidence, based on rigorous methodologies, that elucidates the relationship between social factors and health outcomes, as well as the underlying theory, in order to synthesise such empirical findings into a cohesive model. I will argue that the dual nature of this challenge also is demonstrable in the context of Aboriginal health modelling.

Aboriginal people and 'race'

Before proceeding to unpack the substantive argument in this chapter, I want to make a brief diversion and clarify concepts such as 'Aboriginality' and 'race'. Until very recently, there has been very little debate in the public health literature, both in Australia and internationally, about the use of 'race' as a scientific construct. It has, however, received considerably critical attention in social science literature. It is now recognised that the concept of 'race' originated within particular socio-political contexts and served an ideological function within the social processes of colonialism (Cooper and David 1986; Williams, Lavizzo-Mourey, and Warren 1994; La Veist 1996; Williams 1997). The scientific credibility of this construct is undermined by the observation that the genetic variation within so-called racial groups is greater than the variation between the 'races'. Modern population genetics does not focus on identifying discrete racial categories of people, but rather on identifying 'the clines', or distribution of gene frequencies. In fact, to use 'race' in the context of this current discussion, with its implications of biological determinism, would be contradictory to the development of explanatory models that attempt to integrate social and biological determinants of health.

Where 'race' is still used in public health literature, it tends to be used in a way that implies a 'socially identified population'. Some of the methodological and theoretical challenges this poses will be explored towards the end of the chapter. However, at this point, I want to be clear that 'Aboriginality' is used in the sense of a social identity that has been produced through a complex set of historical, social and political contexts.

Modelling in social epidemiology and Aboriginal health policy

In this section, I want to explore the potential relevance of modelling in social epidemiology to Aboriginal health policy. In order to do this, I will use the framework developed by Turrell and Mathers (2000) as a map of potential policy interventions. Oldenburg et al. (2000) used this particular model to map out a whole-of-government strategy for addressing the determinants of health. Accordingly, governments can potentially achieve health outcomes by influencing the social, physical, economic and environmental determinants of health through policies (economic, welfare, health, housing, transport and taxation) that produce outcomes in education; employment, occupation, income, working conditions, housing and area of residence. In addition, policy interventions can be aimed at the mid-stream level through strategies to improve access to effective health care or reduce individual risk factors. The specific question that I wish to address in this context, is to what extent does Commonwealth policy in Aboriginal health comply with the map provided in the macro and intermediate levels of this model?

Since 1995, the Commonwealth health portfolio has administered the Commonwealth program in Aboriginal health. From the early 1970s, the national program in Aboriginal health had been the administrative and policy responsibility of the Aboriginal affairs portfolio. Arguably, this realignment in responsibility has subtly transformed the development and implementation of national Aboriginal and Torres Strait Islander health policy and strategy. In particular, there has been a greater focus on the development and utilisation of health portfolio mechanisms, structures and policy levers to achieve Aboriginal health outcomes through strategies that improve capacity and performance in the health sector. Other sectors of government, such as housing, environmental and public health infrastructure and education, are acknowledged to play an essential role in achieving outcomes in indigenous health. These sectors are drawn into this health-focused framework through a number of formal and informal inter-sectoral structures (Anderson 1999; Anderson et al. 2001).

One of the key elements in this strategic approach is a series of negotiated intergovernmental agreements (the Framework Agreements in Aboriginal Health). These agreements commit signatories to collaborate in developing specific structures and processes that will provide infrastructure to coordinate the implementation of national strategy in Aboriginal health. These agreements were signed by representatives of the Aboriginal and Torres Strait Islander Commission (ATSIC) and the Aboriginal community-controlled health sector, in addition to the relevant Commonwealth and State/Territories Ministers for Health. Specifically, the Framework Agreements provide the development of national and state/territory planning forums whose focus is to improve Aboriginal primary health care capacity and reduce barriers to access mainstream services. The Commonwealth Department of Health and Aged Care identified the following key developmental priorities in national Aboriginal health strategy (DHAC 1999):

- developing the infrastructure and resources necessary to achieve comprehensive and effective primary health care for indigenous peoples;
- addressing some of the specific health issues and risk factors affecting the health status of indigenous peoples;
- improving the evidence base which underpins the health interventions; and
- improving communication with primary health care services, Aboriginal and Torres Strait Islander peoples and the general population.

There is evidence to support the priority given to the development of the capacity of Aboriginal primary health care services. For instance, a recent analysis of acute hospital separation data compared Aboriginal and nonAboriginal separations for ambulatory sensitive diagnostic related groups. These are groups of conditions for which it is thought that high-quality, appropriate primary health service, deliverable under ideal circumstances, may potentially reduce or eliminate the need for hospitalisation. For this study, age-specific acute hospital separation rates for ambulatory sensitive conditions were 1.7 to 11 times higher for the Aboriginal and Torres Strait Islander people than other Australians (Stamp et al. 1998). Expenditure and utilisation data relating to Aboriginal access of primary health care services is currently patchy in quality and lacking in specificity. Nevertheless, these data tend to support the general view that the capacity to deliver effective needs-based primary health care services to Aboriginal people is relatively poorly developed nationally (see Anderson et al. 2001).

There is also a growing body of evidence that demonstrates an association between effective primary health care and specific Aboriginal health outcomes. Systematic reviews have collated and analysed the quality of existing evidence about effective primary health care delivery (Couzos et al. 1999; Couzos et al. 1998). They suggest that the quality and organisation of health care at the primary level can be critical factors in achieving outcomes. This has been demonstrated for some communicable diseases such as Haemophilus influenza type B (HIB)(Bower et al. 1998); prevention of secondary complications of chronic illnesses, such as the reduction of ischaemic heart disease risk for Aboriginal people with noninsulin-dependent diabetes mellitus (Rowley 2000); and maternal and child health outcomes, such as low birth weight (Mackerras 1998)). However, while it possible to identify discrete health outcomes from health program interventions, there is not a clear consensus about the population health gain that would result from the sum effect of an appropriately resourced and well-organised system of health care.

Recent national policy in Aboriginal health has also focused on the development of specific disease or health risk strategies. In some cases, such as the National Indigenous Australians Sexual Health Strategy, primary care services were conceived as the institutional vehicles through which this strategy would be implemented. In this instance, it was argued that primary health care capacity was critical to achieve the delivery of a regionally-based and integrated clinical, population health and health promotion strategy in sexual health (Anderson and Simmonds 1999). Other disease or risk reduction strategies have addressed social determinants of health through strategies to regulate the supply of particular commodities, such as food or alcohol (Taylor 1999). An accurate map of how national Aboriginal health policy and strategy currently addresses the social determinants of health would need to examine these disease and risk reduction strategies in detail. Nevertheless, the focus of disease and risk-specific strategies reflects the broader focus in Aboriginal policy on improving health sector performance.

The policy link between housing and environmental health infrastructure and health is well established. The National Aboriginal Health Strategy (NAHS 1989), for instance, advocated that a strategic link be maintained between these different sectors. Survey work, such as the National Trachoma and Eye Health Program, had previously demonstrated an association between housing quality and the prevalence of a range of indicators of infectious disease such as nasal discharge, cicatricial trachoma, follicular trachoma, skin infections and otitis media (Royal Australian College of Ophthalmologists 1980). In fact, nearly 70% of the budget appropriated to support the implementation of the NAHS was allocated to housing and community infrastructure programs (DHFS 1994). Following the transfer of administrative responsibility to the health portfolio in 1995, a memorandum of understanding was developed between ATSIC and the Commonwealth health portfolio that identified ATSIC's ongoing role in the delivery of environmental health programs (ATSIC and Commonwealth Department of Health and Human Services 1995). The Commonwealth health portfolio also has continued to collaborate with ATSIC in program delivery on initiatives to improve the environmental health infrastructure in Aboriginal communities (DHFS 1997).

It is apparent from this survey of key health policy and strategy documents that coordinated cross-sectoral strategies have only been developed to a limited extent, with the exception of housing and environmental health. While the importance of effective cross-sectoral approaches in Aboriginal health is frequently acknowledged, very little detail is provided about approaches taken to building collaborations with sectors involved in transport, economic, education or taxation policy. For example, the relationships between Aboriginal economic development, employment programs and health were flagged in the National Aboriginal Health Strategy (1989), but there is no detail provided on how this relationship was to be developed. More recent Commonwealth Aboriginal health strategy documents also do not provide any reporting of policy action in this domain (for example, DHFS 1997; DHAC 1999). Cross-sectoral action with respect to education remains focused on the development of the indigenous health workforce (DHFS 1994, 1997; Schwabb and Anderson 1998). However, there is a growing interest in further developing and strategically focusing policy on the relationship between education and health outcomes (Boughton 2000). In comparison with the whole of government strategy suggested by the Turrell and Mathers model, the Commonwealth strategy in Aboriginal health seems to be quite limited. However, there are some significant clarifications that need to be made at this point.

First, we need to consider what is strategically possible in developing policy interventions that address those social factors implicated in health outcomes. We need to acknowledge that Government policy can influence, to varying degrees, the social determinants of health. So, for example, it may be that we also need to take into consideration those areas of policy where governmental interventions have been relatively successful. It may be that investing in good cross-sectoral strategy in Aboriginal health and education policy is more likely to influence outcomes than, say, investing in economic policy. Here, our interest is not in the relative importance of different social factors in the production of health inequalities, but in the relative effectiveness of interventions to improve outcomes. What is needed in this regard is evidence about effective interventions in an Aboriginal context. What types of economic development also support health gain? How are education services best aligned to produce health gain? Answers to questions such as these would greatly enhance our capacity to attune these models to intervention.

Health policy interventions are conceived in terms of a limited set of tools, such as regulation and standard setting, resource allocation, program development and legislation. The context in which these tools are deployed is critical in determining outcomes. In other words, there are a great many diverse institutional contexts in which a relatively limited set of policy tools may be used to varying effect. The critical issues are the context and strategy through which such tools are deployed. Reform of education policy, taxation policy or transport policy requires the advocacy of the health sector. The capacity of the health sector policy-maker to do this effectively depends on the institutional relationship between the two sectors. Furthermore, Aboriginal health policy development occurs within a particular institutional location within the health sector. Arguably, it may be possible to influence taxation policy through mainstream health sector advocacy. Yet it is unlikely that Aboriginal health interests could achieve such reform in isolation from a broader cross-sectoral engagement, unless the issue was highly discrete with no broader repercussions. Similarly, it is likely that reform in transport policy might be one path by which Aboriginal access to health and social services could be improved. However, the potential health gains from such a strategic approach to reforming policy need to balanced against the resources (political and other) required to achieve policy reform.

The significance of these issues is not developed in the Turrell and Mathers model, which too seamlessly embeds policy and institutional structures in health within the global influences on health. A policy-relevant model would need to provide an elaborated structure that disentangles the relationship between institutions of government and the social determinants of health.

Finally, Aboriginal health interventions are developed in a context of social diversity. How should this be taken into account in explanatory models in social epidemiology? The models we have considered here tend to presume a culturally homogenous population. Are there further social factors or relationships that we need to take account in developing interventions specifically for Aboriginal people? Finally, in these models how do we take into account the relationship between individuals (in whom disease is expressed) and social phenomena? I shall conclude by opening up some of these issues for further theoretical development.

Aboriginal people, racism and health outcomes

Internationally, there has been a reexamination of the role played by 'ethnicity' or 'race' in the production of illness. In part, this reflects increasing dissatisfaction with epidemiological models that explain health inequalities for social minorities as the sum of particular biological and environmental health risks. One approach to reformulating theory in this regard is to draw on a foundational premise in sociology: that 'social facts' are relational. In other words, social phenomena are not just attributes of individuals. They represent attributes or qualities of the relationships among individuals within a population. Social facts are population level phenomena, the sum outcome of individual interactions, rather than average of individual tendencies. This requires a focus on the study of:

> . . . population-level influences on health. Such factors, intrinsically difficult to characterize, are neither the mere aggregation of individual risk factors nor the directly connected upstream determinants of proximate factors. Rather, there appear to be constitutional properties of population, such as herd immunity, income inequality, and social morale, that affect health processes at a supra-individual level, in addition any manifestation of risk that they might induce at the individual level. (McMichael 1999, p 893)

This is relevant as I have framed 'Aboriginality' or 'race' as a social phenomenon in that 'Aboriginality' is an identity that is socially reproduced within a particular cultural, political and historical context. This is not just a theoretical concern. There is empirical work that suggests that the social relations implicated in the production of such social identities also influence the production of health outcomes even when other known social determinants of health are taken into account (see for example Krieger et al. 1993). In other words, racism is a social phenomenon that should be taken into account within explanatory models in social epidemiology. Williams, for example, developed a framework for the study of the effects of 'race' on health (see figure 18.1). This model is based on the premise the 'race' is a:

complex multidimensional construct reflecting the confluence of biological factors and geographical origins, culture, economic, political and legal factors, as well as racism. . . . Social-status categories reflect, in part, differential exposure to risk factors and resources that ultimately affect health through biological pathways. (Williams 1997, p.325)

There is another component of the Williams (1997) model that is potentially significant. He makes a further distinction (drawing on Link and Phelan, 1995) between basic and surface causes. Basic causes he defines as 'factors responsible for generating a particular outcome; changes in these forces create change in the outcome. In contrast, surface causes are related to the outcome, but change in these factors does not produce corresponding change in the outcome'. I interpret this to mean that that changes in surface causes may cause change in the expression of disease, but not alter the key social factors driving the unequal production of disease. Surface factors, such as health risk behaviours, and access to health care are, in this model, also shaped by social phenomena. While this may be a useful way of framing policy priorities, this particular set of concepts deserves exploration in greater detail than is possible in this context.

There are some social epidemiologists who have argued that there are significant methodological limitations in the study of the relationship between race and health outcomes (Kauffman and Cooper 1999, Cooper and Kauffman 1999). Kauffman and Cooper argue that

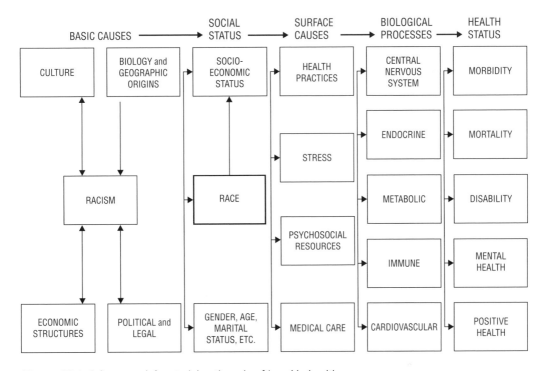

Figure 18.1 A framework for studying the role of 'race' in health

Source: Williams 1997, p328. Copyright 1997, with permission from Elsevier Science.

epidemiological method is based on 'counterfactual argument'. Counterfactual argument is based on the premise that the average causal effect of an exposure could be determined if it was possible retrospectively to change only the individual's exposure status and determine the effect of this on health outcomes. This premise is tenuous at best with respect to social facts, which 'are often attributes of individuals and are components of structured social relations' (Kauffman and Cooper 1999, p 113). Using examples of 'race', gender and class, Kauffman and Cooper argue that this method is unsuited for the analysis of social factors as risk factors. In considering Aboriginal health, these issues are relevant as it could not be argued that an Aboriginal or an otherwise socially disadvantaged person would be the same person if we could somehow extract their 'Aboriginality' or social disadvantage. 'Aboriginality' cannot be disentangled from social factors such as employment, income, and experience of education or marginalisation. Sociological analyses of the production of Aboriginal ill-health illustrate the complex interplay of political, social and economic processes that have historically shaped the Aboriginal social contexts (see, for example, Saggers and Gray 1991; 1998). However, while Kauffman and Cooper consider this problem in basically methodological terms, Mutaner, on the other hand, contends that this problem is theoretical, reflecting the 'lack of *social* theory development, due mainly to the reluctance of epidemiologists to think about social mechanisms (eg, racial exploitation)' (his emphasis, 1999, p 121). However, it is unlikely that theory and methods could be so neatly partitioned, and in fact, both aspects of this problem will require further study.

Nevertheless, for these reasons, care needs to be taken in using constructs such as 'Aboriginality' in explanatory frameworks in social epidemiology. However, from a policy perspective this issue is quite important. For instance, the Williams model suggests that, within whole-of-government strategies in Aboriginal health, it is necessary to develop a focus on strategies that address racism and promote reconciliation between Aboriginal and non-Aboriginal Australians.

Finally, in the representation of the relationship between social phenomena and health outcomes, it is critical that we understand the dynamics of the relationship between individuals and social processes. There is a tendency to obscure the role of individual action in these explanatory models. In the model proposed by Brunner and Marmot (1999), the relationship between social phenomena and individuals is obscured by the lack of a clearly designated category for the 'individual'. Presumably, within this framework, the individual inhabits the space between social structure and social environment and the pathophysiological environment. Similarly, the individual is obscured within Williams' 'race'-specific model. A more clearly delineated multi-level framework overcomes some of these problems. The upstream and midstream factors in Turrell and Mathers (2000) multilevel framework are connected with bold authoritative arrows inferring that all the interconnected relationships are essentially the same. What is required in these explanatory models is a reformulated relationship between individual action (or agency) and societal phenomena. In this way we should consider culture, class or gender as societal phenomena, that exist external to individuals, influence individual action, yet, at the same time, are actively engaged, transformed and socially reproduced as a consequence of individual action. A consequence of this is that social constructs (or social facts) such as culture or class, are all reproduced through individual action. They are ignored or heeded depending on how that particular individual responds to a particular set of social circumstances.

This is not just a narrow theoretical concern – it has implications for how people think about developing strategies in health. Rendering individuals as passive products of their social categories lends itself to mechanistic, top down approaches to achieving health change. Understanding the social dynamics that shape the way in which people actively engage with and respond to health and other social challenges is critical if we are to conceive of policy interventions within terms of social processes. This way, we can better take into account the social processes associated with the implementation of programs and better understand the issues undermining their efficacy.

Conclusion

The development of multi-level explanatory frameworks in social epidemiology promises to provide a more systematic and evidence-based approach to policy development in complex areas of health policy such as Aboriginal health. These multilevel explanatory models organise sets of empirical observations, and structure the relationship between these observations. The structure conferred on these explanatory models is in part an outcome of the evidence at hand, but theories of society also play a critical role in shaping such models.

The explanatory models developed to date in social epidemiology can provide a useful guide to policy development. They may be of particular value in the development of health strategy that engages sectors other than health. However, if they are to be further developed in a way that is more attuned to issues in Aboriginal health, the models need also to elaborate the role of governmental and policy interventions in health change and the relationship between Aboriginal interests, government, other institutions and social processes. Further development would be needed to investigate the potential role of social processes such as racism in the production of health outcomes. Ultimately, however, all interventions in policy will only impact on population health outcomes if they impact on individuals or the relations between individuals. Understanding how individuals engage with social phenomena and vice versa is a theoretical challenge that underlies the development of more effective strategies for health gain.

Further Reading

Australian Bureau of Statistics and Australian Institute of Health and Welfare 1999, The Health and Welfare of Australia's Aboriginal and Torres Strait Islander Peoples, Commonwealth of Australia, Canberra.
   – *Biennial report that contains the most up to date collation of data and information on the health and welfare of indigenous Australians.*
Anderson, I 1997, The National Aboriginal Health Strategy, in Gardner, H (Ed.), Health Policy in Australia, Oxford University Press, Melbourne.

– *Containing a descriptive overview of the content and implementation of the National Aboriginal Health Strategy – the key national policy initiative in Aboriginal health to date. This strategy is currently being reviewed. It is likely that its key principles will remain unchanged.*

Reid, J & Trompf, P 1991, The Health of Aboriginal Australia, Harcourt Brace and Jovanovich, Sydney.

Saggers, S & Grey, D 1991, Aboriginal Health and Society: The traditional and contemporary struggle for better health, Allen and Unwin, North Sydney.

– *These are the two most current generic texts on Aboriginal health that provide a comprehensive overview of issues.*

19

Does our limited analysis of the dimensions of poverty limit the way we seek solutions?

Elizabeth Harris, Don Nutbeam and Peter Sainsbury

Introduction

Poverty is rarely about one thing – it is about having no money, no voice, no infrastructure and no opportunities. Voices of the Poor (World Bank 2000).

Poverty and other forms of social disadvantage are multidimensional in their manifestations, multifactoral in their causes, and complex in the pathways through which they operate on health and well-being. However, there is a danger that the high level of interest in the public health community in the statistical relationship between unequal income distribution and health may lead to an oversimplification of both the nature of poverty and the action required to address health inequality. Also, a preoccupation with describing associations and developing models for explaining causal pathways leaves public health workers open to criticism of developing a research industry that has few tangible benefits for those whose health is most vulnerable.

This paper raises issues that need to be considered as complex notions of poverty and social disadvantage are transferred from (often complex) sociological to (often relatively simple) public health frameworks. For instance:
- Are measures of income and income distribution simply proxies for a more complex and systemic web of disadvantage?
- Is poverty better understood as a set of issues affecting an individual, family network or community rather than as a single entity in itself?
- Does the current emphasis on relative poverty blind us to the absolute paucity of resources and life chances experienced by some Australians?
- Is our limited analysis of the dimensions of poverty preventing a more sophisticated approach to solutions?
- And most importantly, if, as some argue, the prime cause of health inequalities in developed countries is the very unequal income distribution, and the remedies for this lie so clearly

outside the mandate of the health system, are health workers released from any responsibility to act?

Additionally, we reflect on the limitations of the income inequality argument that are emerging in the literature, and examine the ways in which an analysis that is based on simple, strong statistical associations between income inequality and health may be limiting effective action to reduce health inequalities. It is not our purpose to throw the baby out with the bath water. We do not dispute the observed relationship between income inequality and health but seek to reflect on the limitations of this approach in understanding the origins of health inequality and in taking action to redress these inequalities.

Poverty, income inequality, social capital and health

The evidence of a relationship between poverty and health is as old as public health. What is often forgotten is that this evidence led to action by the founders of public health, often opposed by vested interests, that resulted in significant improvements in the health of the most vulnerable in society at that time (Chadwick 1842; Frazer 1947; Hammond and Hammond 1947). Action by governments and communities over many generations has ensured that the most grinding effects of poverty have been reduced through the development of public health infrastructure, public education systems, safe living and working environments and income support systems. So successful have these efforts been that poverty is now often seen as a relative rather than an absolute shortage of resources in many western industrialised countries.

Absolute poverty is 'severe deprivation of basic human needs, including food, safe drinking water, sanitation facilities, health, shelter, education and information. It depends not only on income but also on access to services' (United Nations 1995, p 57). In essence it involves having inadequate resources to maintain subsistence. It is relatively rare in industrialised countries now but still very common in developing countries.

Relative poverty involves being unable to afford the goods, services and activities (eg, housing, food, clothes, recreation, social obligations) that allow people to play the roles, participate in the activities and relationships and follow the customary behaviours that are considered normal in society and are expected of people by virtue of their membership of society (Townsend 1993, chapter 2). Because it is conceptualised relative to the rest of the society in which it occurs, the definition of relative poverty varies among societies and over time; it is also vigorously debated. Once defined, it is difficult to operationalise and measure. However, relative poverty is quite common in most industrialised countries.

Despite the successful elimination of absolute poverty and its effects, the gap in health between rich and poor remains in many western nations (Townsend and Davidson 1982; Mathers 1994).

Over the past 15 years, there has been a growing body of evidence to suggest that societal patterns of health inequality are strongly related to the levels of income inequality within societies, rather than simply individual income levels. The initial interest in this issue arose from an empirical demonstration of a strong association ($p<0.001$) between income inequality and life expectancy in eleven OECD countries (Wilkinson 1986). Wilkinson actually credits Mildred Blaxter with suggesting the association to him (Wilkinson 1986, p 110). One can, however, also identify other reasons for the spurt of interest in income inequality:

- The consistent demonstration of a gradient throughout the whole of society in the relationship between health status and socio-economic status. This can be taken to indicate that the relationship between health and socio-economic resources is a concern for not only the most impoverished but also for the whole society, and hence related to the way society is organised.

- The persistence of the relationship between health status and socio-economic status. Even after the diseases traditionally associated with poverty (particularly the highly fatal infectious diseases) have been largely eliminated in western nations and replaced with chronic non-infectious diseases associated with lifestyle and an ageing population (conditions that have sometimes misleadingly been referred to as diseases of affluence), poorer people have poorer health.

- An increased awareness by all, as a result of extensive media coverage and greater superficial contact between the very wealthy and the rest of society, of the wealth (and its trappings) and the inequalities in wealth that exist in society. A recent Australian NEWSPOLL survey demonstrated that 83% agree that 'in Australia the rich are getting richer and the poor are getting poorer'. Additionally, 55% think that 'the distribution of wealth in Australia' is less fair than it was ten years ago, and 70% would prefer 'the gap between the rich and the poor to get smaller' compared with 28% who would prefer 'the overall wealth of Australia to grow as fast as possible' (NATSEM 2000b).

- Reduced acceptance of religious sanctioning of poverty and a social hierarchy and of religious promises regarding an afterlife. For instance, few people these days believe in the divine right of monarchs or that 'Blessed are the poor in spirit: for theirs is the kingdom of heaven' (St Matthew 5:3) or that 'It is easier for a camel to go through the eye of a needle, than for a rich man to enter into the kingdom of God' (St Matthew 19:24) or in the sentiments of C F Alexander's verse: 'The rich man in his castle, / The poor man at his gate, / God made them, high and lowly, / And ordered their estate'.

Since Wilkinson's (1986) initial finding, the association between income inequality and health among western nations has been developed in more sophisticated analyses (Wilkinson 1996a) and has been demonstrated within the USA (Kennedy, Kawachi and Prothrow-Stith 1996; Kawachi et al. 1997a). Although a recent study comparing the Canadian provinces did not find an association (Ross 2000), overall the evidence suggests that:

- the distribution of income within society matters as much for the society's health and wellbeing as the absolute standard of living once a modest level of economic development has been achieved; and

- an individual's health is affected not only by her or his own income but also by the scale of inequality in the society as a whole (Kawachi et al. 1999a).

Based on these findings, it has been argued that it is relative rather than absolute income that is the more important influence on health status and that a wider income gap between rich and poor results in poorer health for everyone. Wilkinson (1997b and 1999c) argues that social capital, or social cohesion, mediates the influence of income inequality on health through the psychosocial reactions of people to their perceived place in society. For instance, negative emotions such as shame and distrust may induce harmful biological consequences via psychoneuroendocrine processes and/or harmful behaviours, or negative social consequences via antisocial behaviour and/or reduced community participation:

> Health inequalities therefore are not simply the direct result of exposure to material forces like bad housing and diet. Instead, low social status leads to chronic anxiety, permanent increase in stress . . . and poorer immunity. . . . The most important reason why egalitarian societies are healthier seems to be that they enjoy a better quality of social relations (Wilkinson 1999c).

These ideas have not been without their critics, with questions based on methodological and measurement issues (such as the use of ecological data and the lack of standardised measurement instruments), the observation that life expectancy is increasing even in countries where there are wide income inequalities, and the inadequate attention given to the structural and material causes and social context of inequality (Gravell 1998; Judge 1995; Lynch et al. 2000b).

The significance of the debates

The current debates in the literature on the relative importance of absolute and relative poverty and the effects of reduced social capital arising from income inequality on health (Lynch et al. 2000b; Baum 2000; Wilkinson 2000) are important for three reasons. First, they are potent reminders that theoretical models can only ever partly explain the complexity of the factors related to, and the ways in which, poverty influences health. It is therefore to be expected that from time to time the models will need to be substantially redeveloped. Second, the debates challenge public health workers to look beyond large data sets of overly simplified variables to find more sophisticated ways of understanding the causes of health inequality.

Third, the debates challenge us to rethink the dimensions of poverty. The recent World Bank Report, *Voices of the Poor*, provides important insights into the ways people living with poverty view the forces that shape their lives (World Bank 2000). According to the World Bank, poverty is multi-dimensional and is about:

- No money
- No voice
- No infrastructure
- No opportunities

While we need to be cautious in uncritically adopting a World Bank analysis, we should recognise that their interest in the experiences of poor people comes from failed attempts at tackling poverty without an understanding of the historical, social and political environments in which poverty is embedded. Such an understanding demands a more sophisticated analysis of the problem and identification of its component parts, therefore guiding public health workers to develop more complex approaches to solutions.

Introducing context into the income inequality and health debate

Turrell and Mathers (2000) have proposed a framework for understanding the social determinants of health that links the upstream (macro-level) factors, such as broad economic, social and political forces, with what they call midstream and downstream factors. Midstream factors include access to health services, psychological factors and individual behaviours that may lead to increased health risk, and downstream factors include physiological and biological reactions that result in poor health and decreased quality of life. This framework identifies a broad range of social factors, including income, which partially describes the context in which people live their lives. Coburn argues that the lack of consideration of the broad social context presents a major limitation to the income inequality argument (Coburn 2000). According to Coburn, it results in Wilkinson seeing income distribution as resulting in reduced social cohesion rather than both income inequality and reduced social cohesion as stemming from more fundamental social processes.

Without a broader context into which the association between income inequality and health can be placed, there is a real danger that interventions based on these observations will be futile or victim blaming. On one hand, there will be calls for redistribution of income within and between societies which will generally be seen as unacceptable and/or impractical (at least in the short term). On the other hand, the focus will turn inward on social capital and cohesion to explore ways in which people and communities themselves create (and could, even should, solve) their own problems.

Lynch, who has played a major role in developing an understanding of the relationship between income inequality and health, has recently proposed an interpretation of income inequality and health that recognises the broader context in which income inequality emerges. He argues that it is important to differentiate between the health effects of income inequality (which are, of course, manifest in individuals) and reductions to community infrastructure (Lynch 2000). This interpretation recognises that historical, social and political forces create economic systems that result in health-damaging or health-promoting changes to social capital, income distribution, and physical and social infrastructure. Generally, this interpretation assumes that the currently dominant neoliberalism of many developed countries generates mainly health-damaging changes. Lynch's approach recognises that it is not only individual resources but also communal resources (such as community infrastructure) that affect health and opportunities for health.

A local perspective on a national debate

A feature of western industrialised societies is the geographic concentrations of disadvantage within cities and rural areas (Gregory and Hunter 1995; NATSEM 2000(a)). Yet, many public health researchers appear to have little direct professional or personal experience of people living in poverty. Their understandings are largely drawn from epidemiological studies and literature reviews. Poor people can be seen as being 'just like us only with less money'. This often blinds public health workers to the consequences of the desperate lack of resources that many people face in their day-to-day lives. In contrast, through fact, fiction and advertising in the electronic and printed media and as a result of increased geographic mobility, the bulk of society is probably more aware now than ever of the lifestyles of the rich.

Some insights into the forces that shape health inequality can be found by looking at a very disadvantaged part of Sydney. This community (let's call it Waldonville) has become notorious in the adjacent area because of house fires, murders and drug dealing. Thirty percent of the households in Waldonville live on less than $300 per week compared with 14% of households in the whole local government area (LGA). Twenty-seven percent of households earn more than $500 per week compared with 61% in the LGA. Compared with the whole LGA, children in Waldonville are almost twice as likely to be admitted to hospital for bronchiolitis in the first year of life, to have more dental caries, lower levels of immunisation and increased hearing problems at school entry, and are more likely to be notified as 'at risk' of child abuse and neglect (SWSAHS 2000). Poor health and low income clearly go hand in hand in Waldonville.

A household survey conducted in Waldonville in late 1997 found evidence of high levels of stress, and low levels of social support and social connectedness. Specifically:

• Fifty percent of mothers with children under five would not be sorry to leave Waldonville, compared with 11% of similar mothers in a comparable survey conducted in the whole LGA.
• Eleven percent of mothers with children under five in Waldonville had no one to turn to, compared with one to two percent in the LGA.
• Twenty-six percent of mothers with children under five in Waldonville 'fairly often' or 'very often' had problems piling up so high that they felt they could not overcome them, compared with six percent in a statewide survey.
• Thirty-three percent of residents found it 'unpleasant' or 'very unpleasant' to walk around Waldonville, compared with eight percent in a statewide survey (Waldon et al. 1998).

At a personal and local level, these results confirm the association, not only between low income and poor health, but also between poor social cohesion and high stress and poor health. But what do we lose if we stop our search for associations at this point?

The public housing estate in Waldonville was developed over two decades ago as part of a NSW Planning Strategy to attract manufacturing industry to the west of Sydney by ensuring the availability of an affordable workforce. However, not only was there a subsequent collapse in the manufacturing industry but also changes to public housing allocation policies meant that fewer people looking for employment were housed on the estate. Isolated by a six lane freeway from the nearest railway line and major shopping centre, the residents had been promised an expanded local shopping centre and a swimming pool for many years. These were eventually built in a more prosperous neighbouring suburb with which there was no direct public transport connection. Not only did this leave this already disadvantaged community without infrastructure and opportunities for a wide range of activities (essential, pleasurable and potentially health promoting), but also it made many Waldonville residents feel as if they had been abandoned.

Today in Waldonville:
• There is only one public phone and this is not available once the local shop closes.
• There is no bank.

- The buses operate poorly on weekends and stop after dark, and are thought to be unreliable. Buses terminate near the railway station, which then necessitates a long walk to the shopping centre and banks.
- To get to the hospital (including for antenatal care) requires two buses and often takes two hours. By car, it takes less than 10 minutes.
- The Police and other emergency services are reluctant to enter the area, and there can be long delays in getting assistance.
- Local take-away pizza and Kentucky Fried Chicken deliverers and taxis will not enter the area.
- There is no fruit shop or butcher. Limited supplies are available through the local shop.
- The local football club for kids is closed because there was no coach.
- Women report that they have no access to credit. Consequently, if their fridge or washing machine breaks down, it remains unfixed for long periods. Access to washing machines has been identified as a major need in Waldonville.
- The local youth and neighborhood centres are operating on ever decreasing budgets as funds are directed to more 'targeted services' across the wider region to deal with 'high risk' groups.
- The local general medical practice is finding it difficult to survive on Medicare bulk-billing payments only and has opened clinics in other areas, effectively decreasing the general medical cover to Waldonville.
- Many residents report difficulties in receiving help from government departments such as Centrelink and the Department of Housing. Both of these organisations are offering more services through call-centres, an arrangement that requires extended access to a phone you can call out on.

Many of the people in Waldonville feel excluded from mainstream society as the broad social, political and economic trends of Australia are played out in very local, very personal and very diverse ways. Individually and collectively, they have limited access to resources and infrastructure that many of us take for granted. The extent to which it is useful to understand this as 'relative poverty' is open to debate. Yes, the residents of Waldonville are aware that others are better off than they are but they are even more conscious of the effects of the marked shortage of personal and community resources on their daily lives and health.

Limitations of public health research methods

If the public health community accepts that poverty is multi-dimensional and that its effects are felt across the life courses of individuals, communities and generations, then many of the current public health methods that search for strong associations between simple variables measured at one or two levels over limited periods will be found wanting. Shaping complex situations into variables that are transparent and easy to measure often leads to overly simple analyses and solutions, as illustrated by this quote from Putnam:

> The bottom line from this multitude of studies: As a rough rule of thumb, if you belong to no groups but decide to join one, you cut your risk of dying over the next year in half. If you smoke and belong to no groups, it's a toss up statistically whether you should stop smoking or start

joining. These findings are in some ways heartening: it's easier to join a group than to lose weight, exercise regularly, or quit smoking (Putnam 1998).

But in what ways do current public health research methods and approaches need to be developed that will allow us to understand poverty in the terms suggested by the World Bank: no money, no voice, no infrastructure and no opportunities? And how can we, public health workers, utilise our current (very incomplete) knowledge to initiate justifiable remedial action now, while simultaneously shifting the research emphasis from description and aetiology to the development and evaluation of more effective interventions?

We argue that there are two directions in which research needs to change. First, public health needs to develop more sophisticated ways of measuring and modelling the complexity of factors that exist within individuals and their environments that create and sustain health inequalities. Appropriate methods (eg, longitudinal studies that follow individuals through different life stages, composite indicators that allow several factors to be captured simultaneously, participative action research, interventions with very long evaluation periods, multi-level analysis, a focus on 'place') are increasingly being used in public health research. They need, however, to be refined and more systematically applied to understanding the relationship between poverty, income distribution and health, especially in the evaluation of interventions.

Second, by involving the people who live in poverty and documenting their experiences and their explanations of the causes of ill-health and inequality, the voices of those most affected by health inequalities should become central in understanding the processes affecting their lives and how these can be changed (Blaxter 1997; Popay et al. 1998; Popay 2000). Popay et al. (1998) suggest two main reasons for this. First, lay knowledge, rooted in the geographical and physical places where people spend their lives, in their daily experiences and beliefs, and in the experiences of their life up to that point, has significance for understanding the causes of health inequalities and the 'porosity' between different layers of explanation. Second, lay knowledge presents a 'privileged' form of expertise about inequalities in health which may challenge not only the views of those who claim research or policy expertise but also the ways that traditional experts generate their information and explanations, and characterise events, needs and relationships. Thus, the inclusion of the voice of the disadvantaged will influence not only the form, implementation and likelihood of success of local interventions, but also the much broader (upstream) research agendas, policies and programs, and the interactions between interventions at different levels.

So is the health sector off the hook?

Whether low income or income inequality is seen as the fundamental cause of health inequalities, much of the action required to tackle the root cause is outside the control of the health sector. So, are health workers off the hook? Is there nothing that the health sector can do to prevent or reduce the effects of (absolutely or relatively) low income on health? We emphatically argue that, 'No, *public health workers are not off the hook. And yes, there is plenty the health system can do, and is doing, to militate against, and mitigate the effects of, low income*'.

There is increasing pressure within the heath system in Australia and overseas to take action to reduce health inequalities (Acheson 1998; Turrell et al. 1999; NSW Health 2000; Oldenburg et al. 2000) and there is already action at the local level in many parts of Australia. The real danger, though, is that simple analysis will be used to develop simple solutions. Unless we accept that the task of reducing health inequality is complex and political we may find ourselves unable to act in ways that will bring about change.

Whitehead (1990) observed four areas where interventions to reduce health inequalities had been tried:

- Strengthening individuals in disadvantaged circumstances. These interventions can have a behavioural or an empowerment focus. They try to build knowledge, competency and skill to enable people to alter their behaviour, cope better with stress, or take action to improve their life circumstances.
- Strengthening disadvantaged communities. These interventions recognise the importance of community cohesion and try to assist people in disadvantaged communities to join together for mutual support and collective action to reduce health hazards.
- Improving access to essential facilities and services. These interventions ensure better access to the prerequisites for health, such as clean water, safe and fulfilling employment, and nutritious food.
- Encouraging macro-economic and cultural change. These interventions tend to cover several sectors and work across the whole population, for instance to reduce poverty, promote equal opportunities and control environmental hazards.

Whitehead's findings confirm that much of the required action lies outside the health system. However, the health sector does have clear responsibility for improving access to quality health services, improving health literacy, and working with communities to tackle problems that are affecting health. Additionally, the health sector has a responsibility to conduct research and to base action on a sound understanding of the problem and the evidence about effective interventions. This will require:

- a re-orientation of research from describing patterns of health inequality to explaining the patterns and how they can be reduced;
- a commitment by those undertaking interventions to reduce health inequality within the health system to have their activities evaluated; and
- partnerships among researchers, practitioners and communities to build a sound evidence base for practice.

The health sector also has a traditional mandate to advocate for change in other sectors and for social and economic policy changes that promote health and reduce inequalities. Action at the local level, while necessary, will reap a very limited harvest unless the broader social, political and economic forces promote equality throughout society.

Conclusion

It is important to remember that history suggests that it is possible to change social structures and environments in ways that will reduce poverty and improve health. The current public health challenge is five-fold:

- First, to develop research methods and models of understanding that are capable of unraveling the complex, multi-layered social problems that underlie ill health and inequalities in health.
- Second, to shift the research emphasis from describing the problem, to developing and evaluating interventions.
- Third, to develop partnerships among researchers, practitioners and the community that will link evidence of the nature and causes of health inequality with evidence of effective solutions.
- Fourth, to be effective advocates for change outside the health sector's traditional areas of influence.
- Fifth, and most importantly, to ensure that success is judged not just in terms of improvements in the health of the most disadvantaged but also in the narrowing of the health gap between rich and poor.

Further Reading

Kawachi, I, Kennedy, B P & Wilkinson, R G 1999a, Introduction to Inequality and Health, The Society and Population Health Reader, vol.1, The New Press, New York.
  – *Extensive readings over several decades on the development of the income inequality thesis.*
Lynch, J W, Davey Smith, G, Kaplan, G A, House, J S 2000b, Income inequality and mortality: importance to health of individual income, psychosocial environment and material conditions, British Medical Journal 320: 1200–1204.
  – *A short critical overview of causative pathways at the macro (societal) level.*
Bartley, M, Blane, D, & Davey Smith, G. (Eds) 1998, The Sociology of Health Inequalities, Blackwell Press, Oxford.
  – *Contains several articles on a variety of topics related to inequalities in health from a sociological perspective.*

20

Developmental prevention in a disadvantaged community

Ross Homel, Gordon Elias and Ian Hay

The need for a focus on disadvantaged communities

Crime and violence have been near the top of the political agenda in Australia for the past quarter-century. The main response has been punishment – more police and more prisons. Slammed doors and a one-way ticket to 'somewhere else' characterise this time-hallowed and universally popular reaction to malignancy and turpitude.

In the past decade, a number of related problems with a more obvious 'health' flavour have risen in the charts. These problems, which include illicit drug abuse (manifested particularly in deaths from 'overdoses') and child behaviour problems, have not dislodged punishment from its pre-eminent position – indeed, in some respects, they have entrenched its use – but they have had the singular virtue of at least opening the door to a public health policy response.

Drug abuse well illustrates this point. Harm minimisation was, after a brief struggle, accepted in 1985 in Australia (but not the United States) as the overriding principle informing national drug strategy (Homel and Bull 1996). For this reason, it has been harder for governments faced with the drug problem simply to diagnose moral failing and prescribe law enforcement and punishment, notwithstanding recent trends. Harm minimisation requires some focus on prevention and at least a nodding acquaintance with risk and protective factors, something that until recently has been notably lacking from the crime arena (Developmental Crime Prevention Consortium 1999). More generally, the emerging evidence that much the same risk and protective factors underlie juvenile crime, child behaviour problems, mental and physical health, injury and drug use (Davison et al. 2000; Durlak 1998; Marshall and Watt, 1999) strongly suggests that there should be 'joined up solutions' to such 'joined up problems.'

The rise to prominence of crime and health problems in a period of great economic prosperity perhaps illustrates 'modernity's paradox' (Keating and Hertzman 1999, p 1) – improving economic indicators combined with deteriorating indicators of health and well-being, particularly for children and youth. Although evidence for deteriorating outcomes in Australia is patchy (Zubrick et al. 1999), available data do indicate that the health and well-being of children and young people in Australia and in other developed countries at the end of the 20th century is worse than it was in the 1950s and 60s (Eckersley 1998b; Rutter and Smith 1995a). Most of the damage appears to have been done in the 1970s and 1980s, with less marked negative trends in the 90s in some indicators such as serious assaults (Eckersley 1998b; Homel and Mirrlees-Black 1997).

An intensifying 'gradient effect' (a steepening relationship over time between socioeconomic status and outcomes such as literacy or life expectancy) is advanced by Keating and Hertzman (1999) and others as one explanation for the trends. Other hypotheses focus on the increased prevalence of family risk factors such as parental conflict, separation and neglect; changes in adolescent transitions (eg, increased isolation of young people from adults as the result of a stronger youth culture); and cultural shifts (eg, breakdown in frameworks providing values, purpose, and a sense of belonging) (Smith and Rutter 1995).

Evidence for the social gradient hypothesis seems largely lacking in Australia. It is not even clear that all relevant distances along the horizontal axis (ie variation in socioeconomic status) have increased. For example, while a number of studies do suggest an increasing gap between upper and middle-income families (eg, Harding 1997; 2000), this does not necessarily mean that more children are living in poverty. If the Henderson poverty line is used, the percentage of children in poverty has certainly increased markedly in the past 25 years (Harding and Szukalska 1999). However, if the more methodologically rigorous half average poverty line is used, there was between 1982 and 1995/96 'a dramatic one-third drop in before-housing child poverty' (Harding and Szukalska 1999, p iii). This is in sharp contrast to experience in 12 other industrialised countries (Bradbury and Jantii 1998, cited in Harding and Szukalska 1999, p 30). The other hypotheses advanced by Rutter and Smith (1995b), although all plausible, are equally difficult to substantiate from available Australian data.

One thing that does seem clear is that the marked geographical variations in socioeconomic status across Australia documented recently by Glover et al. 1999) have persisted for many years, and may indeed have increased (Harding 2000). Moreover, specific areas have been 'high risk' in terms of a range of social, health and economic indicators for at least a quarter of a century (compare Vinson and Homel 1975 and Vinson 1999). Vinson and Homel's original work demonstrated a coincidence of social, health and crime problems in a small number of urban areas, but the same is undoubtedly true in country regions, particularly in Aboriginal communities (Aboriginal and Torres Strait Islander Women's Task Force on Violence 1999). Such persistent and marked concentrations of crime and disadvantage in specific localities suggest that whatever preventive initiatives are developed at a whole of population level, there is a special need for joined up solutions in the most disadvantaged communities.

The need for a special focus on high risk localities is underlined by recent large scale research in the United States. Pollard et al. (1999) demonstrated in an analysis of questionnaire data from more than 80,000 high school students that there is a strong curvilinear relationship between level of risk (aggregated across individual/peer, family, school and community) and the prevalence of substance use, school problems, and delinquency. Involvement in the less prevalent activities, such as taking a gun to school or delinquency, was particularly high in the highest risk category, leading the researchers to conclude that 'preventive interventions should be focused on geographical areas or populations exposed to high overall levels of risk' (p 156).

Significantly, their data also showed that high scores on protective factors were not sufficient to nullify the impact of a high risk score, although in the two highest risk categories, protective factors did have an ameliorative effect. Their conclusion was that a simple focus on 'strengthening assets' without also attending to risk exposure is 'incomplete as a strategy for reducing the prevalence of problem behaviors' (p 156).

This conclusion is consistent with findings from a recent analysis of the Pittsburgh Youth Study (Wikström and Loeber 1999), which found that living in a very high risk neighbourhood overwhelmed the effects of individual and family protective factors, leading to late-onset serious offending by young adolescents who were previously conforming, well-adjusted children. Neighbourhood status had no direct independent effect on early onset offending, but as the authors note, probably had substantial indirect effects via its impact on families and the development of 'individual dispositions' in early childhood (p 19). An important implication of this study is that adolescent-limited offending (Moffitt 1993) in high risk areas may not be prevented by early intervention programs that strengthen protective factors in individuals, families or even contexts like schools unless these programs also influence the dynamics of peer groups and the public settings inhabited by adolescents (see also Wright et al. 1999).

The creation of more 'child-friendly neighbourhoods' through 'whole of community' approaches, together with early intervention and cross-sectoral collaboration, has gradually been recognised as a critical ingredient for successful child maltreatment prevention programs (Tomison and Wise 1999). Adolescents and their families have naturally been less prominent in these models than families with young children. The recent research evidence suggests that if the child-friendly focus in disadvantaged areas were to be expanded to encompass adolescents and their environments, the potential crime prevention benefits (incorporating *short-term* as well as long-term results) might be substantially increased.

Perhaps surprisingly, despite a century of research on neighbourhoods, many criminologists have been slow to catch up with these trends in prevention research, which have been strongly influenced by human development scholars such as Bronfenbrenner (1979) and Garbarino (1995). One of the main aims of the Developmental Crime Prevention Consortium (1999) in their *Pathways to Prevention* report published by the Federal Government was to bring these fields closer together.[1]

Developmental prevention

The overall goal of the *Pathways* report was to translate developmental prevention planning and implementation from the 'laboratory' to the community. On the one hand, there is the world of science, which includes the results of a small number of carefully designed, thoroughly implemented and rigorously evaluated field interventions. On the other hand, there is the 'real world' of disadvantaged communities and routinely delivered government and non-government programs which have wide reach but are seldom if ever evaluated and are only imperfectly influenced by the scientific literature.

The report of the US Committee on Integrating the Science of Early Childhood Development, titled *From Neurons to Neighborhoods* (Shonkoff and Phillips 2000), is the most recent and most comprehensive review of the scientific research on early childhood, including the intervention literature. The 'classic' interventions include the Perry Preschool Project (Weikart and Schweinhart 1992), the Elmira Prenatal/Early Infancy Project (Olds et al. 1999), and the Seattle Social Development Project (Hawkins et al. 1999). Beginning with the insights from the classic studies, the Consortium's major task was to integrate diverse theoretical and research literatures to construct a framework for *thinking from a developmental perspective* about the prevention of crime and associated problems at the local level. The resulting 'policy framework' (p 18) consisted of a series of steps for planning locality-based crime prevention, especially in multi-problem areas.

These steps involve more than 'risk-focused prevention' (Hawkins and Catalano 1992), although this is extremely important, but also the skills to apply developmental thinking creatively in complex local situations. If, for example, one intervenes to alter the route to social status for adolescents away from involvement in gangs or deviant peer groups, alternative pathways to respect must be created (see Developmental Crime Prevention Consortium 1999, p 86). How are alternative pathways blocked when inflexible school systems or other institutions shut doors in the face of children or adolescents, perhaps reflecting the 'one mistake and you're out!' approach to behaviour management? What can be done, on the basis of developmental and other research, to facilitate movement between life phases, such as the transition to school, especially for ethnic and racial minorities? The questions are endless, but the underlying issues always relate to time and to timing, and to the opening up of alternative routes for participation in and control over mainstream institutions.

It will be apparent that a definition of developmental prevention that encompasses all the concepts elaborated in *Pathways* poses quite a challenge. Nevertheless, a succinct statement that builds on but goes beyond definitions that centre on 'criminal potential in individuals' or on risk and protective factors would have value both for practitioners and for researchers. We have found the following description useful:

> Developmental prevention involves intervention early in *developmental pathways* that lead to crime and related problems, emphasising investment in *child-friendly institutions, communities and social policies* and the manipulation of *multiple risk and protective factors* at different levels of the *social ecology* and at crucial *transition points*, such as around birth, the commencement of school, or graduation from primary to high school.

Certain principles flow from this description:

- 'Early intervention' means 'early in the pathway,' not necessarily early in life. Thus, there is room within a developmental framework for adolescent-focused early interventions.
- Context is always vital. Changing social policies, institutions or neighbourhoods, difficult as this is, is as important as changing individual behaviours.
- Focus on transition points. No one program can cover the waterfront, especially in its early stages, so organising one's thinking around one, or at most two, key life transitions simplifies the planning task while increasing the chances that interventions will have a high uptake by the target population.
- Risk and protective factors do matter, although they are complex to conceptualise and measure, and interventions should be selected that have a good chance of shifting a few of

them. (How many in one project? A rule of thumb seems to be up to six, but this needs a stronger practice base to substantiate it.)

The final step or recommendation of the policy framework proposed in *Pathways* (Recommendation 16) was that Australia should move toward the design of a community-based project that could demonstrate the application of all the steps and the principles in a small number of disadvantaged areas. A whole-of-community approach incorporating a range of programs and services was envisaged, rather than a focus on a single program. The 'move toward' aspect was emphasised, since the authors expressed doubts that either funding or planning for a major project of this kind could be achieved within a single electoral cycle. Inspiration for the demonstration project idea came from several sources.

The evidence on 'what works' in early intervention was of course fundamental, but there were caveats. One problem is that many well-designed programs have a poor take-up rate in disadvantaged areas. The evidence. in this regard has become even more compelling than it was in 1997 when *Pathways to Prevention* was prepared. For example, Durlak and Wells (1997) in a meta-analytic review of primary prevention mental health programs found that parent training failed to achieve results because very few eligible parents participated. A large-scale community intervention in the US called *Children at Risk* (Welsh and Farrington, 1999) also failed due to a very low participation rate. Most worrying, a special issue of the journal *Future of Children* (1999 vol. 9, Issue 1) compiled recent evidence on the impacts of variety of home visiting programs throughout the United States. In an overview, Gomby, Culross and Behrman (1999) observed that there were very wide variations in results with no large or consistent benefits in child development or health behaviours. Key program elements were hard to identify, and there were generally immense problems with implementation and attrition. They concluded that modest expectations for these kinds of programs are appropriate, and that generalisation across contexts and population groups is not possible.

A further, perhaps more fundamental, question is whether even successful US programs could ever achieve the same results in Australia, given that the most deprived groups in these studies (amongst whom the most dramatic results are often achieved) are probably worse off than any part of the Australian population, with the probable exception of Aborigines (Foley et al. 2000). This highlights the need to develop *and* evaluate home-grown initiatives.

A second influence on our thinking was the literature on community organisation or mobilisation, particularly the *Communities That Care* (CTC) model pioneered in the US by Hawkins and Catalano (1992) and now being implemented in the UK (Communities That Care (UK), 1997) and in Australia (Toumbourou 1999). CTC is a highly rational 'public health' approach that involves the systematic identification and measurement of risk and protective factors in a selected community (utilising mainly official data and a standard questionnaire completed by adolescents), and the selection, implementation and evaluation of appropriate evidence-based interventions by a community prevention board. It is a model that is sufficiently flexible to involve all sectors of a community, and if implemented rigorously should achieve substantial results. CTC has not yet been evaluated as an overall model, although a large-scale evaluation of the CTC program in three communities in the UK is currently underway.

One potential criticism of CTC, whether justified or not, is that it could be rather 'top-down' and 'formula' driven, involving community influentials rather than the 'grass-roots'. A further concern is that the conceptualisation and measurement of key risk and protective factors is a complex business, perhaps not easily accomplished through surveys or official statistics. For example, both risk and resilience are best viewed not as traits but as *processes*, 'determined by the impact of particular life experiences on persons with particular conceptions of their own life history or personal narrative' (Cohler in Rutter 2000a, p 657). Community development, the third inspiration for Recommendation 16, is one traditional model for community action that explicitly attempts to resist the tendency to top down approaches and the collection of data that are not grounded in the life histories of local people.

Community workers seek through participatory processes to redress inequality and exclusion, with a focus on groups seen to be marginalised socioeconomically, culturally or politically (Lane and Henry 2000). The community development approach has the potential to reach these marginalised groups and collect information in ways that often elude more formal programs, perhaps even of a sophisticated variety like CTC. Given the evidence that the most marginalised groups are often most at risk and are the hardest to reach, the blending of community development and developmental prevention models may produce a powerful brew.

It is important to remember, however, that community development cannot be viewed just as a clever technique to enhance program penetration rates or to collect more meaningful data. It must be taken on its own terms and used to empower, not to manipulate, disadvantaged groups. Subject to this qualification, community development theory and practice might benefit enormously from an infusion of fresh ideas from the growing literature on human development, and from a sharp focus on risk and protective factors and on appropriate methods of measurement and evaluation. Essentially this means bringing a new kind of resource to disadvantaged communities – the fruits of scientific research. Such research can be a powerful tool facilitating the empowerment of marginalised people, provided resulting programs are understood by, accepted and preferably managed by the relevant groups.

A toe in the deep end – planning for a community project

In this concluding section, we describe briefly some aspects of the development of a project in a disadvantaged area of Brisbane. Since at the time of writing, project implementation had not begun, the area is not identified in this chapter. A very real aspect of the disadvantage experienced by residents in the selected area is stigmatisation simply on the basis of address. Managing this image problem will be one of the many challenges to face the project team.

The aim is to implement some of the recommendations of the *Pathways* report, including a 'scaled down' version of Recommendation 16. The overall theme (and the name of the project) is simply *Pathways*, reflecting not only our starting point but also (hopefully) a positive orientation connoting a rich variety of possibilities and opportunities.

The project, which at the time of writing (mid-2000) was in a planning and data collection phase, involves a collaboration of Griffith University academics, the national welfare agency Mission Australia, and five state government departments, with input from an expert advisory group drawn from Australia and overseas. The next phase will involve the appointment of project staff and the development of links with the community, with a view to gaining local participation and representation on the project management group. An initial three-year project life is envisaged.

The project began because of a 'seeding grant' to Mission Australia by the John Barnes Foundation. The conditions of the grant were that the project should be carried out through schools in disadvantaged areas in Queensland, and that it should 'make a difference.' We drew for possible sites from the 12 disadvantaged areas in Queensland designated by the state government as community renewal areas, comparing crime rates and other indicators to make a final choice. It is possible that a second community will be selected if funds become available. The request to work in schools meant that an initial focus for planning has been the six state schools in the selected area and the attached preschools, together with the associated families.

The education focus is a useful point of entry. Hertzman (1999, p 34), in describing the 'pathways model' of human development, underlines the pivotal role of readiness for school and behaviour problems in school. The review of research by Buchanan (1998) confirmed that emotional and behavioural problems increase the risks of educational failure and social exclusion in childhood, and unemployment, mental ill-health and criminal activity in adult life (see also Pavaluri et al. 1996). Others have noted that school problems 'characterise 80% or more of serious delinquent youth' (Huizinga and Jakob-Chien 1998, p 409). Similarly, findings of the report of the American Psychological Association Commission on Violence and Youth (1993) underscored the relationship between educational failure and antisocial behaviour. In this regard, McCoy and Reynolds (1999) point out that:

- children with language and reading disabilities are at high risk of developing social and emotional problems; and
- studies of children with behaviour problems have found a high incidence of language disorders. That is, there is a high likelihood of the co-occurrence of reading problems, language difficulties and behaviour problems.

This research has influenced our thinking about possible interventions based in preschools and schools.

The area

The study community is one of the poorest urban areas in Queensland, with half of all dwellings currently Housing Commission stock. Sole-parent families are a third of the total, nearly a quarter of the workforce is unemployed, and median household weekly income in 1996 was only $412, one of the lowest levels in Queensland. Nearly one person in five is a child under the age of 10. The community is also multicultural, with substantial Vietnamese, Pacific Islander and indigenous populations, and there are tensions and sometimes fighting between different groups of ethnic young people. Significantly, the juvenile crime rate is more than three times higher than any other community renewal area, although the child abuse notification rate is not the highest in Brisbane. Exactly half of all convicted juvenile offenders are indigenous, although they comprise fewer than 10% of the population.

Despite the poverty, the community does have considerable strengths. There is a sense of pride in the area amongst many residents; parks and gardens are attractive, although the sense of 'safety' is less than desirable; school staff are extremely dedicated and committed to the well-being of the community; and, there are many community and recreational facilities, although according to the teenage population, 'there's not enough to do'. Designation as a community renewal area means that state government resources for building physical and social infrastructure will increasingly become available, with a consultant's report on the suburb and an action plan almost complete. There is also an extremely active network of local service providers and community workers who have compiled extensive data on the community and on the needs of families and children. The existence of several reports on the area means, effectively, that much of the essential data collection and appraisal of community resources has already been completed.

Interestingly, no official data on participation rates in formal preschool programs were available. Our initial estimate from our own survey is that, perhaps surprisingly, around 80% of Year 1 children have attended preschool, often the one attached to their primary school. However, our impression is that the participation rates of indigenous and Pacific Islander children are somewhat lower. Generally, we are finding that schools and preschools are a 'pressure point' in terms of the impact of poverty and multiculturalism. Schools have to employ bilingual teacher aides, as many of the children have limited skills in English. Many also have learning difficulties in their first language, and a number of children are significantly below state norms when they commence preschool. The nutrition of children is also a perennial issue. The schools organise meetings with parents to discuss appropriate food, and frequently provide sandwiches for children to ensure they get a proper meal. School excursions, of course, despite being low cost, often do not involve the children who could benefit the most.

The evolving model: child, family, school and community

Without further extensive consultation with parents from all ethnic groups and also with service providers and community workers, it is not possible to state with certainty what programs will be introduced. However, our preliminary work suggests that the general model that is evolving will be acceptable and useful, complementing existing and planned programs in the area. The current project focus is children aged three to six years and their families, preschools, childcare centres, schools and, where possible, the wider community. Thus the transition to school is the immediate focus, with enhanced readiness for school a specific goal. We envisage a set of programs divided into two broad, inter-related categories: family programs and preschool/school programs.

The family programs are conceptualised as consisting of overlapping layers, moving from informal, broad-based programs such as play groups, parenting training, and education forums, to formal support services such as parenting support groups or toy libraries, through to intensive family support and assistance, such as individual and family counselling (including intensive work with families with one or more members in jail or juvenile detention) (Nocella 1996). Some of these services already exist in the area. Many need to be better resourced, while others (as few as possible) will need to be built from scratch.

One resource we hope to bring to the community is a research base consisti
mising or 'proven' Australian programs. Some programs of this type were reviewed
Developmental Crime Prevention Consortium (1999) and have developed further sin
the audit (late 1997). Some have now been evaluated. One example is *TUFF – Together for
Under Fives and Families*. This project was established in 1995 in Coonamble, New South
Wales. It is a joint project between the departments of Health, Community Services and
School Education, and is part of a broader program known as the *Schools as Community Centres
Program*. The aim of this program is to promote a healthy positive start for children entering
school, through inter-agency collaboration and provision of support to families. Outcomes in
Coonamble include (amongst many):

- a significant increase in enrolments in transition-to-school programs, with early identification of at-risk children;
- increased emergent literacy behaviours;
- increased involvement of Aboriginal families and workers in developing strategies to meet
family needs; and
- increased age-appropriate immunisation. (Updated information on TUFF kindly provided
by the Coonamble project team.)

There is a growing consensus amongst researchers that appropriate early learning experiences can act as protective factors, with positive effects upon the cognitive and social
development of preschool children to prevent, or allay, serious educational and behaviour
problems (Golly et al. 1998; Schweinhart and Weikart 1997; Sylva and Colman 1998).
Research findings have made it clear, however, that not all intervention programs are equally
effective in addressing the problems of children with emotional and behaviour difficulties
(Barlow 1998). Analyses of successful programs have revealed that significant elements incorporate a curriculum focus on the specific factors detrimentally affecting social adjustment and
educational progress (Sylva and Colman 1998), and, as we have seen, a focus on key transition
points in the life of the child (Golly et al. 1998). Other significant program elements (as in the
Schools as Community Centres example) involve intervention at the ecological levels of the
parents, family and the wider community, as well as parent and teacher education components
(Barlow 1998;Wasserman and Miller, 1998).

In the light of these significant elements, we are developing a program at the preschool-to-
school transition point that has been piloted in Brisbane and subjected to a preliminary
qualitative evaluation that showed positive results (Elias and Taylor 1995). The research literature strongly suggests that parent-oriented intervention facilitates improved language and
literacy outcomes (Edwards 1995; Snow et al. 1999; Whitehurst et al. 1994). Consequently, a
major component of the proposed program is the enhancement of parent–child and
teacher–child interaction patterns through modifying the adults' interactive style. In particular,
the modifications to adult interactive styles focus on factors relating to children's development of
communication and language skills. It has frequently been pointed out that children's oral
language skills underpin the development of literacy (Bowey 1995; O'Connor et al. 1995), and
that children from low-income families are often disadvantaged with respect to skills essential to
literacy acquisition in a school system dominated by middle-class expectations and practices. In
the light of these findings, relevant program elements include training parents in adult–child

in the use of conversational styles of interaction that enhance the
d language (Dickinson and Smith 1994).

nmunication enhancement groups will be conducted in a number
teacher with specialist qualifications in this field, but later by other
cialist in the methods. These groups will involve parents with their
ill focus on the development of communication skills in play, con-
ding contexts. Allied to this, play groups with similar language and
communica ill be conducted for younger children with their mothers. Communication programs will be developed suited to the particular needs of the parents and children in
the various preschool communities (eg, to meet the needs of non-English-speaking parents).
All this will be fully integrated with the family support activities, including such practical (but
vital) elements as assistance with transport and childcare. The aim is not a narrow focus on
one domain, such as cognitive skills, but on broad aspects of the social and emotional development of children and parents.

Conclusion

The locality matters, especially for families with young children. Disadvantaged communities,
given their concentration of poverty, crime and child maltreatment, matter even more,
whatever the larger societal trends toward greater or lesser inequality. Moreover, the impact of
neighbourhood organisation and social climate on children and young people, independent of
the characteristics of individuals and families, suggests that programs need to be directed to
the community itself, not just to the individuals living in it.

The combination of community development and developmental prevention
approaches has promise as a way of enhancing the impact of programs in the poorest areas, and
genuinely facilitating the move toward independent living by the most disadvantaged families
and their children. This 'transition to a new research mode' is fraught with risks – after all, few
seem to have gone before, few can provide guidance along the way. So a team effort is
required, pooling the skills and insights from many disciplines. There must be, as well, a willingness to take risks and make mistakes. But the journey does seem worth undertaking.

Note

1 The Developmental Crime Prevention Consortium comprised (at the time the Pathways
report was prepared) the convenor, Ross Homel (Griffith University), Judy Cashmore (NSW
Child Protection Council), Linda Gilmore (UQ), Jacqueline Goodnow and Alan Hayes
(Macquarie University), Jeanette Lawrence (Univ. of Melbourne), Marie Leech (Uniya),
Ian O'Connor, John Western and Jake Najman (UQ) and Tony Vinson (UNSW).

Further Reading

Developmental Crime Prevention Consortium. 1999, Pathways to Prevention: Developmental and Early Intervention Approaches to Crime in Australia, National Crime Prevention, Canberra.
  – *The first major attempt in Australia to think systematically about crime prevention, especially in disadvantaged communities, from a developmental perspective.*
Shonkoff, J P & Meisels, S J (Eds) 2000, Handbook of Early Childhood Intervention (2nd edition), Cambridge University Press, Cambridge, UK.
  – *A rich resource for understanding everything from the neurobiological bases of early intervention to the sociology of community development in disadvantaged neighbourhoods.*
Shonkoff, J P & Phillips, D A (Eds) 2000, From Neurons to Neighbourhoods: The Science of Early Childhood Development, National Academy Press, Washington, DC.
  – *A comprehensive review of the scientific research on early childhood, including the intervention literature.*

21
Rethinking evaluation for policy action on the social origins of health and well-being

Beverly Sibthorpe and Jane Dixon

> Health inequalities exist in every country in which they have been assessed but action to tackle them has, with a few exceptions, been conspicuous by its absence (McKee and Jacobson 2000, p 668).

Introduction

We are entering the 21st century with two bodies of evidence that raise fundamental issues about the role of governments and scientists in promoting health and well-being. The first reveals enormous gains made during the 20th century in extending life expectancy for a majority of citizens in the world. At the same time, numerous studies confirm the persistence of social gradients of health for many diseases, as well as increasing social gradients for diseases for which the gap had been narrowing in the 1970s and 1980s. Woodward and colleagues (this volume) provide one illustration, with evidence of a recent mortality cross-over between Australia and New Zealand, due to uneven health improvements of different ethnic groups in New Zealand compared to the average improvement made by Australia's population. This loss of hard-won health gains by some New Zealanders is not confined to that country, with similar findings being reported for parts of Eastern Europe and for regions in rural Australia (Bobák et al. 2000a; Burnley 1998).

In the last couple of years, bodies like the International Society for Equity in Health, the International Poverty and Health Network and the Global Equity Gauge Initiative have been established by scientists and public health practitioners (International Society for Equity in Health Constitution 2000; Heath et al. 2000; Rockefeller Foundation 2000). These action groups are responding to a general lack of government commitment in the area of health inequalities. They share a common aim to produce evidence on which to base interventions that will reduce inequalities in health within and between countries.

Their attention is well directed. A search of the literature for evidence of systematic attempts by governments in this area reveals few examples. (Finland, the Netherlands and, very recently, the UK are notable exceptions.) What it does reveal is enormous national variation with respect to policy (in) action (Hupalo and Herden 1999; Acheson 1998; WHO 2000; New Zealand Ministry of Health 2000b; Mackenbach et al. 1999). In this chapter, we attempt to summarise the underlying reasons for this inaction, with a particular focus on what we see as a key element, namely lack of evidence on which a broad-based reform agenda could be built. The inaction, it seems, has as much to do with uncertainty about how to act as with political resistance.

We begin by drawing out the main themes in the literature on action to address health inequalities that amply demonstrate the need to break the current evidence-to-action impasse. We then go on to examine in detail the central conundrum that faces governments everywhere: that in an increasingly 'evidence-based' world, there is very little evidence to guide population health policy. Why? We argue that, paradoxically, our approaches to evaluation have become a major impediment to progress in accumulating evidence on the effectiveness of broad-based interventions to address inequalities.

We propose that, by rethinking the common distinction between monitoring and research, we can gather evidence, appropriate in scale and relevance, for government action on the structural determinants of health. By harnessing the strengths of both monitoring and research and orienting them to policy evaluation, we will be better able to gather the evidence on which broad-based agendas for change can be built. We put forward this proposal, fully recognising that evidence alone will not lead to government action. Getting issues onto the policy agenda is fundamental to any public policy response, and there remains the perennial task of convincing opinion leaders and others that the evidence before them cannot be ignored (Walt 1998; Tarlov 1999).

The underlying reasons for inaction and disappointing progress

Contemporary accounts of interventions that are successful in reducing health inequalities (Gepkens and Gunning-Shepers 1996; Pettigrew and Macintyre 2001; Oldenburg et al. 2000) are frequently making claims in relation to trials of interventions to change individual health behaviours or small-scale targeted interventions providing heating to cold houses, milk to children, or ante-natal visits to pregnant women. They are usually not talking about evidence on government-level interventions designed to have major structural or whole-of-population effects. Even then, they are outnumbered by those that lament the disappointing record on successful intervention (Graham 2001; Shaw et al. 1999; Syme 1996b; chapters in Marmot and Wilkinson 1999). In its thorough review of interventions to reduce health inequalities, the Evaluation Group established under the UK Independent Inquiry into Inequalities in Health was forced to propose 'promising policies' as opposed to what would generally be considered evidence-based policies, due to a dearth of studies in the area (Pettigrew and Macintyre 2001).

Researchers offer a mix of reasons why so little progress has been made (Shaw et al. 1999; Heymann 2000; Whitehead 1995; Syme 1998). They fall into two broad categories – barriers to policy action and reasons for limited impacts (see table 21.1).

Table 21.1 Barriers to policy action and reasons for limited impacts

Barriers to policy action	Reasons for limited impacts
• Policy inertia • Different worldviews of researchers and policy makers • Lack of appropriate evidence	• Poor implementation of policies • Poor program design • Limited understanding of structure and agency or of risk conditions and risk factors • 'Soundbite' interventions

Barriers to policy action

The major barriers to policy action appear to be three-fold. The first could be called policy inertia, a phrase describing government inability or unwillingness to respond to evidence. Generally, inertia results from government assessments that the policy options before it are too financially or politically costly or that they would require a revolution in administrative arrangements. Conclusions that health inequalities could be substantially reduced through poverty elimination (Howden-Chapman and O'Dea, this volume) or the elimination of racial discrimination (Anderson, this volume) obviously raise the spectre of significant economic and political costs. Similarly, solutions that require different forms of governance – whether of a global nature (Butler et al.; Legge, this volume) or of a community nature (Homel et al., this volume) – are problematic for national governments for administrative reasons. One form of governance promoted in public health circles is intersectoral action, but achieving collaboration among government, non-government not-for-profit, commercial and religious sectors is, in our experience, rare. Similarly, 'joined-up' ways of working in which different government portfolios champion the same policy and contribute resources to achieve shared outcomes are underdeveloped. While it is recognised that health portfolios incur significant health system costs due to social problems generated in the taxation, employment and other ministries, it has not proven easy in Australia, at least, to achieve intergovernmental action on health issues. Time and again, public policy texts confirm Charles Lindblom's assertion that when offered difficult choices, policy-makers retreat to incremental changes based on 'successive limited comparisons' (Howlett and Ramesh 1995, p 143; Colebatch 1998).

McKee and Jacobson (2000) have identified another factor which, in our opinion, encourages policy inertia – the different worlds inhabited by public health practitioners and researchers. They note that the public health field as a whole is weakened because of different training and the few professional opportunities for contact and sharing of ideas between practitioners and researchers. Gill Walt goes a step further, describing how the advice offered by researchers is invariably viewed as irrelevant by policy-makers. She argues that the latter are receptive to research findings that 'they find palatable, viable, persuasive or gratifying' (Walt 1998, p 187). Policy-makers are simultaneously attracted by scientific certainty and by research that acknowledges political exigencies. Unfortunately, the social-determinants-of-health field is riddled with research findings that are highly contingent upon the context of the study – too ambiguous for some – and that fly in the face of political palatability.

A third obstacle to policy action is reflected in arguments about lack of appropriate evidence on which to base a broad-based reform agenda. This debate demonstrates the dominance of reductionist science in the health inequalities field. Australia's National Health and Medical Research Council (2000) has outlined three dimensions to evidence: strength (consisting of level or the study design, quality or bias minimisation and statistical precision), size of effect and relevance of evidence. The evidence-based medicine movement, which adopts uncritically these dimensions to evidence, exercises considerable influence within the health sciences and government health departments in Australia and elsewhere at present (Rychetnik and Frommer 2000, pp 9–10). This means that the movement's preferred study design, a systematic review of randomised control trials (RCTs) is the favoured approach in all study contexts. But when one examines meta-reviews of interventions to reduce health inequalities, based solely on evidence produced through RCTs, the limited options before government become only too obvious (Arblaster et al. 1996). Thus, while we wait for the trials to produce 'Level 1 evidence', decisions about intervention can be deflected. This is a central conundrum to which we return below.

Reasons for limited impact

Complementing the analyses of why there has been so little policy action to redress health inequalities, are commentaries that focus on why the actions which have been taken have had such a marginal impact on health gradients. In a study of the social health policies administered by the Finnish government over three decades, Sihto and Keskimaki (2000) argue that poor policy implementation rather than lack of policies is to blame for increasing health inequalities in that country. Despite years of equitable social and health policies, Finland has relatively equitable incomes accompanied by high health inequalities. The authors argue that even though health equity targets were emphasised, the intersectoral action needed to achieve them was missing, and that there was a *laissez-faire* attitude as to how to aim at the targets. They noted that the Finnish Health For All program implementation failed because of '1) universal fear of change, 2) inadequately developed social change technologies, and 3) the failure to plan implementation' (Sihto and Keskimaki 2000, p 283).

Inadequate policy implementation may be accompanied by the poor design of programs, although it is sometimes unclear whether disappointing outcomes are the result of program design failure or of evaluation design failure. Nowhere is this more apparent than in the numerous reflections on the major cardiovascular disease (CVD) prevention programs. While there is widespread disagreement on why well-funded CVD studies, like Stanford and Minnesota, are producing inconsistent results, there is greater consensus that the experimental designs have been flawed (Susser 1995; Winkelby 1994). (The Stanford Five-City Project began in 1978, and the Minnesota Heart Health Program was funded in 1980.) The faults extend to inadequate sample size and exposure to the intervention and inability to control for secular trends and other confounders. One risk of the critical appraisals of community-based interventions is that intervening at the population level becomes identified with failure. This encourages a retreat into the clinic and an emphasis on individual risk factors, exemplified by preventative screening and tailor-made behaviour modification programs. In essence, the evaluation methods of clinical epidemiology legitimise interventions that trivialise the causes of social problems.

A related reason for poor outcomes in respect of health inequalities could well be naivety about risk factors, risk conditions (another term for the social environment) and interventions (Syme 1996b; Mustard 1996). If good program design relies on theoretically grounded assumptions about the nature of the variables, then inadequate conceptualisation will inevitably lead to poor design. It is possible to reinterpret the Finnish case-study and argue that the failure to arrest growing health inequalities in that country has little to do with inadequate policy implementation. Instead it might be due to inadequate program design based on poor conceptualisation of 'lifestyle', a point mentioned in passing by the authors. This is also a likely reason for the lack of success of CVD prevention programs for addressing health inequalities (Winkelby 1994).

The chapters by Powles and Eckersley (this volume) distinguish between culturally and socio-economically determined behaviours. While we see these as much more closely interdependent, we support the central point that factors in addition to income and income inequality contribute to the adoption of habits and attitudes that produce and reproduce social hierarchies. (Leonard Syme (1998) has proposed that the persistence of health inequalities could be due to 'the persistence of hierarchy'.) Income alone cannot distinguish social status. Other dimensions of social class or social group affiliation such as education, ethnicity and religion, are also important.

So-called 'lifestyle choices' are shaped by these dimensions of affiliation (the structural element), whose constraints individuals have some capacity to accept, reject or modify (the element of agency). What so often goes unacknowledged is the extremely important insight offered by French sociologist Pierre Bourdieu (1984) that individual choices are in fact the unconsciously performed, taken-for-granted actions of everyday life that reflect social position.

The structure–agency theory adopted by sociologists and anthropologists informs us that lifestyle patterns may be differentially adopted, thereby creating differently patterned conditions of risk, or social environments, that must be understood in their own right and separately from individual risk factors. For example, decisions by groups to adopt the bicycle rather than the motor car as their primary means of transport, or to adopt dietary customs based on 'slow food' as opposed to fast food, foster particular social environments. These environments, in turn, structure or encourage the adoption or rejection of behaviours and attitudes, which affect individual risk factors. Reflecting Bourdieuan thinking, 'in assessing health and disease data, we still should consider the extent to which limits in capacity, energy and poor health affect work, earnings, and status positions in social structures as well as the reverse' (Mechanic 2000, p 294).

If lifestyle is reduced to individual risk factors, then the resulting interventions will not be designed to impact on the social environment that gives rise to lack of physical activity, over-nutrition, excess alcohol consumption and violent behaviour. In other words, if more effective interventions are desired then greater theoretical sophistication is required in the area of 'status, opportunity, privilege, power, and authority' (Tarlov 1999, p 292). This point is also made in the previous chapter by Homel and colleagues.

Finally, the tendency for governments to develop what we are terming 'soundbite interventions' (a term inspired by reading Heymann 2000) does not help. These are programs aimed at electorate-based population groups that can be explained on the evening news. Australia is awash with government-funded health programs for rural and remote populations that are of this nature. While these programs may play a part in reducing urban–rural health differentials, they are characterised by easily measured outcomes, such as numbers of new general practitioners in the bush, households with access to tele-medicine technologies and patient access to high-tech diagnostic facilities. They are not based on any evidence of a relationship between per capita expenditure on healthcare and life expectancy or any other health outcome, but on a current Australian bureaucratic adage: 'what gets measured, gets done'. In short, interventions that are designed around measurability or evaluability criteria are rarely based on a sound appreciation of theories of causation or of a history of public health interventions. Powles' (this volume) description of public health's 'success without intervention' is a salutory reminder that popular adaptations to knowledge about the causes and management of disease are as important as professionally driven interventions.

This assessment of the reasons why so little progress has been made in addressing health inequalities highlights the need for a circuit-breaker to the evidence–action impasse. At the heart of the problem is the interweaving of policy inertia and reductionist science, with its hierarchy of evidence that privileges particular study designs. We believe that the equity in health and well-being agenda will be better served by other kinds of research more suited to the task at hand. In the remainder of the paper, we make a case for recasting the source and nature of the evidence base needed for an agenda to systematically address health inequalities.

Obtaining the evidence

Berkman and Kawachi (2000) characterise the study of the social determinants of health as 'social epidemiology'. Its interest in understanding the determinants of health inequalities in terms of social structures and processes, and its orientation towards social action, places it squarely within the traditions of critical social science, which is characterised by a belief that:

> [P]eople are constrained by the material conditions, cultural context and historical conditions in which they find themselves . . . [They] live in a world of structures and processes that limit their options and shape their beliefs and behavior but are not locked into an inevitable set of structures, relationships or laws, . . . [because] they can develop new meanings or ways of seeing that enable them to change these structures, relationships and laws. (Neuman 1994, p 69)

Thus, social epidemiology's theoretical roots are anchored much more in Marx and Durkheim than in medicine. And interventions building on the knowledge generated by social epidemiologists will most often have to address structural factors in communities, rather than behaviours in individuals. Yet, when we come to think about evaluating these interventions, we tend to slide inexorably into positivist ways of thinking (Lomas 1998). This pushes us relentlessly towards positivist experimental methods: measuring intervening factors and the (precisely defined) elements of the intervention, clearly delineating and measuring outcomes, controlling for background effects, holding the intervention constant, studying and carefully selecting (and excluding) individual participants, and relying heavily on statistical analysis

(Ovretveit 1998). We cling to this approach, calling for (Dixon and Leeder 2000) and privileging (Arblaster et al. 1996) randomised controlled trials, even when we know, that in this context, they are extremely difficult to conduct and often unhelpful in terms of the information they produce.

The *main reason* such trials are extremely difficult to conduct and unhelpful is that people interested in the social determinants of health seek improved understanding of the impacts of (changes to) social structures and processes on communities, and these cannot be properly elucidated using positivist methods. As Swales (2000, p 324) puts it: 'the reductionist logic of the randomised controlled trial cannot easily be applied to social policy'. From this fundamental mismatch between paradigm and method, many of our problems arise. We grapple with the fact that human communities are enormously complex and subject to the impacts of local, regional, national and international social, economic and political change. We struggle for precise definition and constancy knowing that interventions to reduce inequalities have to be multi-faceted, flexible and dynamic, continuously adapting to new knowledge (Powles, this volume). We agonise over measurement, knowing that much of what is central to what we are trying to do does not lend itself to measurement and that there are likely to be many unanticipated (and thus unmeasured) impacts. We worry about controlling for background effects, knowing that randomisation is often not an option and, even if it were, that there are likely to be problems with dilution bias (Lindholm and Rosen 2000) and confounding. We talk about the importance of long, even multi-generational timeframes for follow-up, knowing that the vast majority of intervention evaluations will never have this luxury. And the few that do face the very real possibility that, over time, changes in the political, economic, social and environmental conditions may render the interventions or their evaluations, or both, obsolete. (Ashton (2000, p 724) caricatured such research as the tendency to receive funding and 'disappear for three to five years, only coming back with the answer when the question [has] changed'.) We wrestle with what is in part an ethical dilemma: that rigorous experimental evaluations are expensive and drain scarce dollars from program delivery in needy communities. And we know, that because they are so expensive, they are seldom going to be funded adequately, particularly not by governments who often, rightly, have other imperatives. Even when such studies are properly funded, we know they often will not provide very satisfactory answers. This makes both evaluators and those wanting to draw on the evidence they produce increasingly suspicious about the usefulness and value for money of the evaluations – and the interventions! Generalisability is often such an issue that findings may never be taken up to anything like the extent the cost of the evaluation might warrant. So, it is not surprising that evaluation of community-based interventions to address the up-stream social determinants of health is increasingly the subject of comment and scepticism (eg, Feinleib 1996; Judge 2000; Lindholm and Rosen 2000; Puska 2000; Homel et al., this volume).

All this leads us and others (Lomas 1998; Smith PJ et al. 1997) to conclude that the current pre-occupation with pursuing community-based interventions that have rigorous experimental or quasi-experimental designs is inappropriate. Indeed, a world in which future social policies and programs are based on amassed evidence from social intervention 'experiments' is quite fanciful. For the kinds of issues we are concerned about and the type and scale of the interventions that need to be conducted, these are quite simply the wrong methods.

Not only are they the wrong methods for specific interventions, but they also militate against obtaining evidence from the natural 'experiments' embodied in government policies and programs that will in many, if not most, cases be *the* major interventions in health inequalities.

So how can we most effectively and efficiently accumulate knowledge to inform decision-making to reduce health inequalities? We can do this by rethinking the orthodox divide between monitoring and research, and harnessing them both for evaluation purposes.

What is monitoring?

Monitoring is defined by Last (2001) as 'the intermittent performance and analysis of routine measurements aimed at detecting changes in the environment or health status of populations' but also 'episodic measurement of the effect of an intervention on the health status of a population or environment'. The measurements are often called indicators, one of the earliest definitions of which is given by Bauer (1966, p 1) as 'statistics, statistical series and all other forms of evidence that enable us to assess where we stand and are going *with respect to our values and goals*, and to evaluate the specific programs and determine their impact' [emphasis added]. Salvaris et al. (2000, p 57) define an indicator as 'a measurement of something important or valuable'. Monitoring in this sense is not to be confused with program monitoring, which is more narrowly concerned with ongoing oversight of program performance (Last, 2001; Rossi and Freeman 1993).

According to Bauer (1966), expanded interest in monitoring social indicators in the US grew out of recognition of the need to monitor the impact on society of federal programs. As a movement, it has had its critics. In the 1980s, Hogwood and Gunn wrote that:

> [A]spirations of this 'social indicators movement' have not been met, nor is it likely that they will be. This reflects problems over values (disagreements about the normative implications of changes in indicators), problems over our knowledge of social processes (which is necessary if we are to be able to assess the impact of government programs on indicators) and also more technical problems of measurement (selecting indicators which are both valid ie, meaningful measurements of the problem with which we are concerned and reliable ie, will consistently reflect changes in the problem) (Hogwood and Gunn 1984, p 81).

In spite of this, monitoring of social indicators both nationally and internationally is well in train. Indeed, population health monitoring provides the information on which much of Australia's current knowledge about the nature and scope of inequalities is based. And there is growing interest and activity at all levels of government in a broader array of indicators, for example for social capital, sustainable development, citizenship, income inequality, subjective well-being, biological diversity and many more topics (Eckersley 1998a). The potential for synergy between monitoring and evaluation is immediately obvious. By expanding what we monitor to include indicators that reflect our understanding of the social determinants of health, and by undertaking research to investigate the relationships between various types of intervention and shifts in selected indicators, we can gather evidence about both intended and unintended impacts. The sum of this activity is evaluation: the passing of judgement about the worth of policies and programs, or more prosaically, the answer to Neuman's (1994, p 23) question, '*Does it work?*'

The use of monitoring data for evaluative purposes is not new. It happens all the time. Social and political critique commonly involves interrogation of the relationships between indicators and changes occurring in international, national, regional or local conditions. For example, an academic researcher may assess the impact of an employment scheme on the economic status of a disadvantaged group (Altman and Gray 2000), or social trends may be qualitatively 'mapped' to suicide rates and other indicators to investigate possible relationships between the two (Eckersley 1998b). (Journalists also carry out such studies, although often with less theoretical grounding or empiricism.) However, such research is usually not considered evaluative, a term much more narrowly linked to experimental studies of 'an intervention'. But why? Changes to welfare entitlements, the establishment of more family-friendly workplaces, or the introduction of new taxes are all, in effect, interventions. Indeed, they are exactly the kinds of broad-based interventions advocated by social determinists, and interrogation of the shifts in indicators that map their impacts on populations are, in effect, evaluative.

The monitoring

All OECD countries have many of the elements of a mechanism for national monitoring of the social condition already in place. In Australia, the infrastructure provided by the Australian Bureau of Statistics (ABS) and the Australian Institute of Health and Welfare (AIHW), and data from registers, from routine surveys undertaken by the ABS (eg, census, household expenditure, labour force and health surveys) and from other collections (see Turrell et al. 1999) already provide a basis for monitoring activities with temporal depth. In Australia, resources such as HealthWIZ and the Social Health Atlas (Glover et al. 1999) make accessible data for a number of different sectors including health, population census, social security, and child-care. Importantly, attempts are being made to expand what we monitor, as demonstrated by the inclusion of indicators of access to health services and community involvement in health policy, planning and program implementation in the National Aboriginal Health Performance Indicators (AIHW 2000) (these indicators are far from perfect, and much of the developmental work on their validity and practicability is yet to be done, but they constitute a significant first step in expanding the meaning and role of monitoring in Aboriginal health) and consideration by the ABS of including indicators of phenomena such as social capital (ABS 2000c).

Many countries including the USA, Canada and UK are pouring resources into greatly expanded monitoring. Canada has embarked on an ambitious population health initiative that will, significantly, be monitored by Statistics Canada.

Under the US *Healthy People* initiative, 467 national objectives with associated indicators have been developed, with a subset of 12 considered to be the highest priority for reporting. These have been picked up, modified or changed by individual states. An often-cited example is the Oregon Legislative Assembly's *Oregon Shines* initiative, which includes 92 indicators relating to the economy, education, civic engagement, social support, public safety, community development, and the environment (Oregon Progress Board, 1999). All jurisdictions are required to report annually on their respective indicators.

Developing a set of robust indicators obviously requires some entity to be given responsibility and long-term funding to coordinate a national (and international) effort. Health inequalities policy evaluators will want to draw on indicators from a range of areas, such as housing, education, justice and welfare, as well as health, and will need to get involved in the development of appropriate indicators across this range. Beyond this however, a set of national indicators does not necessarily require much intersectoral collaboration, since sectors can be held responsible both for the data collection and reporting mechanisms within their sectors – thus the education, health and justice systems can work relatively independently. Where the innovation would lie, at least in Australia, is in bringing together and making widely accessible key indicators from a range of different sectors to provide a much more comprehensive overview of the social condition than is currently available. Where cross-sectoral work would need to be done is in the research area – interrogating the meaning not only of trends in the indicators but also of possible cross-linkages between them, for example, between health and education, or between crime rates and trust.

To provide an effective framework for evaluation, indicators have to be available at regular intervals, some quite frequent. This means that much greater effort needs to be invested in collection, quality assurance, collation and timely reporting of data from a range of jurisdictions and sectors. This effort is required anyway, for better monitoring of the condition of the nation, for accountability and, increasingly, for benchmarking. It can also provide a basis for the evaluation of community interventions.

In order to address some of the key questions exercising the minds of health (and social) inequalities interventionists, we will undoubtedly need to expand what we monitor. A starting point for identifying indicators for health inequalities monitoring is to return to the 'pathways stories', explicated in the earlier chapters of this volume, particularly Turrell's chapter, and receiving fuller treatment in other texts (Marmot and Wilkinson 1999; Berkman and Kawachi 2000). Each pathway contains theories about cause and effect relationships as well as concepts underpinning the theories. If there is interest in monitoring the impact of particular risk conditions (rather than individual risk factors) on social gradients for CVD, for example, attention can be paid to one pathway or to the composite impact of several pathways. To date, the neo-materialist pathway has been studied through indicators that include individual and area poverty levels, degree of income inequality, housing type and environmental hazards. Social support and demand-control in the workplace are the indicators frequently used by pyscho-social pathway researchers to describe the way individuals respond to their social environment. The Whitehall studies on the effect of work organisation on CVD have used indicators from both pathways and are now extending the data collected to biological pathways (Brunner and Marmot 1999).

Once the pathways have been selected, further theoretical and technical issues arise with the choice of indicators. For example, whether social capital is to be measured on the basis of it being a property of individuals or of a social unit is an epistemological question surrounded by much debate (Kawachi and Berkman 2000). The answer to the question has implications for the indicators best able to operationalise the concept, with repercussions for the unit of measurement. If social capital is considered to be embodied in individuals, then aggregate variables are appropriate, and surveys are the logical data collection instruments. If, however, social capital is thought to reside in social units, integral variables are required with observational techniques being the principal means of capturing them (Kawachi and Berkman 2000). The latter are underdeveloped compared to individual unit aggregation, however, some progress is being made particularly by those focusing on the social properties of localities (Macintyre and Ellaway 2000). The observational techniques used are familiar to qualitative researchers and include community network analysis, textual analysis of public documents, geographic mapping of services and journeys to work, and ethnographic accounts of leadership and behaviours in workplaces and communities. Their use is well illustrated in the chapter by Harris et al. (this volume).

The chapters by Woodward, and Butler and colleagues show how advantageous it is to be able to compare indicators across nations by manipulating national data collections. Even better is the ability to draw on international longitudinal studies, such as the World Values Survey undertaken by the Inter-University Consortium for Political and Social Research. In a positive development, the European Union has commissioned Erasmus University's Department of Public Health to develop indicators of health that can be standardised across the Union and to develop indicators appropriate for each country's monitoring purposes.

It is possible that national indicators may not allow fine-grained assessment of the impacts on small communities within countries. However, NZ experience with a deprivation index is salutary in this respect. This index has been under development for over a decade, the latest version being NZDep96. NZDep96 is an area-based measure of deprivation on a scale of 1(least deprived) to 10 (most deprived) that combines nine variables from the 1996 census that reflect eight dimensions of deprivation, such as education, income and occupation (Crampton 1999; Health Funding Authority 2000). It can be applied to a 'meshblock', which is a small geographical unit comprising a median of just 90 people (Crampton 1999). Data show that those at the lower (more deprived) end of the scale have a marked increase in avoidable mortality rates over those at the most advantaged end (Health Funding Authority 2000). The index is now used in a number of health-related research and policy settings, demonstrating the usefulness of macro indicators in assessing differences between groups at the micro level.

The research

Under an 'evaluation-through-monitoring-and-research' approach, evaluation dollars will be spent on rigorous and systematic research to investigate the relationships between interventions and shifts in the relevant indicators. This will have to involve triangulation of epidemiological, sociological, anthropological, economic and policy analysis. Its purpose will be to investigate, through 'creative study designs' (Lomas 1998, p 1185), specific research questions, the answers to which would flesh out our understanding of the relationships, including intermediate effects, between intervention and outcome. Much of this interrogative work will, of necessity, be qualitative (see example below). This will give rise to a change in emphasis in the training, methods and theoretical orientations of the health intervention evaluation workforce, away from the current heavy reliance on conventional epidemiology to inclusion of a range of other disciplines and methods and a heavy emphasis on good policy analytical skills. Public health historians have much to contribute, as the chapter by Powles illustrates. Being able to draw on a century or more of data and recognising multiple social processes lends depth to the inferences that can be drawn between interventions and population health outcomes. Those with conventional epidemiological skills will also still have an important role to play, not only in the ongoing development and interrogation of the validity of the indicators, but also in the analysis of the quantitative data incidentally available or purpose-collected that will be an integral part of the exploration of plausible links.

Evaluation through monitoring and research

The proposed approach, then, is evaluation through the systematic and rigorous use of a range of research methods to understand the (causal) links between structural reforms and shifts in health indicators. We use a hypothetical example to illustrate the approach. Suppose that empirical and theoretical work has established that 'trust', an element of social capital, is positively associated with a number of health outcomes including self-rated health. Trust is monitored nationally in a periodic social survey and is known to vary widely between communities. The police department decides to address the issue of trust in a cluster of communities with the lowest levels of trust in a major metropolitan area, by making a number of changes to policing arrangements. It wants to evaluate the impact of the changes, which are likely to take about five years for their full effects to be felt. Their evaluators advise that, rather than trying to undertake a long, costly experimental or quasi-experimental study, they plan to use the trust indicator from the social survey as their outcome, and ask, 'What is the relationship between changes to policing arrangements (the intervention) and changes in trust between date x and date y?' To answer this question, they draw up a research plan that involves analysis of:

- retrospective and prospective analysis of quantitative data from the police department in this and neighbouring jurisdictions on expenditure, police coverage, arrests, and types of crime etc;
- qualitative data from key informant interviews, focus groups and community meetings;
- written material including policy documents, reports, newspapers, and community newsletters; and
- international data from a number of countries in Europe that have a range of different but nevertheless comparable policing arrangements.

They may also have access to published data from other surveys conducted in the area during the intervening years that have elements that are pertinent to their question. By rigorous analysis and interpretation of data from all these sources, they attempt to assess the links between the changes to policing arrangements and shifts in levels of trust (and thus social capital) after five years.

The example is represented diagrammatically in figure 21.1.

The evaluation of the folate fortification policy by the Australian Food and Nutrition Monitoring Unit is a more concrete example. Folate fortification of foods is one of the interventions for which there is substantial evidence of a health benefit (reduction in birth defects) and the potential to reduce health inequalities. The Unit was asked to compile existing data to evaluate the policy after developing a conceptual framework to identify the variables of interest (the indicators), and to organise the information by level of evaluation (process, impact and outcome). Information came from routine data collections for baseline and subsequent data, reworking of older data to allow for comparability over time, several purpose-built, one-off surveys conducted by different government bodies for their own purposes, information supplied by the food industry and modelling of data when particular collections ceased (Abraham and Webb 2000). Interestingly, one of the key findings of the evaluation was the

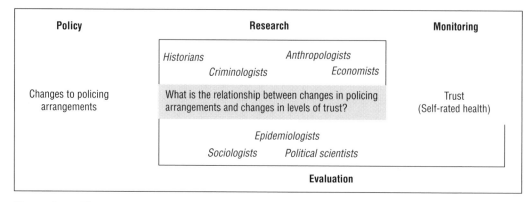

Figure 21.1 Diagrammatic representation of evaluation through monitoring and research

inadequacy of the data sets in the food and nutrition area to enable accurate monitoring of the policy implementation, as well as the health outcomes. For example, birth defects were substantially under-enumerated in the current system.

The work of Ichiro Kawachi and colleagues in the US on the way in which social capital affects health demonstrates the triangulation of monitoring data from different sources. They cross-referenced data from two questions, one on per capita membership in voluntary associations, and another on levels of interpersonal trust, in the General Social Surveys with data on self-rated health from a national Behavioral Risk Factor Survey (Kawachi and Berkman 2000). This sort of research should be able to be replicated in Australia in a few years with the inclusion of social capital questions in the General Social Survey cross-referenced to other routine collections such as the Crime and Safety Survey (ABS 1998b).

The proposed approach will not get us to causation as (narrowly) defined by epidemiology. But this is anyway extremely difficult in complex open systems (Judge 2000) and, in the context of social epidemiology, is itself the subject of critique (Armstrong 1999; Kreiger 1994). What investigations of the relationships between changes in social conditions and shifts in indicators can do is draw increasingly plausible explanations of the links between the two, or, in the words of Lomas (1998, p 1185) 'tell compelling causative stories from associative data'.

Strengths of the approach?

We believe the proposed approach constitutes a more effective and efficient way of evaluating broad-based health inequalities interventions for the following reasons:

- It will reduce the overall costs of evaluation per se. It could be argued that it would just shift some evaluation costs to better monitoring. To some extent this is true, but because monitoring data can be used for multiple evaluations, and over time, as well as for other purposes, there are clearly economies to be achieved.
- So long as we have the right indicators, it will establish a framework for the evaluation of all interventions. Having the right indicators means ensuring that they have cross-cultural validity and importance.

- It will increasingly impose the use of standard measures of impact and outcome, in place of the current proliferation that renders cross-comparisons between evaluations a distant dream in most cases. Through use and interrogation, the robustness and political respectability of the measures will increase over time, an important issue in terms of the political processes involved in achieving change.
- Because no jurisdiction will be able to afford the cost of senseless monitoring, it will force us to focus, over time, on the most important indicators.
- It better accommodates the layering of analysis and interpretation both of aggregated individual and community indicators, as well as other types of information from a range of different sources that is necessary to understand social structures and processes, and their impacts on individuals.
- It lends itself well to consideration of cross-portfolio impacts – for example on health, education and crime – of broad-based interventions.
- It allows the all-important reporting of time trends, giving much greater temporal depth to our evaluation efforts (currently sadly lacking).
- It will allow comparisons between communities at local, regional, national (and international) levels – critical to an endeavour concerned with relativities (something many of our current program evaluations fail to address).
- It opens the way for benchmarking, again addressing relativities, and allowing governmental and other instrumentalities to be held accountable for levels achieved.
- It encourages interventions to adapt in response to program learning or changes in economic or political conditions, and frees evaluators from the often pointless pursuit of measurement of both elements of the intervention, and of trying to hold their interventions constant in the face of good evidence to do otherwise.
- By virtue of the centrality of qualitative approaches, it allows individuals and communities a much greater voice in identifying both the *felt* impacts of social change and possible solutions.
- It allows governments to act now on indicator development and reporting, based on current and rapidly accumulating evidence about what it is important to monitor, thus doing something tangible with long-term benefits and without constraints of trying to envisage what kinds of interventions may be implemented now or in the future.
- To a significant extent, publicly available routine data collections allow evaluative activities to take place wherever and whenever there are researchers and other critics with the means to undertake the interrogative work, whether or not it is formally embodied in and funded through an 'intervention' or is endorsed by interest groups, including governments and other entities. In a very real sense, evaluation that proceeds through a credible national monitoring system can hold itself above the vagaries of politics. (Though still open to challenge are the interpretations of the plausible links drawn by various commentators, including evaluators.) Importantly, community groups can have accessible impact and outcome information to provide them with the basis for comment and political action.

Of course, the monitoring framework will only be as good as the scope and quality of its 'basket of indicators' (a term used by the UK government in its recent health inequalities reduction targets announcement). In order adequately to assess the impact of interventions to reduce health inequalities, we clearly have to expand what we monitor. This process will have to be ongoing but have obvious limits, perhaps exceeded already by the US's *Healthy People 2020* with its hundreds of indicators. It will require national leadership and a very long time-frame. The indicators will need to be valid and reliable. Eventually, in order to be manageable and affordable, monitoring systems may need to drop old indicators in order to add new ones, which will interrupt the analysis and interpretation of time trends. It would be hoped that the indicators that were lost were considered expendable for good, empirical reasons. Even then it must be remembered that, in Biderman's words,

> Statistical data about society are themselves institutional products. They are products of major and costly social undertakings; of elaborate institutions. As such, they are influenced and constrained by the principles that pertain to all complex institutions in society, including some that also shape the phenomena they measure . . . Therefore . . . attempts to use social indicators to direct social change will greatly profit by subjecting social statistics to the same kinds of detached, sociological scrutiny that we give other institutional products (Biderman 1966, pp 69–70).

Such scrutiny would have to be an integral part of our evaluation efforts.

Conclusion

In concentrating on the contribution that research can make to reducing health inequalities, we do not wish to convey an impression that a better approach to evaluation alone will result in successful action. We would, however, argue that it will greatly alleviate the paradoxical condition in which we currently find ourselves – that our approach to evaluation is the major impediment to the collection of evidence.

We believe that a better approach to evaluation hinges on the development and use of a basket of indicators of health and well-being. These become the intervention outcomes, applicable to multiple interventions in different places (international down to local) at different times. They apply equally to policies and programs specifically designed to reduce health inequalities as well as those that are not. As Turrell et al. (1999, p 65) argue, such data cannot be expected to tell us much about the processes and mechanisms underpinning the observed patterns in health inequalities. But this is not, as they argue, because 'they were not designed for research purposes per se'. It has little to do with the inherent attributes of the data. It is because the next step that we are advocating – the use of a range of research methods to help understand the mechanisms lying behind the trends in the indicators – has not been done in a systematic way.

If we do not take a fresh approach to evaluation, away from the current obsession with experimental and quasi-experimental methods, it is difficult to see how we can escape our current predicament. There will be continuing policy inertia and, inevitably, an emphasis on interventions that focus on (more manageable) downstream factors that are politically less problematic and allow better control and more precise measurement. Thus, the limitations of our evaluation methods will drive intervention, a highly undesirable outcome. If there is now sufficient evidence that best practice approaches to addressing inequalities need to be ecological in their approach, intersectoral, and have multiple entry points, aiming for simplification would be flying in the face of the evidence!

It will not be an easy task to come up with plausible explanations of the relationship between interventions and changes in health inequalities using this approach. Evaluators will not be able to retreat behind the fortress of test statistics and p values to defend their arguments. There will need to be true interdisciplinarity in the research effort, and a recognition of the equally valuable and important contribution that different disciplines have to make. Epidemiologists will need to restrain themselves from denigrating explanations of 'causality' that are defined in ways other than those they are used to. And robust debate about analysis and interpretations will have to be actively encouraged and engaged in by those both within and outside academic circles, especially including members of communities about whom the debates are being had.

We believe that value judgements about interventions to reduce health inequalities can be made through the rigorous and systematic marrying of monitoring and research. The development of robust indicators, on which the whole approach rests, will require national leadership and coordination, probably best set in the context not just of health inequalities, but of social inequalities more broadly. The mindset will have to be one of developing and implementing a system that will last for decades to come. And indicator developers will have to be cognisant of international developments, so that ultimately we will be able to make and understand local through to global comparisons of health inequalities.

We are grateful to Dr Jerry Schwab for his helpful critique of earlier drafts of this manuscript and to Dr Karen Webb for her insights into monitoring for policy purposes.

Further Reading

Swales, J 2000, Inequalities: a challenge to science and politics, New Zealand Medical Journal 11 August: 324–5.
  – *A thought-provoking discussion, both of the limits of conventional evaluation methods when applied to social programs, and what role epidemiologists might play in social advocacy.*
Armstrong, D 1999, 'Controversies in epidemiology', teaching causality in context at the University at Albany, School of Public Health. Scandinavian Journal of Public Health 27: 81–4.
  – *Argues that the way in which the conceptualisation of disease processes is restricted to the current causal paradigm, which is based on socially determined ideas of individualism, reductionism, monocausality and the legitimacy of social inequalities, is a fundamental assumption underlying conventional epidemiological debates of causality and must be challenged.*

Bibliography

Aardal-Eriksson, E., Karlberg, B.E. & Holm, A.C. 1998, Salivary cortisol: an alternative to serum cortisol determinations in dynamic function tests, Clinical Chemistry and Laboratory Medicine 36: 215–22.

Abbasi, K. 1999, Free the slaves. Debt relief for the world's poorest is feasible but may not happen [editorial], British Medical Journal 318: 1568–9.

Aboriginal and Torres Strait Islander Commission and Department of Health and Human Services 1995, Memorandum of Understanding between the Department of Health and Human Services and the Aboriginal and Torres Strait Islander Commission (ATSIC), Schedule 1, Definitions.

Aboriginal and Torres Strait Islander Women's Task Force on Violence 1999, Report. Department of Aboriginal and Torres Strait Islanders, Brisbane, Qld.

Abraham, B. & Webb, K. 2000, An interim evaluation of the voluntary folate fortification policy, Australian Food and Nutrition Monitoring Unit, University of Queensland, <www.sph.uq.edu.au/nutrition/monitoring>

Acheson, D. 1998, Independent Inquiry into Inequalities in Health Report, The Stationery Office, UK.

Acheson, E.D. 1993, Behold a pale horse: a view from Whitehall, PHLS Microbiology Digest 10: 133–40.

Ackerman, A., Ramanathan, V., Toon, O.B., Stevens, D.E., Heymsfield, A.J. & Welton, E.J. 2000, Reduction of tropical cloudiness by soot, Science 288: 1042–7.

Adler, N.E., Boyce, T., Chesney, M.A., Cohn, S., Folkman, S., Kahm, R.L. & Syme, S.L. 1994, Socioeconomic status and health: the challenge of the gradient, American Psychologist 49(1): 15–24.

Adler, N.E., Marmot, M., McEwen, B.S. & Stewart, J. (Eds) 1999, Socio-economic Status and Health in Industrial Nations: social, psychological, and biological pathways, Annals of the New York Academy of Sciences vol.896, Academy of Sciences New York, NY.

Aggarwal, A. & Narain, S. 1991, Global warming in an unequal world: a case of environmental colonialism, Earth Island Journal 6 (2): 39–40.

Aghion, P., Caroli, E. & Garcia-Penalosa, C. 1999, Inequality and economic growth: the perspective of the new growth theories, Journal of Economic Literature 37: 1615–60.

Akanji, A.O., Ezenwaka, C., Adejuwon, C.A. & Osotimehin, B.O. 1990, Plasma and salivary concentrations of glucose and cortisol during insulin-induced hypoglycaemic stress in healthy Nigerians, African Journal of Medicine and Medical Science 19: 265–9.

Akerstedt, T. 1998, Shiftwork and disturbed sleep/wakefulness, Sleep Medicine Reviews 2: 117–28.

Akerstedt, T., Kecklund, G., Olsson, B. & Lowden, A. 2000, New working time arrangements, performance and health, in Isaksson, K., Hogstedt, C., Eriksson, C. & Theorell, T. (Eds), pp. 207–14.

Allen, M.R., Stott, P.A., Mitchell, J.F.B., Schnur, R. & Delworth, T.L. 2000, Quantifying the uncertainty in forecasts of anthropogenic climate change, Nature 407: 617–20.

Altman, J.C. & Gray, M.C. 2000, The effects of the CDEP scheme on the economic status of Indigenous Australians: some analyses using the 1996 Census. Discussion Paper No.195, Centre for Aboriginal Economic Policy Research, The Australian National University, Canberra.

American Psychological Association, Commission on Violence and Youth 1993, Violence and Youth: Psychology's Response, Vol 1. Washington DC.

Amick, B.C., Levine, S., Tarlov, A.R. & Chapman Walsh, D. (Eds) 1995, Society and Health, Oxford University Press, New York.

Anand, S. & Chen, L. 1996, Health implications of economic policies: a framework of analysis, United Nations Development Programme, New York.

Andersen, R.M. 1995, Revisiting the behavioral model and access to medical care: Does it matter? Journal of Health and Social Behaviour 36 (March): 1–10.

Anderson, I. 1997, The National Aboriginal Health Strategy, in Gardner, H. (Ed.), Health Policy: Development, Implementation, and Evaluation in Australia, Melbourne, Oxford University Press, pp. 119–35.

Anderson, I. 2000(a), Critical issues in national Aboriginal and Torres Strait Islander health policy and strategy, in Galbally, R., Krupinski, J. (Eds), Reform Redesign Revolution, Health Agendas for the 21st Century, Australian International Health Institute, The University of Melbourne, Melbourne.

Anderson, I. 2000(b), Problematic paradigms, social epidemiology and the health of Aboriginal and Torres Strait Islanders, Australasian Epidemiologist 7: 32–5.

Anderson, I., Simmons, S. 1999. HIV prevention and Aboriginal and Torres Strait Islander primary health care, Health Promotion Journal of Australia 9: 44–8.

Anderson, I., Young, H., Markovic, M. & Manderson, L. 2001, Aboriginal Primary Health Care in Victoria: Issues for policy and regional planning, VicHealth Koori Health Research and Community Development Unit, Discussion Paper, No 1, Centre for the Study of Health and Society, University of Melbourne.

Anderson, N.B. & Armstead, C.A. 1995, Toward understanding the association of socioeconomic status and health: a new challenge for the biopsychosocial approach, Psychosomatic Medicine 57: 213–25.

Andrain, C.F. 1998, Public Health Policies and Social Inequality, New York University Press, New York.

Aneshensel, C.S. & Pearlin, L.I. 1987, Structural contexts of sex differences in distress, in Aneshensel, C.S. & Pearlin, L.I. (Eds), Gender and Stress, Free Press, New York, pp. 75–95.

Anonymous. 1994(a), Structural adjustment too painful? [editorial]. Lancet 344: 1377–8.

Anonymous. 1994(b), Apocalypse soon, The Economist July 23: 29–30.

Anonymous. 1997, Plenty of gloom, The Economist December 20: 19–21.

Antonovsky, A. 1967, Social class, life expectancy and overall mortality, Milbank Memorial Fund Quarterly XLV: 31–73.

Arblaster, L., Lambert, M., Entwistle, V., Forster, M., Fullerton, D., Sheldon, T. & Watt, I. 1996, A systematic review of the effectiveness of health service interventions aimed at reducing inequalities in health. Journal of Health Services Research and Policy 1 (2): 93–103.

Argyle, M. 1997, Is happiness a cause of health? Psychology and Health 12: 769–81.

Ariouat, J.F. & Barker, D.J. 1993, The diet of girls and young women at the beginning of the century, Nutrition and Health 9(1): 15–23.

Armstrong, B.K., Margetts, B.M., Masarei, J.R. & Hopkins S.M. 1983, Coronary risk factors in Italian migrants to Australia, American Journal of Epidemiology 118(5): 651–8.

Armstrong, D. 1999, Controversies in epidemiology, teaching causality in context at the University at Albany, School of Public Health, Scandinavian Journal of Public Health 27: 81–4.

Arnetz, B.B. 1984, The potential role of psychosocial stress on levels of hemoglobin A_{1c} (HbA_{1c}) and fasting plasma glucose in elderly people, Journal of Gerontology 39: 424–9.

Aronsson, G. 1999, Influence of worklife on public health, Scandinavian Journal of Work Environment and Health 25: 597–604.

Ashton, J.R. 2000, Public Health Observatories – the key to timely public health intelligence in the new century, Journal of Epidemiology and Community Health 54: 724–5.

Atkinson, A.B. 1983, The Economics of Inequality (2nd edition), Clarendon Press, Oxford.

Atkinson, A.B., Rainwater, L. & Smeeding, T.M. 1995, Income distribution in OECD countries: evidence from the Luxembourg Income Study, OECD Social Policy Studies, 18.

Atkinson, A.B. 1999, The distribution of income in the UK and OECD countries in the twentieth century, Oxford Review of Economic Policy 15, 4: 56–75.

Auslander, W.F., Bubb, J., Rogge, M. & Santiago, J.V. 1993, Family stress and resources: potential areas of intervention in children recently diagnosed with diabetes, Health and Social Work 18: 101–13.

Australian and New Zealand Food Authority 1999, Food Safety Standards, Costs and Benefits, Commonwealth of Australia, Canberra.

Australian Bureau of Statistics & Australian Institute of Health and Welfare 1999, The health and welfare of Australia's Aboriginal and Torres Strait Islander peoples, ABS 4704.0, Australian Bureau of Statistics, Canberra.

Australian Bureau of Statistics 1986, Australian Standard Classification of Occupations: standard classification (1st edition), Cat. 1222.0, Australian Bureau of Statistics, Canberra.

Australian Bureau of Statistics 1994, Apparent determinants of private health insurance, Canberra, Australian Bureau of Statistics, Canberra.

Australian Bureau of Statistics 1998(a), Australian Social Trends 1998, Cat. 4102.0, Ausinfo, Canberra.

Australian Bureau of Statistics 1998(b), Crime and Safety Survey, Australian Bureau of Statistics, Canberra.

Australian Bureau of Statistics 1998(c), Social Atlas Series, Cat. 2030.0–2030.8, Australian Government Publishing Service, Canberra.

Australian Bureau of Statistics 1999, Income Distribution Australia, 1997–8, Cat. 6523.0, Australian Government Publishing Service, Canberra.

Australian Bureau of Statistics 2000(a), Household Expenditure Survey: Detailed expenditure items, Australia. Cat No.6535.0, Australian Bureau of Statistics, Canberra.

Australian Bureau of Statistics 2000(b), Labour Force May 2000, ABS Product No 6291.0.40.001, Australian Bureau of Statistics, Canberra.

Australian Bureau of Statistics 2000(c), Measuring Social Capital: Current Collections and Future Directions, Discussion Paper, Canberra.

Australian Centre for Industrial Relations Research and Training (ACIRRT) 1999, Australia at Work: Just Managing? Prentice Hall, Sydney.

Australian Institute of Health and Welfare 1998, Australia's Health 1998, Australian Institute of Health and Welfare, Canberra.

Australian Institute of Health and Welfare 2000, Australia's Health 2000, Australian Institute of Health and Welfare, Canberra.

Axinn, W., Duncan, G. & Thornton, A. 1997, The effects of parental income, wealth and attitudes on children's completed schooling and self-esteem, in Duncan, G.J. & Brooks-Gunn, J. (Eds), 1997, Consequences of Growing up Poor, Russell Sage, New York.

Backlund, E., Sorlie, P.D. & Johnson, N.J. 1996, The shape of the relationship between income and mortality in the United States: evidence from the National Longitudinal Mortality study, Annals of Epidemiology 6: 12–20.

Banks, K. 1997, The social capital of self-help mutual aide groups, Social Policy (Fall): 30–8.

Barber, J.G. 2001, Relative misery and youth suicide, Australian and New Zealand Journal of Psychiatry 35(1): 49–57.

Barbone, F., Filiberti, R., Franceschi, S., Talamini, R., Conti, E., Montella, M. & La Vecchia, C. 1996, Socioeconomic status, migration and the risk of breast cancer in Italy, International Journal of Epidemiology 25(3): 479–87.

Barefoot, J.C. & Schroll, M. 1996, Symptoms of depression, acute myocardial infarction and total mortality in a community sample, Circulation 93: 1976–80.

Barefoot, J.C., Larsen, S., von der Lieth, L. & Schroll, M. 1995, Hostility, incidence of acute myocardial infarction, and mortality in a sample of older Danish men and women, American Journal of Epidemiology 142: 477–84.

Barefoot, J.C., Peterson, B.L., Dahlstrom, W.G., Siegler, I.C., Anderson, N.B. & Williams, R.B.J. 1991, Hostility patterns and health implications: correlates of Cook-Medley Hostility Scale scores in a national survey, Health Psychology 10: 18–24.

Barker, D.J. 1992, The fetal origins of adult hypertension, Journal of Hypertension [10(7)] Supplement: 539–44.

Barker, D.J. 1995, The Welcome Foundation Lecture, 1994, The Fetal Origins of Disease, Proceedings of the Royal Society of London. Series B: Biological Sciences 262 (1363): 37–43.

Barker, D.J., Gluckman, P.D., Godfrey, K.M., Harding, J.E., Owens, J.A. & Robinson, J.S. 1993, Fetal nutrition and cardiovascular disease in adult life, Lancet 341 (8850): 938–41.

Barker, D.J.P. & Martin, C.N. 1992, The maternal and fetal origins of cardiovascular disease, Journal of Epidemiology and Community Health 46: 8–11.

Barker, D.J.P. 1991, The intrauterine origins of cardiovascular disease and obstructive lung disease in adult life: the Marc Daniels Lecture 1990, Journal of the Royal College of Physicians, London 25: 129–33.

Barker, D.J.P. 1994, Mothers, Babies and Health in Later Life (2nd edition), Churchill Livingstone, Edinburgh.

Barlow, J. 1998, Parent-training programmes and behaviour problems: findings from a systematic review, in Buchanan, A. & Hudson, B.L. (Eds), Parenting, Schooling and Children's Behaviour, Ashgate, Sydney, pp. 89–109.

Barrett, G.F., Crossley, T.F. & Worswick, C. 2000, Consumption and income inequality in Australia, in Castles, I. (Ed.), Facts and Fancies of Human Development, pp. 47–54.

Bartley, M., Blane, D. & Davey Smith, G. (Eds) 1998, The Sociology of Health Inequalities, Blackwell, Oxford.

Bartley, M., Ferrie, J. & Montgomery, S.M. 1999, Living in a high unemployment economy: understanding the health consequences, in Marmot, M. & Wilkinson, R.G. (Eds), pp. 81–104.

Barton, J. 1994, Choosing work at night: A moderating influence on individual tolerance to shiftwork, Journal of Applied Psychology 79: 449–54.

Barton, J., Aldridge, J. & Smith, P. 1998, The emotional impact of shift work on the children of shift workers, Scandinavian Journal of Work, Environment and Health 24: 146–50.

Bauer, R.A. 1966, Detection and anticipation of impact: the nature of the task, in Bauer, R.A., Social Indicators, The MIT Press, Massachusetts, pp. 1–67.

Baum, F. & Kahssay, H. 1999, Health development structures: an untapped resource, in Kahssay, H.M. & Oakley, Peter (Eds), Community Involvement in Health development: A Review of the Concept and Practice, WHO, Geneva.

Baum, F. 2000, Social capital, economic capital and power: further issues for a public health agenda, Journal of Epidemiology and Community Health 54: 509–20.

Baum, F., Bush, R., Modra, C., Murray, C., Cox, E., Alexander, K. & Potter, R. 2000, Epidemiology of participation: an Australian community study, Journal of Epidemiology and Community Health 54: 414–23.

Baum, F., Modra, C., Bush, R., Cox, E., Cooke, R. & Potter, R. 1999, Volunteering and Social Capital: an Adelaide Study, Australian Journal on Volunteering, February.

Bauman, Z. 1995. Life in Fragments: Essays in Postmodern Morality, Oxford, Blackwell.

Baume, P. E. 1995. Waiting times for non-urgent specialist appointments, Medical Journal of Australia 162 (19 June): 648–49.

Baumeister, R. F. & Leary, M. R. 1995, The need to belong: desire for interpersonal attachments as a fundamental human motivation, Psychological Bulletin 117 (3): 497–529.

Baxter, J., Emmison, M. & Western, J.S. (Eds) 1991, Class Analysis and Contemporary Australia, Macmillan, Melbourne.

Beaglehole, R., Bonita, R., Jackson, R. & Stewart, A. 1986, Cardiovascular mortality in New Zealand and Australia 1968–1983: how can the diverging trends be explained? New Zealand Medical Journal 99 (794): 1–3

Beaglehole, R., Dobson, A., Hobbs, M.S., Jackson, R. & Martin, C.A. 1989, CHD in Australia and New Zealand, International Journal of Epidemiology, 18(3 Suppl 1): S145–8.

Beaglehole, R., Stewart, A.W., Jackson, R., Dobson, A.J., McElduff, P. & D'Este, K. et al. 1997, Declining rates of coronary heart disease in New Zealand and Australia, 1983–1993, American Journal of Epidemiology 145: 707–13.

Beal, S. 1988, Sleeping position and SIDS [letter], Lancet 2: 512.

Beatty, J. 1999, Sex and the Social Critic, Atlantic Unbound, August 26, <www.theatlantic.com/unbound/polipro/pp9908.htm> (last visited 18.3.01).

Bebbington and Miles. 1989, The background of children who enter Local Authority care, British Journal of Social Work 19: 349–68.

Bedharz, P. 1994, Social Theory: A guide to critical thinkers, Allen & Unwin, London.

Bello, W.F. Cunningham, S. & Rau, B. 1994, Dark victory: the United States, structural adjustment, and global poverty, Pluto, London.

Benabou, R. 1996, Inequality and growth, NEBR Macroeconomics Annual 11: 11–74.

Benediktsson, R., Lindsay, R.S., Noble, J., Seckl, J.R. & Edwards, C.R.W. 1993, Glucocorticoid exposure in utero: a new model for adult hypertension, Lancet 341: 339–41.

Bennett, S.A. 1995, Cardiovascular risk factors in Australia: trends in socioeconomic inequalities. Journal of Epidemiology and Community Health 49: 363–72.

Ben-Shlomo, Y., White I.R. & Marmot, M. 1996. Does the variation in the socioeconomic characteristics of an area affect mortality? British Medical Journal 312: 1013–14.

Berkman, L. & Syme, S.L. 1999, Social networks, social resistance and mortality: a nine-year follow-up study of Alameda County residents, American Journal of Epidemiology 109(2): 186–204.

Berkman, L.F. & Breslow, L. 1983, Health and Ways of Living: The Alameda County Study, Oxford University Press, New York.

Berkman, L.F. & Glass, T. 2000, Social integration, social networks, social support, and health, in Berkman, L.F. & Kawachi, I. (Eds), pp. 137–73.

Berkman, L.F. & Kawachi, I. (Eds) 2000, Social Epidemiology, Oxford University Press, New York.

Berkman, L.F. & Macintyre, S. 1997, The measurement of social class in health studies: old measures and new formulations, in Kogevinas, M., Pearce, N., Susser, M. & Boffetta, P. (Eds), Social Inequalities and Cancer, International Agency for Research on Cancer, IARC Scientific Publications No. 138, World Health Organization, Lyon.

Berry, A., Bourguignon, F. & Morrison, C. 1983, Changes in the world distribution of income between 1950 and 1977, The Economic Journal 370: 331–50.

Biderman, A.D., 1966, Social indicators and goals, in Bauer, R.A. (Ed.), Social Indicators, The MIT Press, Massachusetts, pp. 68–153.

Birch, C. 1999, Biology and the Riddle of Life, University of NSW Press, Sydney.

Bittman, M. & Rice, J. 1999, Are working hours becoming more unsociable? Social Policy Research Centre Newsletter 74: 1–5.

Björntorp, P. 1988, The associations between obesity, adipose tissue distribution and disease, Acta Medica Scandinavica 723 (Suppl.): 121–34.

Björntorp, P. 1999, Neuroendocrine perturbations as a cause of insulin resistance, Diabetes Metabolism Research Review 15: 427–41.

Björntorp, P., Holm, G. & Rosmond, R. 1999. Hypothalamic arousal, insulin resistance and type 2 diabetes mellitus, Diabetic Medicine 16: 373–83.

Black, D., Morris, J.N., Smith, C., Townsend, P. & Whitehead, M. 1988, Inequalities in Health: The Black Report, Penguin, London.

Blair, T. & Schroder, G. 1999, Europe: The Third Way – Die Neue Mitte, Labour Party and SPD, London.

Blakely, T., Kiro, C. & Woodward, A. 2001, Unlocking the numerator–denominator bias. II: Adjustments to mortality rates by ethnicity and deprivation during 1991–94. New Zealand Medical Journal (in press).

Blane, D., Brunner, E. & Wilkinson, R. (Eds) 1996, Health and Social Organisation: Towards a health policy for the 21st century, Routledge, London and New York.

Blane, D., Davey Smith, G. & Bartley, M. 1993, Social selection: what does it contribute to social class differentials in health? Sociology of Health and Illness 15: 1–15.

Blaxter, M. 1990, Health and Lifestyles, Tavistock/Routledge, London.

Blaxter, M. 1997, Whose fault is it? People's own conceptions of the reasons for health inequalities, Social Science & Medicine, 44: 747–56.

Blum, R.W., Beuhring, T., Shew, M.L., Bearinger, L.H., Sieving, R.E. & Resnick, M.D. 2000, The effects of race/ethnicity, income, and family structure on adolescent risk behaviours, American Journal of Public Health 90: 1879–84.

Bobák, M., Brunner, E., Miller, N.J, Škodová, Z. & Marmot, M. 1998, Could antioxidants play a role in high rates of coronary heart disease in the Czech Republic? European Journal of Clinical Nutrition 52: 632–6.

Bobák, M., Jha, P., Nguyen, S. & Jarvis, M. 2000(a), Poverty and smoking, in Tobacco control in developing countries, Jha, P. & Chaloupka, F. (Eds), Oxford University Press, New York, pp. 41–61.

Bobák, M., Hynek, P., Rose, R., Hertzman, C. & Marmot, M. 2000(b), Socioeconomic factors, material inequalities, and perceived control in self-rated health: cross-sectional data from seven post-communist countries, Social Science & Medicine 51: 1343–50.

Boisjoly, J., Duncan, G. & Hofferth, S. 1995, Access to social capital, Journal of Family Issues 16: 609–931.

Borrell, C., Plasencia, A., Pasarin, I. & Ortun, V. 1997, Widening social inequalities in mortality: the case of Barcelona, a southern European city, Journal of Epidemiology and Community Health 51: 659–67.

Bosma, H., Marmot, M.G., Hemingway, H., Nicholson, A., Brunner, E.J. & Stansfield, S. 1997, Low job control and risk of coronary heart disease in the Whitehall II (prospective cohort) study, British Medical Journal 314: 558–65.

Bosma, H., Peter, R., Siegrist, J. & Marmot, M. G. 1998, Alternative job stress models and the risk of coronary heart disease, American Journal of Public Health 88: 68–74.

Boughton, B. 2000, What is the connection between Aboriginal education and Aboriginal health, Cooperative Research Centre for Aboriginal and Tropical Health, Occasional Papers Series Number 2.

Bourdieu, P. 1977, Outline of a Theory of Practice, Cambridge University Press, London.

Bourdieu, P. 1984, Distinction: A Social Critique of the Judgement of Taste, Routledge, London.

Bower, C., Condon, R., Payne J., Burton, P., Watson, C. & Wild, B. 1998, Measuring the impact of conjugate vaccine on invasive Haemophilus influenza type b infection in Western Australia, Australian and New Zealand Journal of Public Health 22: 67–72.

Bowey, J.A. 1995, Socioeconomic status differences in preschool phonological sensitivity and first-grade reading achievement, Journal of Educational Psychology 87: 476–87.

Boxall, P. 1997, Models of employment and labour productivity in New Zealand: an interpretation of changes since the Employment Contracts Act, Industrial Relations 18: 113–24.

Boyce, W.T., Adams, S., Tschaan, J.M., Cohen, F., Wara, D. & Gunnar, M.R. 1995(a), Adrenocortical and behavioural predictors of immune responses to starting school, Pediatric Research 38: 1009–17.

Boyce, W.T., Champoux, M., Suomi, S.J. & Gunnar, M.R. 1995(b), Salivary cortisol in nursery-reared rhesus monkeys: reactivity to peer interactions and altered circadian activity, Developmental Psychobiology 28: 257–67.

Boyce, W.T., Chesney, M., Alkon, A., Tschann, J.M., Adams, S., Chesterman, B., Cohen, F., Kaiser, P., Folkman, S. & Wara, D. 1995(c), Psychobiological reactivity to stress and childhood respiratory illnesses: results of two prospective studies, Psychosomatic Medicine 57: 411–22.

Boyce, W.T., Jensen, E.W., Cassel, J.C., Collier, A.M., Smith, A.N. & Ramey, C.T. 1977, Influence of life events and family routines and childhood respiratory tract illness, Pediatrics 60: 609–15.

Boyer, M. C. 1983, Dreaming the Rational City: The myth of American city planning, MIT Press, Cambridge, Mass.

Boyer, R. & Drache, D. (Eds) 1996, States Against Markets: the limits of globalisation, Routledge, London and New York.

Brasure, M., Stearns, S.C., Norton, E.C. & Ricketts III, T. 1999, Competitive behavior in local physician markets, Medical Care Research and Review 56(4): 395–414.

Bremner, J.D., Randall, P., Vermetten, E., Staib, L., Bronen, R.A., Mazure, C., Capelli, S., McCarthy, G., Innis, R.B. & Charney, D.S. 1997, Magnetic resonance imaging-based measurement of hippocampal volume in posttraumatic stress disorder related to childhood physical and sexual abuse – a preliminary report, Biological Psychiatry 41: 23–32.

Bronfenbrenner, U. 1979, The Ecology of Human Development: Experiments by Nature and Design, Harvard University Press, Cambridge, Mass.

Bronnum-Hansen, H. & Juel, K. 2000, Estimating mortality due to cigarette smoking: two methods, same result, Epidemiology 11: 422–6.

Brooks-Gunn, J., Duncan, G.J. & Britto, P.R. 1999, Are socioeconomic gradients for children similar to those for adults? Achievement and health of children in the United States, in Keating, D. & Hertzman, C. (Eds).

Brooks-Gunn, J., Duncan, G.J. & Maritato, J. 1996, Poor families, poor outcomes: the wellbeing of children and youth, in Duncan, G.J. & Brooks-Gunn, J. (Eds), 1996, Consequences of Growing Up Poor, Russell Sage Foundation, New York, pp. 1–17.

Brooks-Gunn, J., Guo, G. & Furstenberg, F.F., Jr. 1993, Who drops out and who continues beyond high school? A 20-year follow-up of black urban youth, Journal of Research on Adolescence 3: 271–94.

Broom, D.H. 1986, The occupational health of houseworkers, Australian Feminist Studies 2: 15–34.

Brosnan, P. & Walsh, P. 1998, Employment security in Australia and New Zealand, Labour and Industry 8: 23–41.

Broussard, E.R. 1995, Infant attachment in a sample of adolescent mothers, Child Psychiatry and Human Development 25: 211–19.

Brown, M.C. 1999, Policy-induced changes in Maori mortality patterns in the New Zealand economic reform period, Health Economics 8: 127–36.

Brummett, B.H., Babyak, M.A., Barefoot, J.C., Bosworth, H.B., Clapp-Channing, N.E., Siegler, I.C., Williams, Jr, R.B. & Mark, D.B. 1998, Social support and hostility as predictors of depressive symptoms in cardiac patients one month after hospitalization: a prospective study, Psychosomatic Medicine 60: 707–13.

Brunner, E. & Marmot, M. 1999, Social organisation, stress, and health, in Marmot, M. & Wilkinson, R.G. (Eds), pp. 17–43.

Brunner, E. 1996, The social and biological basis of cardiovascular disease, in Blane, D., Brunner, E. & Wilkinson, R. (Eds), pp. 272–99.

Brunner, E. 1997, Socioeconomic determinants of health: Stress and the biology of inequality, British Medical Journal 314: 1472–6.

Brunner, E.J., Marmot, M.G., Nanchahal, K., Shipley, M.J., Stansfeld, S.A., Juneja, M. & Alberti, K.G.M.M. 1997, Social inequality in coronary risk: central obesity and the metabolic syndrome: evidence from the Whitehall II study, Diabetologia 40: 1341–9.

Bryan, J.H., Foley, D.H. & Sutherst, R.W. 1996, Malaria transmission and climate change in Australia, Medical Journal of Australia 164: 345–7.

Buchanan, A. 1998, A consensus, in Buchanan, A. & Hudson, B.L. (Eds), Parenting, Schooling and Children's Behaviour, Ashgate, Sydney, pp. 178–91.

Bulgaria National Statistical Institute 1989, Budgeti na domakinstvata v Republica Bulgaria [Household budgets in the Republic of Bulgaria] 1987. Izdatelstvo i Pechatnitca [Publishing and Printing House], Sofia.

Bunker, J.P. 1995, Medicine matters after all, Journal of the Royal College of Physicians of London 29: 105–12.

Burford, G. & Hudson, J. (Eds) 2000, Family Group Conferences: New Directions in Community-Centered Child and Family Practice, Aldine De Gruyter, New York, pp. 242–52.

Burnley, I.H. 1998, Inequalities in the transition of ischaemic heart disease mortality in New South Wales, Australia, 1969–1994, Social Science & Medicine, 47(9): 1209–22.

Burrows, C., Brown, K. & Gruskin, A. 1993, Who buys health insurance? A survey of two large organisations, Australian Journal of Social Issues 28: 106–23.

Burt, R. 1997, The contingent value of social capital, Administrative Science Quarterly 42: 339–65.

Butler, C.D. & Smith, L. 1999, Changes in global exchange adjusted income inequality from 1990–97. Economics Society of Australia, La Trobe University, Melbourne.

Butler, C.D. 1994, Overpopulation, overconsumption and economics, Lancet 343: 582–4.

Butler, C.D. 1997, The consumption bomb, Medicine Conflict and Survival 13: 209–18.

Butler, C.D. 2000(a), Inequality, global change and the sustainability of civilisation, Global Change and Human Health 1: 156–72. <www.baltzer.nl/naphtml.htm/GLOBI>

Butler, C.D. 2000(b), Entrapment: global ecological and/or local demographic? Reflections upon reading the British Medical Journal's 'six billion day' special issue, Ecosystem Health 6: 171–80.

Butler, C.D., 2001, Epidemiology, Australians and global environmental change, Australasian Epidemiologist 8(1); 13–16.

Butler, D. 1998, British BSE reckoning tells a dismal tale, Nature 392: 532–3.

Calle, E.E., Thun, M.J., Petrelli, J.M., Rodriguez, C. & Heath, C.W., Jr. 1999, Body-mass index and mortality in a prospective cohort of US adults, New England Journal of Medicine 341: 1097–105.

Callister, P. 1996, Ethnic and labour force classification in couple families: some methodological issues in the use of census data, NZ Population Review 22: 83–7.

Callister, P. 1998, 'Work-rich' and 'work-poor' individuals and families: changes in the distribution of paid work from 1986–1996, Social Policy Journal of New Zealand 10: 101–21.

Cameron, A.C. & McCallum, J. 1996, Private health insurance choice in health: the role of long-term utilisation of health services, in Economics and Health, 1995, School of Health Services Management, UNSW, Sydney, pp. 143–57.

Cameron, A.C. & Trivedi, P.K. 1991, The role of income and health risk in the choice of health insurance: evidence from Australia, Journal of Public Economics 45: 1–28.

Cameron, A.C., Trivedi, P.K., Milne, F. & Piggott, J. 1988, Microeconometric model of the demand for health care and health insurance in Australia, Review of Economic Studies 55: 85–106.

Cameron, J.L. 1997, Stress and behaviorally induced reproductive dysfunction in primates, Seminars in Reproductive Endocrinology 15: 37–45.

Cameron, M. & Newstead, S. 1996, Mass media publicity supporting police enforcement and its economic value, Monash University Accident Research Centre, Melbourne, <www.general.monash.edu.au/muarc/media/media.htm> (accessed 20/10/99).

Campbell, D.T. 1975, On the conflicts between biological and social evolution and between psychology and moral tradition, American Psychologist, December: 1103–26.

Cannon, W.B. 1929, Bodily Changes in Pain, Hunger, Fear, and Rage, Appleton & Lange, East Norwalk.

Cantor, C.H., Neulinger, K. & De Leo, D. 1999, Australian suicide trends 1964–1997 – youth and beyond, Medical Journal of Australia 171: 137–41.

Capitanio, J.P. & Lerche, N.W. 1998, Social separation, housing relocation, and survival in simian AIDS: a retrospective analysis, Psychosomatic Medicine 60: 235–44.

Carlson, M. & Earls, F. 1997, Psychological and neuroendocrinological sequelae of early social deprivation in institutionalized children in Romania, Annals of the New York Academy of Science 807: 419–28.

Carroll, D., Davey Smith, G., Sheffield, D., Shipley, M.J. & Marmot, M.G. 1997, The relationship between socioeconomic status, hostility, and blood pressure reactions to mental stress in men: data from the Whitehall II study, Health Psychology 16(2): 131–6.

Cashmore, J. & Paxman, M. 1996, Wards Leaving Care: A Longitudinal Study, NSW Department of Community Services, Sydney.

Cassel, J. 1976, The contribution of the social environment to host resistance, American Journal of Epidemiology 104: 107–23.

Cassis, G. 1998, Biodiversity loss: a human health issue [editorial], The Medical Journal of Australia 169: 568–9.

Castles, I. 2000, Reporting on human development: Lies, damned lies and statistics, in Castles, I. (Ed.), Facts and Fancies of Human Development, Academy of the Social Sciences in Australia, Canberra, pp. 55–82.

Cavelaars, A., Kunst, A., Geurts, J. et al. 1998, Differences in self-reported morbidity by income level in six European countries, in Cavelaars, A., Cross-National Comparisons of Socio-economic Differences in Health Indicators, Erasmus University, Rotterdam, pp. 49–66.

Chadwick, E. 1842, The Sanitary Conditions of the Labouring Populations of Great Britain. Republished (1965, ed. M.W. Flynn) by Edinburgh University Press, Edinburgh.

Chaing, T-L. 1999, Economic transition and changing relation between income inequality and mortality in Taiwan: regression analysis, British Medical Journal 319: 1162–5.

Chaloupka, F.J., Hu, T.-W., Warner, K.E., Jacobs, R. & Yurekli, A. 2000, The taxation of tobacco products, in Jha, P. & Chaloupka, F. (Eds), Tobacco Control in Developing Countries, Oxford University Press, New York, pp. 237–72.

Chapin III, F.S., Zavaleta, E.S., Eviner, V.T., Naylor, R.L., Vitousek, P.M., Reynolds, H.L., Hooper, D.U., Lavorel, S., Sala, O.E., Hobbie, S.E., Mack, M.C. & Díaz, S. 2000, Causes, consequences and ethics of biodiversity, Nature 405: 234–42.

Chaturvedi, N., Jarrett, J., Shipley, M.J. & Fuller, J.H. 1998, Socioeconomic gradient in morbidity and mortality in people with diabetes: cohort study findings from the Whitehall study and the WHO multinational study of vascular disease in diabetes, British Medical Journal 316: 100–5.

Checkley, S. 1996, The neuroendocrinology of depression and chronic stress, British Medical Bulletin 52: 597–617.

Cheung, Y.B. 2000, Marital status and mortality in British women: a longitudinal study, International Journal of Epidemiology 29 (1): 93–9.

Chichlinisky, G. & Head, G. 1998, Economic returns from the biosphere, Nature 391: 629–30.

Chossudovsky, M. 1997, The globalisation of poverty. Impacts of IMF and World Bank reforms, Third World Network, Penang.

Chrousos, G.P. & Gold, P.W. 1992, The concepts of stress and stress system disorders, Journal of the American Medical Association 267: 1244–52.

Chrousos, G.P. 1998, Stressors, stress, and neuroendocrine integration of the adaptive response, Annals of the New York Academy of Science 851: 311–35.

Chrousos, G.P., McCarty, R., Pacak, K., Cizza, G., Sternbery, E., Gold, P.W. & Kvetnansky, R. (Eds) 1995, Stress: basic mechanisms and clinical implications, Annals of the New York Academy of Sciences, vol. 771, The New York Academy of Sciences, New York.

Cicerone, R. J. 1988. Methane linked to warming, Nature 334: 198.

Cichetti, D. 1996, Child maltreatment: implications for developmental theory and research, Human Development 39: 18–39.

Cirulli, F., Pistillo, L., Acetis, L.D., Alleva, E. & Aloe, L. 1998, Increased number of mast cells in central nervous system of adult male mice following chronic subordination stress, Brain Behaviour and Immunity 12: 123–33.

Clarke, R., Shipley, M., Lewington, S., Youngman, L., Collins, R., Marmot, M. & Peto, R. 1999, Underestimation of risk associations due to regression dilution in long-term follow-up of prospective studies, American Journal of Epidemiology 150(4): 341–53.

Clements, A.D. & Parker, C.R. 1998, The relationship between salivary cortisol concentrations in frozen versus mailed samples, Psychoneuroendocrinology 23: 613–16.

Cobb, C., Halstead, T. & Rowe, J. 1995, If the GDP is up, why is America down? Atlantic Monthly 277: 61–78.

Coburn, D. 2000, Income inequality, social cohesion and the health status of populations: the role of neoliberalism, Social Science & Medicine 51: 135–46.

Coe, C.L. 1999, Psychosocial factors and psychoneuroimmunology within a lifespan perspective, in Keating, D. & Hertzman, C. (Eds), pp. 201–19.

Coie, J.D., Watt, N.F., West, S.G., Hawkins, J.D., Asarnow, J.R., Markman, H.J., Ramey, S.L., Shure, M.B. & Long, B. 1993, The science of prevention: a conceptual framework and some directions for a national research program, American Psychologist 48: 1013–22.

Cold, S., Hansen, S., Overvad, K. & Rose, C. 1998, A woman's build and the risk of breast cancer, European Journal of Cancer 34: 1163–74.

Cole, S.W., Kemeny, M.E. & Taylor, S.E. 1997, Social identity and physical health: accelerated HIV progression in rejection-sensitive gay men, Journal of Personality and Social Psychology 72: 320–35.

Colebatch, H.K. 1998, Policy, Open University Press, Buckingham.

Coleman, J.S. 1988, Social capital in the creation of human capital, American Journal of Sociology 94 (Supplement): S95–S120.

Coleman, J.S. 1990, Foundations of Social Theory, Harvard University Press, Harvard.

Coleman, J.S. 1993, Properties of rational organisation, in Lindenberg, S. & Schneider, H. (Eds), Interdisciplinary Perspectives on Organisation Studies, Pergamon Press, Oxford, pp. 79–90.

Commonwealth Department of Health and Aged Care (DHAC) 1999, Commonwealth Jurisdictional Report for Australian Health Ministers Conference on progress made un the Aboriginal and Torres Strait Islander Framework Agreement, Australian Health Ministers Conference, Canberra.

Commonwealth Department of Health and Family Services (DHFS) 1994, The National Aboriginal Health Strategy, An Evaluation, Commonwealth Department of Health and Family Services, Canberra.

Commonwealth Department of Health and Family Services (DHFS) 1997, Submission from the Commonwealth Department of Health and Family Services, in 'House of Representatives Standing Committee on Family and Community Affairs: Inquiry into Indigenous Health, Submissions authorised for publication, Volume One, National Organisations', Standing Committee on Family and Community Affairs, Canberra volume 1, pp. 215–316.

Connell, R.W. 1977, Ruling Class, Ruling Culture, Cambridge University Press, Melbourne.

Constantino, J.N. 1996, Intergenerational effects of the development of aggression: a preliminary report, Journal of Developmental and Behavioral Pediatrics 17: 176–82.

Contoyannis, P. & Forster, M. 1999, Our healthier nation? Health Economics 8: 289–96.

Cooper, R. & David, R. 1986, The biological concept of race and its application to public health and epidemiology, Journal of Health Politics, Policy and Law 11(1): 97–116.

Cooper, R.S. & Kauffman, J.S. 1999, Is there an absence of theory in social epidemiology? The authors respond to Muntaner, American Journal of Epidemiology 150: 127–8.

Coote, B. 1992, The Trade Trap: Poverty and the Global Commodity Markets, Oxfam, London.

Corin, E. 1994, The social and cultural matrix of health and disease, in Evans, R.G., Barer, M.L. & Marmor, T.R. (Eds), pp. 93–132.

Corin, E. 1995, The cultural frame: context and meaning in the construction of health, in Amick, B.C., Levine, S., Tarlov, A.R. & Chapman Walsh, D. (Eds), pp. 272–304.

Costanza, R., Daly, H., Folke, C., Hawken, P., Holling, C.S., McMichael, A.J., Pimental, D. & Rapport, D. 2000, Managing our environmental portfolio, BioScience 50: 149–55.

Costanza, R., d'Arge, R., de Groot, R., Farber, S., Grasso, M., Hannon, B., Limburg, K., Naeem, S., O'Neill, R.V., Paruelo, J., Raskin, R., Sutton, P. & van den Belt, M. 1997, The value of the world's ecosystem services and natural capital, Nature 387: 253–60.

Couto, R.A. & Guthrie C.S. 1999, Making Democracy Work Better: mediating structures, social capital and the democratic prospect, The University of North Carolina Press, Chapel Hill.

Couzos, S. & Murray, R. 1999, Aboriginal Primary Health Care, an Evidence-based Approach, Oxford University Press, South Melbourne.

Couzos, S., Metcalf, S., Murray, R. & O'Rourke, S. 1998, Systematic Review of Existing Evidence and Primary Care Guidelines on the Management of Non-insulin Dependent Diabetes, Commonwealth of Australia, Canberra.

Cox, A.D., Pound A., Mills, M., Puckering, C., Owen, A.L. 1991, Evaluation of a home visiting and befriending scheme for young mothers – Newpin, Journal of the Royal Society of Medicine 84: 217–20.

Cox, E. 1995, A Truly Civil Society, ABC Books, Sydney.

Crampton, P. 1999, Third Sector Primary Health Care. A report prepared for the National Health Committee, Department of Public Health, Wellington School of Medicine, Health Services Research Centre.

Crampton, P., Salmond, C., Woodward, A. & Reid, P. 2000, Socioeconomic deprivation and ethnicity are both important for anti-tobacco health promotion, Health Education & Behavior 27, 317–27.

Creedy, J. 1996, Measuring income inequality, The Australian Economic Review, 2nd Quarter: 236–46.

Creedy, J. 1997, Statistics and Dynamics of Income Distribution in New Zealand, Institute of Policy Studies, Wellington.

Crnic, K., Greenberg, M.T., Ragozin, A.S., Robinson, N.M. & Basham, R.B. 1983, Effects of stress and social support on mothers and premature and full-term infants, Child Development 54: 209–217.

Cross, S.E. & Madson, L. 1997, Models of the self: self-construals and gender, Psychological Bulletin 122 (1): 5–37.

Csikszentmihalyi, M. 1999, If we are so rich, why aren't we happy? American Psychologist 54(10): 821–7.

Cummins, R.A. 1998, The second approximation to an international standard for life satisfaction, Social Indicators Research 43: 307–34.

Curran, L.M. Caniago, I. Paoli, G.D., Astianti, D., Kusneti, M., Leighton, M., Nirarita, C.E. & Haeruman, H. 1999, Impact of El Niño and logging on canopy tree recruitment in Borneo, Science 286: 2184–8.

Cutler, D.M. & Katz, L.F. 1991, Macroeconomic performance and the disadvantaged, Brookings Papers on Economic Activity 2: 1–74.

Cynander, M.S. & Frost, B.J. 1999, Mechanisms of brain development: neuronal sculpting by the physical and social environment, in Keating, D. & Hertzman, C. (Eds), pp. 153–84.

D'Espaignet, E.T., Dwyer, T., Newman, N.M., Ponsonby, A.L. & Candy, S. 1990, The development of a model for predicting infants at high risk of sudden infant death syndrome in Tasmania, Paediatric and Perinatal Epidemiology 4: 422–35.

Daedalus 1994, Health and Wealth, 123(4).

Daly, H. 1996, Beyond Growth, Beacon Press, Boston.

Daly, H.E. & Cobb, J.B. 1989, For the Common Good, Beacon Press, Boston.

Daly, M.C., Duncan, G.J., Kaplan, G.A. & Lynch, J.W. 1998, Macro-to-micro links in the relation between income inequality and mortality, The Milbank Quarterly 76: 315–39.

Daniel, M., O'Dea, K., Rowley, K.G., McDermott, R. & Kelly, S. 1999(b), Social environmental stress in indigenous populations: potential biopsychosocial mechanisms, Annals of the New York Academy of Science 896: 420–3.

Daniel, M., O'Dea, K., Rowley, K.G., McDermott, R. & Kelly, S. 1999(a), Glycated hemoglobin as an indicator of social environmental stress among indigenous versus westernized populations, Preventative Medicine 29: 405–13.

Danziger, S.H. & Gottschalk, P. (Eds) 1993, Uneven Tides: Rising Inequality in America, Russell Sage, New York.

Dasgupta, P. & Serageldin, I. (Eds) 2000, Social capital: A Multifaceted Perspective, World Bank, Washington DC.

Dasgupta, P. 1996, The Economics of the Environment, Proceedings of the British Academy 90: 165–221.

Davey Smith, G., Shipley, M.J. & Rose, G. 1990, Magnitude and causes of socioeconomic differentials in mortality: further evidence from the Whitehall Study, Journal of Epidemiology and Community Health 44: 265–70.

Davidson, M.B., Schriger, D.L., Peters, A.L. & Lorber, B. 1999, Relationship between fasting plasma glucose and glycosylated hemoglobin: potential for false-positive diagnoses of type 2 diabetes using new diagnostic criteria, Journal of the American Medical Association 281: 1203–10.

Davis, H. 1993, Counselling Parents of Children with Chronic Illness or Disability, British Psychological Society Books, Leicester.

Davis, P., Howden-Chapman, P. & McLeod, K. 1997, The New Zealand Socioeconomic Index: a census-based occupational scale of socioeconomic status, in P. Crampton & P. Howden-Chapman (Eds), Socioeconomic Inequalities and Health. Proceedings of the Socioeconomic Inequalities and Health Conference, Wellington, 9–10 December 1996, Institute of Policy Studies, Wellington, pp. 131–48.

Davis, P., McLeod, K., Ransom, M. & Ongley, P. 1997, The New Zealand Socioeconomic Index of Occupational Status (NZSEI), Stats NZ Research Report 2, Statistics New Zealand, Wellington.

Davis, P., Graham, P. & Pearce, N. 1999, Health expectancy in New Zealand, 1981–1991: social variations and trends in a period of rapid social and economic change, Journal of Epidemiology and Community Health, 53: 519–27.

Davison, T., Ferraro, L. & Wales, R. 2000, Review of the antecedents of illicit drug use with particular reference to adolescents, Unpublished paper, University of Melbourne.

De Angelis, D., Gilks, W.R. & Day, N.E. 1998, Bayesian projection of the acquired immune deficiency syndrome epidemic, Applied Statistics 47: 449–98.

Deeble, J., Mathers, C., Smith, L., Goss, J., Webb, R. & Smith, V. 1998, Expenditures on health services for Aboriginal and Torres Strait Islander people, AIHW Cat No. HWE 6, Canberra.

Deininger, K. & Squires, L. 1998, A new data set measuring income inequality, World Bank Economic Review 10: 565–91.

Demers, R.Y., Neale, A.V., Wenzloff, N.J. & Gronsman, K.J. 1989, Glycosylated hemoglobin levels and self-reported stress in adults with diabetes, Behavioural Medicine 15: 167–72.

Demine, A.K. 2000, Public health in Eastern Europe, Lancet 356: s49.

Department of Statistics 1995, Labour Market Statistics 1995, Department of Statistics, Wellington.

Department of the Environment, Transport and the Regions 1998, Road accidents Great Britain 1997: the casualty report, The Stationery Office, London.

Developmental Crime Prevention Consortium 1999, Pathways to Prevention: Developmental and Early Intervention Approaches to Crime in Australia, National Crime Prevention, Canberra.

Diamond, J. 1991, The Rise and Fall of the Third Chimpanzee, Radius, London.

Dickinson, D.K. & Smith, M.W. 1994, Long-term effects of preschool teachers' book readings on low-income children's vocabulary and story comprehension, Reading Research Quarterly 29: 105–22.

Diener, E. & Suh, E. 1997, Measuring quality of life: economic, social and subjective indicators, Social Indicators Research 40: 189–216.

Diener, E. 2000, Subjective well-being: the science of happiness and a proposal for a national index, American Psychologist 55(1): 34–43.

Diener, E., Suh, E., Lucas, R. & Smith, H. 1999, Subjective well-being: three decades of progress, Psychological Bulletin 125(2): 276–302.

DiGiacomo, S.M. 1999. Can there be a 'cultural epidemiology'? Medical Anthropology Quarterly 13(4): 436–57.

Dixon, J. & Leeder, S. 2000, HIRC: An assessment and decisions for a forward plan 2001–2003, Unpublished discussion paper for the Health Inequalities Research Collaboration Board.

Dobson, A.J. 1987, Trends in cardiovascular risk factors in Australia, 1966–1986: evidence from prevalence surveys, Community Health Studies 11(1): 2–14.

Dobson, A.J., Gibberd, R.W., Leeder, S.R., O'Connell, D.L. 1985, Occupational differences in ischaemic heart disease mortality and risk factors in Australia, American Journal of Epidemiology 122: 283–90.

Dobson, A.J., McElduff, P., Heller, R., Alexander, H., Colley, P. & D'Este, K. 1999, Changing patterns of coronary heart disease in the Hunter region of New South Wales Australia, Journal of Clinical Epidemiology 52(8): 761–71.

Dodge, K.A., Pettit, G.S. & Bates, J.E. 1994, Socialisation mediators of the relation between socio-economic status and child conduct problems, Child Development 65: 649–65.

Donald, M., Dower, J., Lucke, J. & Raphael, B. 2000, The Queensland Young People's Mental Health Survey Report, Centre for Primary Health Care, School of Population Health and Department of Psychiatry, University of Queensland.

Douglas, R.M. 2000, Sustaining rural and regional Australia, National Centre for Epidemiology and Population Health Paper, ANU, Canberra.

Droomers, M., Schrijvers, C.M.T., Van de Mheen, H. & Mackenbach, J.P. 1998, Educational differences in leisure time physical inactivity: a descriptive and explanatory study, Social Science & Medicine 47(11): 1655–76.

Duckett, S.J. 1984, Structural interests and Australian health policy, Social Science & Medicine 18(11): 959–66.

Duckett, S.J. 1998, Responding to health inequalities in Australia: a proposed strategy, Australian Journal of Primary Health – Interchange 4(2): 9–19.

Dudley, M., Kelk, N., Florio, T., Howard, J., Waters, B., Haski, C. & Alcock, M. 1997, Suicide among young rural Australians 1964–1993: a comparison with metropolitan trends, Social Psychiatry and Psychiatric Epidemiology 32: 251–60.

Duncan, G.J. & Brookes-Gunn, J. 1996, Income effects across the lifespan; integration and interpretation, in Duncan, G.J. & Brookes-Gunn, J. (Eds), Consequences of Growing Up Poor, Russell Sage, New York.

Duncan, G.J. 1996, Income dynamics and health, International Journal of Health Services 26(3): 419–44.

Duncan, G.J., Brooks-Gunn, J. & Klebanov, P.K. 1994, Economic deprivation and early childhood development, Child Development 65: 296–318.

Durkheim, E. 1970, Suicide: A Study in Sociology, London, Routledge and Kegan Paul (first published 1897).

Durlak, J. & Wells, A. 1997, Primary prevention mental health programs for children and adolescents: a meta-analytic review, American Journal of Community Psychology 25(2): 115–52.

Durlak, J.A. 1998, Common risk and protective factors in successful prevention programs, American Journal of Orthopsychiatry 68(4): 512–20.

Dwyer, T., Blizzard, L., Morley, R. & Ponsonby, A-L. 1999, Within pair association between birth weight and blood pressure at age 8 in twins from a cohort study, British Medical Journal 319: 1325–9.

Earle, T.L., Linden, W. & Weinberg, J. 1999, Differential effects of harassment on cardiovascular and salivary cortisol stress reactivity and recovery in women and men, Journal of Psychosomatic Research 46: 125–41.

Easterling, D.R., Meehl, G.A., Parmesan, C., Changnon, S.A., Karl, T.R. & Mearns, L.O. 2000, Climate extremes: observations, modeling, and impacts, Science 289: 2068–74.

Easton, B.H. 1997, In Stormy Seas, The Post-War New Zealand Economy, University of Otago Press, Dunedin.

Eckersley, R. (Ed.) 1998(a), Measuring Progress: Is Life Getting Better? CSIRO Publishing, Collingwood.

Eckersley, R. 1998(b), Redefining progress: shaping the future to human needs, Family Matters 51: 6–12.

Eckersley, R. & Dear, K. (in press), The cultural correlates of youth suicide, Social Science & Medicine.

Eckersley, R. 1993, Failing a generation: the impact of culture on the health and well-being of youth, Journal of Paediatrics and Child Health 29: S16–S19.

Eckersley, R. 1995, Values and visions: youth and the failure of modern western culture, Youth Studies Australia 14(1): 13–21.

Eckersley, R. 1997, Portraits of youth: understanding young people's relationship with the future, Futures 29: 243–9.

Eckersley, R. 1999, Quality of Life in Australia: An Analysis of Public Perceptions, Discussion Paper no. 23, September, The Australia Institute, Canberra.

Eckersley, R. 2000(a), The state and fate of nations: implications of subjective measures of personal and social quality of life, Social Indicators Research 52(1): 3–27.

Eckersley, R. 2000(b), The mixed blessings of material progress: diminishing returns in the pursuit of happiness, Journal of Happiness Studies 1(3): 267–92.

Eckersley, R. 2001, Taking the prize or paying the price? Young people and progress, in Rowling L., Martin, G. & Walker, L. (Eds), Mental Health Promotion and Young People: Concepts and practice, McGraw Hill (in press).

Ecob, R. & Davey Smith, G. 1999, Income and health: what is the nature of the relationship? Social Science & Medicine 48: 693–705.

Edwards, L.B., Livesay, V.T. & Acquaviva, F.A. 1971, Height, weight, tuberculous infection, and tuberculous disease, Archives of Environmental Health 22: 106–12.

Edwards, P.A. 1995, Empowering low-income mothers and fathers to share books with young children, The Reading Teacher 48: 558–64.

Elchardus, M. 1991, Flexible men and women: the changing temporal organisation of work and culture – an empirical analysis, Social Science Information 30(4): 701–25.

Elchardus, M. 1994, In praise of rigidity: on temporal and cultural flexibility, Information sur les Sciences Sociales 33(3): 459–77.

Elias, G. & Taylor, E. 1995, Report of the Review of the Logan West Language Skills Program, Faculty of Education, Griffith University, Brisbane.

Elliott, A. 1995, The postmodern twilight for ethics, The Australian, 6 December, Higher Education, p. 27.

Elliott, P., Stamler, J., Nichols, R., Dyer, AR., Stamler, R., Kesteloot, H. & Marmot, M. 1996, Intersalt revisited: further analyses of 24-hour sodium excretion and blood pressure within and across populations, British Medical Journal 312(7041): 1249–53.

Eng, E. & Parker, E. 1994, Measuring community competence in the Mississippi delta: the interface between program evaluation and empowerment, Health Education Quarterly 21: 199–220.

Engwicht, D. 1992, Towards an Eco City, Envirobooks, Sydney.

Erikson, R. 1992. Social policy and inequality in health: considerations from the Swedish experience, International Journal of Health Services 3(3/4): 215–22.

European Committee for Health Promotion Development. 1999, Reducing inequalities in health – Proposals for health promotion policy and action. Consensus Statement: World Health Organization, Copenhagen.

Evans, R.G., Barer, M.L. & Marmor, T.R. (Eds) 1994, Why are Some People Healthy and Others Not? The determinants of health of populations, Aldine de Gruyter, New York.

Ewertz, M. 1988(b), Risk of breast cancer in relation to social factors in Denmark, Acta Oncologica 27(6B): 787–92.

Ewertz, M. 1998(a), Risk factors for breast cancer and their prognostic significance, Acta Oncologica, 27(6A): 733–7

Farmer, P. 1996, Social inequalities and emerging infectious diseases, Emerging Infectious Diseases 2: 259–68.

Farrington, D.P. 1994, Early developmental prevention of juvenile delinquency, Criminal Behaviour and Mental Health 4: 209–27.

Feinleib, M. 1996, Editorial: New directions for community intervention studies, American Journal of Public Health 86(12): 1696–7.

Felitti, V.J., Anda, R.F., Nordenberg, D., Williamson, D.F., Spitz, A.M., Edwards, V., Koss, M.P. & Marks, J.S. 1998, Relationship of childhood abuse and household dysfunction to many of the leading causes of death in adults, American Journal of Preventative Medicine 14: 245–58.

Fergusson, D.M. 1998, The Christchurch Health and Development Study: An overview and some key findings, Social Policy Journal of New Zealand 10: 154–76.

Ferrie, J.E., Shipley, M.J., Marmot, M.G., Stansfield, S. & Davey Smith, G. 1995, Health effects of anticipation of job change and non-employment: longitudinal data from the Whitehall II study, British Medical Journal 311: 1264–9.

Ferrie, J.E., Shipley, M.J., Marmot, M.G., Stansfield, S.A. & Smith, G.D. 1998, The health effects of major organisational change and job insecurity, Social Science & Medicine 46: 243–54.

Feyer, A.-M., Langley, J., Howard, M., Horsburgh, S., Wright, C., Alsop, J. & Cryer, C. 2001, The work-related fatal injury study: numbers, rates and trends of work-related fatal injuries in New Zealand 1985–1994, New Zealand Medical Journal 114(1124): 6–10.

Fincher, R. & Nieuwenhuysen, J. (Eds) 1998, Australian Poverty: Then and Now, Melbourne University Press, Melbourne.

Firebaugh, G. 2000, Observed trends in between-nation income inequality and two conjectures, The American Journal of Sociology 106: 215–21.

Fiscella, K. & Franks, P. 1997, Poverty or income inequality as a predictor of mortality: longitudinal cohort study, British Medical Journal 314: 1724–6.

Fishbein, M. 1996, Editorial: Great expectations, or do we ask too much from community-level interventions? Americal Journal of Public Health 86(8): 1075–6.

Flegg, A. 1982, Inequality of income, illiteracy, and medical care as determinants of infant mortality in developing countries, Population Studies 36: 441–58.

Fleming, R. 1997, The Common Purse: Income sharing in New Zealand families, Auckland University Press/ Bridget Williams Books, Auckland.

Flinn, M.V. & England, B.G. 1997, Social economics of childhood glucocorticoid stress response and health, American Journal of Physical Anthropology 102: 33–53.

Flugge, G. 1996, Alterations in the central nervous α_2-adrenoceptor system under chronic psychosocial stress, Neuroscience 75: 187–96.

Flugge, G., Ahrens, O. & Fuchs, E. 1997, β-adrenoceptors in the tree shrew brain, II, time-dependent effects of chronic psychosocial stress [125I] iodocyanopindolol binding sites, Cellular and Molecular Neurobiology 17: 417–43.

Fogel, R.W. & Costa, D.L. 1997, A theory of technophysio evolution, with some implications for forecasting population, health care costs, and pension costs, Demography 34: 49–66.

Fogel, R.W. 1993, New sources and new techniques for the study of secular trends in nutritional status, health, mortality and the process of aging, Historical Methods 26: 5–43.

Foley, D., Goldfield, S., McLoughlin, J., Nagorcka, J., Oberklaid, F. & Wake, M. 2000, A Review of the Early Childhood Literature, Department of Family and Community Services, Canberra.

Foley, M. & Edwards, B. 1999, Is it time to disinvest in social capital? Journal of Public Policy 19: 141–73.

Folkard, S. 1997, Black times: temporal determinants of transport safety, Accident Analysis and Prevention 29: 417–30.

Folling, I. 1990, The clinical value of glycated hemoglobin and glycated plasma proteins, Scandinavian Journal of Clinical and Laboratory Investigation 202 (Suppl.): 95–8.

Fonagy, P. 1996, Patterns of attachment, interpersonal relationships and health, in Blane, D., Brunner, E. & Wilkinson, R. (Eds).

Foskett, A. 1991, Canberra – towards a healthy city, Australian Urban Studies 19(4): 1–4 & 13–15.

Francis, D., Diorio, J., Paplante, P., Weaver, S., Seckl, J. & Meaney, J. 1996, The role of early environmental events in regulating neuroendocrine development, Annals of New York Academy of Sciences 794: 136–52.

Francis, D.D. & Meaney, M.J. 1999, Maternal care and the development of stress responses, Current Opinion in Neurobiology 9: 128–34.

Frank, R.H. & Cook, P.J. 1995, The Winner-Take-All Society, Simon & Schuster, New York.

Frankel, S., Elwood, P., Sweetnam, P., Yarnell, J. & Smith, G.D. 1996, Birthweight, body-mass index in middle age, and incident coronary heart disease, Lancet 348(9040): 1478–80.

Frankenberg, R. 1966, Communities in Britain, Penguin, Middlesex.

Fraser-Smith, N., Lesperance, F., Juneau, M., Talajic, M. & Bourassa, M.G. 1999, Gender, depression, and one-year prognosis after myocardial infarction, Psychosomatic Medicine 61: 26–37.

Frazer, W.M. 1947, Duncan of Liverpool. An account of the work of Dr W.H. Duncan Medical Officer of Health of Liverpool 1847–63, Hamish Hamilton, London.

Freire, P. 1972, Pedagogy of the Oppressed, Penguin, Harmondsworth.

Friedland, W.H., Barton, A.E. & Thomas, R.J. 1981, Manufacturing Green Gold, Cambridge University Press, Cambridge.

Frost, L. 1991, The New Urban Frontier: Urbanisation and City Building in Australasia and the American West, University of NSW Press, Sydney.

Frustenberg, F. & Huges, M. 1995, Social capital and successful development among at-risk youth, Journal of Marriage and the Family 57: 580–92.

Fukuyama, F. 1995, Social capital and the global economy, Foreign Affairs 89: 103.

Funkhouser, G.R. 1989, Values changes necessary for a sustainable society, Bulletin of Science, Technology and Society 9: 19–32.

Furlong, A. & Cartmel, F. 1997(a), Risk and uncertainty in the youth transition, Young 5(1): 3–20.

Furlong, A. & Cartmel, F. 1997(b), Young People and Social Change: Individualisation and Risk in Late Modernity, Open University Press, Buckingham.

Galard, R., Gallart, J.M., Catalan, R., Schwartz, S., Arguello, J.M. & Castellanos, J.M. 1991, Salivary cortisol levels and their correlation with plasma ACTH levels in depressed patients before and after the DST, American Journal of Psychiatry 148: 505–8.

Gallie, D. 2000, The polarization of the labour market and exclusion of vulnerable groups, in Isaksson, K., Hogstedt, C., Eriksson, C. & Theorell, T. (Eds), pp. 245–266.

Gallo, L.C. & Matthews, K.A. 1999, Do negative emotions mediate the association between socio-economic status and health? in Adler, N.E., Marmot, M., McEwen, B.S. & Stewart, J. (Eds), pp. 226–45.

Garbarino, J., 1995, Raising Children in a Socially Toxic Environment, Jossey-Bass, San Francisco.

Gascon, C., Williamson, G.B. & da Fonseca, G.A.B. 2000, Receding forest edges and vanishing reserves, Science 288: 1356–8.

Genco, R.J., Ho, A.W., Kopman, J., Grossi, S.G., Dunford, R.G. & Tedesco, L.A. 1998, Models to evaluate the role of stress in periodontal disease, Annals of Periodontology 3: 288–302.

Gepkens, A. & Gunning-Schepen, L. 1996, Interventions to reduce socioeconomic health differences: a review of the international literature, European Journal of Public Health 6: 218–26.

Gibbon, P. (Ed.) 1995, Structural adjustment and the working poor in Zimbabwe: studies on labour, women, informal sector workers and health, Nordiska Afrikainstitutet, Uppsala.

Giddens, A. 1998, The Third Way: The Renewal of Social Democracy, Polity Press, Cambridge.

Giddens, A. 1999, The Third Way and Its Critics, Polity Press, Oxford.

Glover, J., Harris, K. & Tennant, S. 1999, A Social Health Atlas of Australia, Second Edition, Volume 1: Australia, Public Health Information Development Unit, University of Adelaide, Adelaide.

Glyn, A. & Miliband, D. (Eds) 1994. Paying for Inequality: The Economic Cost of Social Injustice, Rivers Oram Press, London.

Godfrey, K.M. & Barker, D.J. 2000, Fetal nutrition and adult disease, American Journal of Clinical Nutrition, 71(5 Suppl): 1344S–52S.

Goldstein, L.H., Trancik, A., Bensadoun, J., Boyce, W.T. & Adler, N.E. 1999, Social dominance and cardiovascular reactivity in preschoolers: associations with SES and health, Annals of New York Academy of Sciences 896: 363–6.

Goldston, D.B., Kovacs, M., Obrosky, D.S. & Iyengar, S. 1995, A longitudinal study of life events and metabolic control among youths with insulin-dependent diabetes mellitus, Health Psychology 14: 409–14.

Golly, A.M., Stiller, B. & Walker, H.M., 1998, First step to success: replication and social validation of an early intervention program, Journal of Emotional and Behavioural Disorders 6(4): 243–50.

Gomby, D.S., Culross, P.L. & Behrman, R.E. 1999, Home visiting: recent program evaluations, Future of Children 9(1): 2–26.

Goodwin, P.E. 1991, Transport: The New Realism, Transport Studies Unit, Oxford University.

Gordon, P. & Richardson, H. 1997, Are compact cities a desirable planning goal?, Journal of the American Planning Association 63(10): 95–106.

Gordon, T. 1975, Parent Effectiveness Training, Peter Wyden, New York.

Gordon, D. 2000, Inequalities in income, wealth and standard of living in Britain, in Pantazis, C. & Gordon, D. (Eds), Tackling Inequalities: Where Are We Now and What Can Be Done? Policy Press, Bristol, pp. 55–8.

Gottman, J. & Declaire, J. 1997, The Heart of Parenting: How to Raise an Emotionally Intelligent Child, Bloomsbury Press, London.

Gould, B.J., Davie, S.J. & Yudkin, J.S. 1997, Investigation of the mechanism underlying the variability of glycated haemoglobin in non-diabetic subjects not related to glycaemia, Clinica Chimica Acta 260: 49–64.

Graham, H. 2001, From science to policy: options for reducing health inequalities, in Leon, D.A. & Walt, G. (Eds), Poverty, Inequality, and Health: An International Perspective, Oxford University Press, pp. 294–311.

Grange, J.M. & Zumia, A. 1999, Paradox of the global emergency of tuberculosis, Lancet 353: 996.

Granovetter, M. 1985, Economic action, social structure and embeddedness, American Journal of Sociology 91: 481–510.

Gravelle, H. 1998, How much of the relation between population mortality and unequal distribution of income is a statistical artefact? British Medical Journal 316: 382–5.

Gray, J. 1999, False Dawn, The Delusions of Global Capital, Granta, London.

Gray, J. 2000, Wild globalisation, Guardian Weekly 163(27): 9.

Gregory, B. 1998, Summing up, in Eckersley, R. (Ed.), Measuring Progress: Is Life Getting Better? 365–70.

Gregory, R. & Hunter, B. 1995, The Macro Economy and the Growth of Ghettos and Urban Poverty in Australia, Discussion Paper 325, Centre for Economic Policy Research, Australian National University, Canberra.

Grossi, G., Ahs, A. & Lundberg, U. 1998, Psychological correlates of salivary cortisol secretion among unemployed men and women, Integrative Physiological and Behavioral Science 33: 249–63.

Grundmann, E. 1992, Cancer morbidity and mortality in USA Mormons and Seventh-day Adventists, Archives d'Anatomie et de Cytologie Pathologiques 40 (2–3): 73–8.

Guilderson, T.P. & Schrag, D.P. 1998, Abrupt shift in subsurface temperatures in the tropical Pacific associated with changes in El Niño, Science 281: 240–3.

Gump, B.B., Matthews, K.A. & Raikkonen, K. 1999, Modeling relationships among socioeconomic status, hostility, cardiovascular reactivity, and left ventricular mass in African American and White children, Health Psychology 18: 140–50.

Haan, M., Kaplan, G.A. & Camacho, T. 1987, Poverty and health: prospective evidence from the Alameda county study, American Journal of Epidemiology 125(6): 989–98.

Hales, C.N. 1997, Non-insulin-dependent diabetes mellitus, British Medical Bulletin 53: 109–22.

Hales, S., Howden-Chapman, P., Salmond, C., Woodward, A. & Mackenbach, J. 1999, National infant mortality rates in relation to gross national product and distribution of income, Lancet 354: 2047.

Hall, W., Ross, J., Lynskey, M., Law, M. & Degenhardt, L. 2000, How many dependent opioid users are there in Australia? Monograph No. 44, National Drug and Alcohol Research Centre, Sydney.

Hallqvist, J., Diderichsen, F., Theorell, T., Reuterwall, C., Ahlbon, A. and the SHEEP study 1998, Is the effect of job strain on myocardial infarction due to interaction between high psychological demands and low decision latitude? Results from the Stockholm Heart Epidemiology Program (SHEEP), Social Science & Medicine 46: 1405–15.

Halpern, D.S. 2001, Morals, social trust and inequality: can values explain crime? British Journal of Criminology 41(2): 236–51.

Hamilton, C. 1994, The Mystic Economist, Willow Park Press, Canberra.

Hamilton, C. 1999, The genuine progress indicator – methodological developments and results from Australia, Ecological Economics 30: 13–28

Hamilton, C. & Dennis, R. 2000, Tracking Well-being in Australia. The Genuine Progress Indicator 2000, The Australia Institute, Discussion Paper 35, Canberra, <www.gpionline.net>

Hammond, J.L. & Hammond, B. 1947. The Bleak Age, Penguin, West Drayton, UK.

Hansen, J.E., Sato, M., Ruedy, R., Lacis, A. & Oinas, V. 2000, Global warming in the twenty-first century: An alternative scenario, Proceedings of the National Academy of Sciences 97: 9875–80.

Harbridge, R. & Hince, K. 1994, Bargaining and worker representation under New Zealand's employment contracts legislation: a review after 2 years, Relations Industrielles 49: 576–94.

Harbridge, R. & Tolich, D. 1992, Collective employment contracts and new working time arrangements in New Zealand, Wellington, Labour, Employment and Work in New Zealand: Proceedings of the Fifth Conference.

Harbridge, R., Crawford, A. & Keily, P. (Eds) 1998, Employment contracts: bargaining trends and employment law update 1997/98, Victoria University of Wellington, Wellington.

Hardes, G., Dobson, A., Lloyd, D., Leeder, S. 1985, Coronary heart disease mortality trends and related factors in Australia, Cardiology 72: 23–8.

Harding, A. & Szukalska, A. 1999. Trends in Child Poverty in Australia: 1982 to 1995–96. Discussion Paper No. 42, National Centre for Social and Economic Modelling, Canberra.

Harding, A. 1997, The suffering middle: trends in income inequality in Australia, 1982 to 1993–94, The Australian Economic Review 30(4): 341–58.

Harding, A. 2000, Opinion: Swill time for those at the top, National Centre for Social and Economic Modelling, Canberra.

Harrington, J.M. 1994, Working long hours and health, British Medical Journal 308: 1581–82.

Hartshorn, G. & Bynum, N. 1999, Tropical forest synergies, Science 286: 2093–4.

Haskett, M.E. & Kistner, J.A. 1991, Social interactions and peer perceptions of young physically abused children, Child Development 62: 979–90.

Hauner, H., Ditschuneit, H.H., Pal, S.B., Moncayo, R. & Pfeiffer, E.F. 1988, Fat distribution, endocrine and metabolic profile in obese women with and without hirsutism, Metabolism 37: 281–86.

Hawe P. 1994, Capturing the meaning of 'community' in community intervention evaluation: some contributions from community psychology, Health Promotion 9: 199–210.

Hawke, A. & Woden, M. 1997, The Changing Face of Australian Industrial Relations, National Institute of Labour Studies, Flinders University, Adelaide.

Hawkins, D. & Catalano, R. 1992, Communities That Care, Jossey-Bass, San Francisco.

Hawkins, J.D., Catalano, R.F., Kosterman, R., Abbott, R. & Hill, K.G. 1999, Preventing adolescent health-risk behaviours by strengthening protection during childhood, Archives of Pediatrics and Adolescent Medicine 153(3): 226–34.

Hawthorne, G. 1991, Pre-driver education: An evaluation of a traffic safety education program for senior students in Victorian post-primary schools. PhD thesis submitted to Monash University 1991, Monash University, Melbourne, Australia.

Hays, S. 1994, Structure and agency and the sticky problem of culture, Sociological Theory 12 (1): 57–72.

Hazledine, T. 1998, Taking New Zealand Seriously, Harper Collins, Auckland.

Health Funding Authority and Ministry of Health 1997, Disability in New Zealand: Overview of the 1996/97 Surveys, Ministry of Health, Wellington.

Health Funding Authority. 2000, Striking a Better Balance: A Health Funding Response to Reducing Inequalities in Health, New Zealand Health Funding Authority.

Health WIZ, <www.prometheus.com.au/healthwiz/hwizf.htm>

Heath, I., Haines, A., Glover, J. & Hetzel, D. 2000, Editorial: Open invitation from the International Poverty and Health Network to all healthcare professionals: help reduce the burden of ill-health due to poverty, Medical Journal of Australia 172: 356–7.

Hedley, O. 1939, Analysis of 5116 deaths reported as due to acute coronary occlusion in Philadelphia 1933–37, Public Health reports (Washington), pp. 972–1012.

Hellhammer, D.H., Buchtal, J., Gutberlet, I. & Kirschbaum, C. 1997, Social hierarchy and adrenocortical stress reactivity in men, Psychoneuroendocrinology 22: 643–50.

Henderson, H. 1981, The Politics of the Solar Age: Alternatives to Economics, Anchor, New York.

Henning, J. 1995, Commentary: The Employment Contracts Act and work stoppages, New Zealand Journal of Industrial Relations 20: 77–92.

Henry, J.P. & Wang, S. 1998, Effects of early stress on adult affiliative behavior, Psychoneroendocrinology 23: 863–75.

Henry, J.P. 1992, Biological basis of the stress response, Integrative Physiological and Behavioral Science 27: 66–83.

Hertzman, C. & Wilkinson, R. 1996, What's been said and what's been hid: population health, global consumption and the role of national data systems, in Blane, D., Brunner, E. & Wilkinson, R. (Eds), pp. 94–108.

Hertzman, C. 1999, Population health and human development, in Keating, D. & Hertzman, C. (Eds), pp. 21–40.

Hertzman, C. 2000, Social change, market forces and health, Social Science & Medicine 51: 1007–8.

Hettne, B. 1995, Development Theory and the Three Worlds, Longman Scientific and Technical, Harlow.

Heymann, S.J. 2000, Health and social policy, in Berkman, L.F. & Kawachi, I. (Eds).

Hiley, C.M.H. & Morley, C.J. 1994, Evaluation of government's campaign to reduce risk of cot death, British Medical Journal 309: 703–4.

Hince, K. & Harbridge, R. 1994, The Employment Contracts Act: an interim assessment, New Zealand Journal of Industrial Relations 19: 235–25.

Hirohata, T. & Kono, S. 1997, Diet/nutrition and stomach cancer in Japan, International Journal of Cancer Suppl.: 1034–6.

Hirschman, A.O. 1982, Rival interpretations of market society, Journal of Economic Literature 20: 1463–84.

Hobbs, M.S.T., Jamrozik, K.D., Hockey, R.L., Alexander, H.M., Beaglehole, R., Dobson, A.J., Heller, R.F., Jackson, R. & Stewart, A.W. 1991, Mortality from coronary heart disease and incidence of acute myocardial infarction in Auckland, Newcastle and Perth, Medical Journal of Australia 155(7): 436–42.

Hoek, H.W., Brown, A.S. & Susser, E. 1998, The Dutch famine and schizophrenia spectrum disorders, Social Psychiatry and Psychiatric Epidemiology 33 (8): 373–9.

Hoghughi, M. 1998, The importance of parenting in child health, British Medical Journal 316: 1545.

Hogwood, B. & Gunn, 1984, Policy Analysis for the Real World, Oxford University Press, Oxford.

Homel, R. & Bull, M. 1996, 'Under the influence': Alcohol, drugs and crime, in Hazlehurst, K. (Ed.), Crime and Justice: An Australian textbook in criminology, Law Book Co., Sydney, pp. 151–78.

Homel, R. & Mirrlees-Black, C. 1997, Assault in Queensland, Queensland Criminal Justice Commission, Brisbane.

Hopkins, S. & Kidd, M.P. 1996, The determinants of the demand for private health insurance under Medicare, Applied Economics 28: 1623–32.

Hopkinson, N. 1999, An African solution? Lancet 353: 1530.

Horber, F.F., Zurcher, R.M., Herren, H., Crivelli, M.A., Robotti, G. & Frey, F.J. 1986, Altered body fat distribution in patients with glucocorticoid treatment and in patients on long-term dialysis, American Journal of Clinical Nutrition 43: 758–69.

Horne, D. 1966, The Lucky Country, Angus & Robertson, Sydney.

Houghton, J., Meira-Filho, L., Callendar, B., Harris, N., Kattenberg, A. & Maskell, K. (Eds) 1996, Climate change 1995: The Science of Climate Change, Cambridge University Press, Cambridge.

House, J., Landis, K. & Umberson, D. 1988, Social relationships and health, Science 214: 540–5.

House, J., Robbins, C. et al. 1982, The association of social relationships and activities with mortality: prospective evidence from the Techumseh community health study, American Journal of Epidemiology 116: 123–40.

Houston, B.K., Babyak, M.A., Chesney, M.A., Black, G. & Ragland, D.R. 1997, Social dominance and 22-year all-cause mortality in men, Psychosomatic Medicine 59: 5–12.

Howden-Chapman, P. & Cram, F. 1998, Social, Economic and Cultural Determinants of Health, Background Paper 1 for National Health Committee, Wellington.

Howden-Chapman, P. & Tobias, M. (Eds) 2000, Social Inequalities in Health: New Zealand, Ministry of Health, Wellington.

Howden-Chapman, P. 2001, Social capital and health in New Zealand, in Pearce, N. (Ed.), Explanations for Socioeconomic Differences in Health, Massey University (in press).

Howlett, M. & Ramesh, M. 1995, Studying Public Policy: Policy Cycles and Policy Subsystems, Oxford University Press, Toronto.

Huizinga, D. & Jakob-Chien, C. 1998, The contemporaneous co-occurrence of serious and violent juvenile offending and other behavior problems, in Loeber, R. & Farrington, D.P. (Eds), Serious and Violent Juvenile Offenders, Sage, London, pp. 47–67.

Humphreys, J.S., Mathews-Cowey, S. & Weinand, H.C. 1997, Factors in accessibility of general practice in rural Australia, Medical Journal of Australia 166: 577–80.

Hupalo, P. & Herden, K. 1999, Health Policy and Inequality, Occasional Papers: New Series No.5, Commonwealth Department of Health and Aged Care, Canberra.

Hyslop, D. 2000, A Preliminary Analysis of the Dynamics of Individual Market and Disposable Incomes, Treasury Working Papers 15.

Ickovics, J.R., Viscoli, C.M. & Horwitz, R.I. 1997, Functional recovery after myocardial infarction in men: the independent effects of social class, Annals of Internal Medicine 127: 518–25.

Ife J. 1995, Community development: Creating Community Alternatives, Vision, Analysis and Practice, Longman, Melbourne.

Industrial Relations Service 1997, Contract: Special Edition, Department of Labour, Wellington.

International Society for Equity in Health 2000, Constitution, <www.iseqh.org>

Isaksson, K., Hellgren, J. & Pettersson, P. 2000, Repeated downsizing: attitudes and well-being for surviving personnel in a Swedish retail company, in Isaksson, K., Hogstedt, C., Eriksson, C. & Theorell, T. (Eds), pp. 85–101.

Isaksson, K., Hogstedt, C., Eriksson, C. & Theorell, T. (Eds), 2000, Health Effects of the New Labour Market, Kluwer Academic/Plenum Publishers, New York.

Israel, B., Checkoway, B., Schulz, A., et al. 1994, Health education and community empowerment: conceptualizing and measuring perceptions of individual, organizational and community control, Health Education Quarterly 21(2): 153.

Jacobs, J. 1965, Death and Life of Great American Cities, Penguin, London.

Jarvis, M.J. & Wardle, J. 1999, Social patterning of individual health behaviours: the case of cigarette smoking, in Marmot, M.G. & Wilkinson, R.G. (Eds), pp. 240–55.

Jeanrenaud, B. 1994, Central nervous system and peripheral abnormalities: clues to the understanding of obesity and NIDDM, Diabetologia 37 (Suppl. 2): S170–8.

Jeebhay, M., Hussey, G. et al. (Eds) 1997, Lighten the burden of Third World health. The new world order: a challenge to Health for All by the Year 2000. Lighten the burden of Third World health, International People's Health Council, National Progressive Primary Health Care Network, The South African Health and Social Services Organisation, Cape Town, South Africa.

Johnson, N.J., Backlund, E., Sorlie, P.D. & Loveless, C.A. 2000, Marital status and mortality: the National Longitudinal Mortality Study, Annals of Epidemiology 10 (4): 224–38.

Johnston-Brooks, C.H., Lewis, M.A., Evans, G.W. & Whalen, C.K. 1998, Chronic stress and illness in children: the role of allostatic load, Psychosomatic Medicine 60: 597–603.

Jones, D. 1999, Quality of Life: What Australians Think and Feel About Their Lives, Communications Research Services, Sydney.

Joos, F., Plattner, G.-K., Stocker, T.F., Marchal, O. & Schmittner, A. 1999, Global warming and marine carbon cycle feedbacks on future atmospheric CO_2, Science 284: 464–7.

Judge, K. 1995, Income distribution and life expectancy: a critical appraisal, British Medical Journal 311: 1282–5.

Judge, K. 2000, Tackling health inequalities: building an effective evidence base. Keynote vignettes, International Society for Equity in Health Inaugural Conference, Havana, 7 pp.

Judge, K., Mulligan, J. & Benzeval, M. 1998, Income inequality and population health, Social Science & Medicine 46(4–5): 567–79.

Kahn, H.S., Tatham, L.M., Pamuk, E.R. & Heath, C.W. 1998, Are geographic regions with high income inequality associated with risk of abdominal weight gain? Social Science & Medicine 47(1): 1–6.

Kaplan, B.H. 1992, Social health and the forgiving heart: the type B story, Journal of Behavioral Medicine 15: 3–13.

Kaplan, G.A. 1995, Where do shared pathways lead? Some reflections on a research agenda, Psychosomatic Medicine 57: 208–12.

Kaplan, G.A. 1996, People and places: contrasting perspectives on the association between social class and health, International Journal of Health Services 26(3): 507–19.

Kaplan, G.A. 1999, What is the role of the social environment in understanding inequalities in health?. In Adler, N.E. et al. (Eds), Socioeconomic Status and Health in Industrial Nations, New York Academy of Sciences, New York.

Kaplan, G.A., Pamuk, E.R., Lynch, J.W., Cohen, R.D. & Balfour, J.L. 1996, Inequality in income and mortality in the United States: analysis of mortality and potential pathways, British Medical Journal 312: 999–1003.

Kaplan, J.R., Adams, M.R., Clarkson, T.B., Manuck, S.B., Shively, C.A. & Williams, J.K. 1996, Psychosocial factors, sex differences, and atherosclerosis: lessons from animal models, Psychosomatic Medicine 58: 598–611.

Kaplan, R.D. 1994, The coming anarchy, Atlantic Monthly 273(2): 44–76.

Karoly, L.A., Greenwood, P.W., Everingham, S.S., Hoube, J., Kilburn, M.R., Rydell C.P., Sanders, M. & Chiesa, J. 1998, Investing in Our Children, Rand, Santa Monica CA.

Kasser, T. & Ryan, R.M. 1993, A dark side of the American Dream: correlates of financial success as a central life aspiration, Journal of Personality and Social Psychology 65 (2): 410–22.

Kasser, T. & Ryan, R.M. 1996, Further examining the American Dream: differential correlates of intrinsic and extrinsic goals, Personality and Social Psychology Bulletin 22 (3): 280–7.

Kasser, T. 2000, Two versions of the American Dream: which goals and values make for a high quality of life? in Diener E. & Rahtz D.R. (Eds), Advances in Quality of Life Theory and Research, vol. 1, Kluwer, Dordrecht, pp. 3–12.

Kauffman, J.S. & Cooper, R.S. 1999, Seeking causal explanations in social epidemiology, American Journal of Epidemiology 150: 113–20.

Kawachi, I. & Kennedy, B.P. 1997(a), The relationship of income inequality to mortality: does the choice of indicator matter? Social Science & Medicine 45(7): 1121–7.

Kawachi, I. & Kennedy, B.P. 1997(b), Health and social cohesion: why care about income inequality? British Medical Journal 314: 1037–40.

Kawachi, I., Kennedy, B.P. & Glass, R. 1999(c), Social capital and self-rated health: a contextual analysis, American Journal of Public Health 89(8): 1187–93.

Kawachi, I. & Berkman, L.F. 2000, Social cohesion, social capital, and health, in Berkman, L.F. & Kawachi, I., (Eds), pp. 174–90.

Kawachi, I. & Marmot, M.G. 1998. Commentary: What can we learn from studies of occupational class and cardiovascular disease? American Journal of Epidemiology 148(2): 160–3.

Kawachi, I. 1999, Social capital and community effects on population and individual health, in Adler, N.E., Marmot, M., McEwen, B.S. & Stewart, J. (Eds), pp. 120–30.

Kawachi, I. 2000, Income inequality and health, in Berkman, L.F. & Kawachi, I. (Eds), pp. 76–94.

Kawachi, I., Kennedy, B.P., Lochner, K. & Prothrow-Stith, D. 1997(a), Social capital, income inequality, and mortality, American Journal of Public Health 87(9): 1491–8.

Kawachi, I., Kennedy, B. & Lochner, K. 1997(b), Long live community: social capital as public health, The American Prospect Nov–Dec 35: 56.

Kawachi, I., Kennedy, B.P.E. & Wilkinson, R.G. (Eds) 1999(a), The Society and Population Health Reader: Income Inequality and Health vol.1, The New Press, New York.

Kawachi, I., Kennedy, B.P. & Wilkinson, R.G. 1999(b), Crime: social disorganisation and relative deprivation, Social Science & Medicine 48: 719–31.

Keating, D.P. & Hertzman, C. (Eds) 1999, Developmental Health and the Wealth of Nations: Social, Biological and Educational Dynamics, Guilford, New York.

Keeling, C. & Whorf, T. 2000, Ocean tides found to influence climate, Proceedings of the National Academy of Science 97: 3814–9.

Kehrer, B.H. & Wolin, C.M. 1979, Impact of income maintenance on low birthweight: evidence from the Gary Experiment, Journal of Human Resources 14: 435–62.

Kelly, P. 2000, Facing the future, The Australian, June 24.

Kelly, S., Hertzman, C. & Daniel, M. 1997, Searching for the biological pathways between stress and health, Annual Review of Public Health 18: 437–62.

Kelsey, J. 1993, Breast cancer epidemiology: summary and future directions, Epidemiologic Reviews 15(1): 256–63.

Kennedy, B.P., Kawachi, I. & Prothrow-Stith, D. 1996, Income distribution and mortality: cross-sectional ecological study of the Robin Hood index in the United States, British Medical Journal 312: 1004–7, (erratum, 312: 1253).

Kennedy, B.P., Kawachi, I., Glass, R. & Prothrow-Stith, D. 1998, Income distribution, socioeconomic status, and self-rated health in the United States: multilevel analysis, British Medical Journal 317: 917–21.

Kenworthy, J., Laube, F., Newman, P., Barter, P., Raad, T., Poboon, C. & Guia, B. 1999, An International Sourcebook of Automobile Dependence in Cities, 1960–1990, University Press of Colorado, Boulder, Colorado.

Kessler, R.C. 1982, A disaggregation of the relationship between socioeconomic status and psychological distress, American Sociological Review 47: 752–64.

Kim, J.Y., Millen, J. et al. (Eds) 2000, Dying for Growth: Global inequalities and the health of the poor, Common Courage Press and Institute of Health and Social Justice, Monroe, Maine.

Kirschbaum, C. & Hellhammer, D.H. 1994, Salivary cortisol in psychoneuroendocrine research: recent developments and applications, Psychoneuroendocrinology 19: 313–33.

Kitagawa, E.M., Hauser, P.M. 1973, Differential Mortality in the United States, Harvard University Press, Cambridge, pp. 17–26.

Kivimaki, M., Vahtera, J., Koskenvuo, M., Uutela, A. & Pentti, J. 1998, Response of hostile individuals to stressful changes in their working lives: test of a psychosocial vulnerability model, Psychological Medicine 28: 903–13.

Knack, S. & Keefer, P. 1997, Does social capital have an economic payoff? A cross-country investigation, Quarterly Journal of Economics 112 (4): 1251–88.

Knutson, T.R., Tuleya, R.E. & Kurihara, Y. 1998, Simulated increase of hurricane intensities in a CO_2-warmed climate, Science 279: 1018–20.

Kochan, T.A., Smith, M., Wells, J.C. & Rebitzer, J.B. 1994, Human resource strategies and contingent workers: the case of safety and health in the petrochemical industry, Human Resource Management 33: 55–77.

Kolvin, I., Miller, F.J.W., Scott, D., Gratzanis, S.R.M. & Fleeting, M. 1990, Continuities of deprivation (ESRC/DHSS Studies in Deprivation and Disadvantages No. 15), Avebury, Aldershot.

Korten, D.C. 1995, When Corporations Rule the World, Kumarian Press, West Hartford, Connecticut.

Kostoff, S. 1991, The City Shaped: Urban Patterns and Meanings through History, Thames and Hudson, London.

Kreitman, N., Carstairs, V. & Duffy, J. 1991, Association of age and social class with suicide among men in Great Britain, Journal of Epidemiology and Community Health 45: 195–202.

Krieger, N. & Smith, G.D. 2000, Seeking causal explanations in social epidemiology, American Journal of Epidemiology 151: 831–2.

Krieger, N. 1994, Epidemiology and the web of causation: has anyone seen the spider? Social Science & Medicine 39(7): 887–903.

Krieger, N. 2000, Epidemiology and social sciences: towards a critical reengagement in the 21st century, Epidemiologic Reviews 22(1): 155–63.

Krieger, N., Rowley, D., Herman, A., Avery, B. & Philips, M. 1993, Racism, sexism, and social class: implications for studies of health, disease, and well-being, American Journal of Preventive Medicine 9(6 sup): 82–122.

Kubzansky, L.D. & Kawachi, I. 2000, Affective states and health, in Berkman, L.F. & Kawachi, I. (Eds), pp. 213–41.

Kubzansky, L.D., Kawachi, I. & Sparrow, D. 1999, Socioeconomic status, hostility, and risk factor clustering in the Normative Aging Study: any help from allostatic load? Annals of Behavioral Medicine 21: 330–8.

Kunitz, S.J. 1994, Disease and Social Diversity. The European impact on the health of non-Europeans, Oxford University Press, New York.

Kunst, A.E. 1997, Cross-national Comparisons of Socio-economic Differences in Mortality, Erasmus University, Rotterdam.

Kunst, A.E., Groenhof, F. & Mackenbach, J.P. 1998, Mortality by occupational class among men 30–64 years in 11 European countries, EU Working Group on Socioeconomic Inequalities in Health, Social Science & Medicine 46: 1459–76.

Labonte, R. 1990, Empowerment: notes on professional and community dimensions, Canadian Review of Social Policy 6: 1–12.

Labonte, R. 1997, Power, Participation and Partnerships for Health Promotion, VicHealth, Melbourne.

Lamond (Eds) 1977, Women, Minorities and Employment Discrimination, Lexington Books, Mass.

Landes, D.S. 1999, The Wealth and Poverty of Nations: Why some are so rich and some so poor, W.W. Norton & Company, New York.

Landsberg, L. 1986, Diet, obesity and hypertension: a hypothesis involving insulin, the sympathetic nervous system, and adaptive thermogenesis, Quarterly Journal of Medicine 61: 1081–1090.

Lane, M. & Henry, K. 2000, Community Development, Crime and Violence: a case study, Unpublished paper, Department of Social Work, Social Policy & Sociology, University of Sydney.

Lantz, P.M., House, J.S., Lepkowski, J.M., Williams, D.R., Mero, R.P. & Chen, J. 1998, Socioeconomic factors, health behaviors, and mortality: results from a nationally representative prospective study of US adults, Journal of the American Medical Association 279: 1703–8.

Lasch, C. 1995, The Revolt of the Elites and the Betrayal of Democracy, W.W. Norton, New York.

Last, T.M., 2001, A Dictionary of Epidemiology (4th edition), Oxford University Press, New York.

Laugesen, M. & Swinburn, B. 2000(a), The New Zealand food supply: trends 1961–1995 and comparison with other OECD countries, New Zealand Medical Journal 113: 311–15.

Laugesen, M. & Swinburn, B. 2000(b), New Zealand's tobacco control programme 1985–1998, Tobacco Control 9 (2): 155–62.

LaVeist, T. 1996, Why we should continue to study race . . . but do a better job: an essay on race, racism and health, Ethnicity and Disease 6: 21–29.

Law, M. & Wald, N. 1999, Why heart disease mortality is low in France: the time lag explanation, British Medical Journal 318: 1471–6.

Law, M.R., Wald, N.J., Wu, T., Hackshaw, A. & Bailey, A. 1994, Systematic underestimation of association between serum cholesterol concentration and ischaemic heart disease in observational studies: data from the BUPA study, British Medical Journal 308(6925): 363–6.

Lawson, J. & Black, D. 1993, Socio-economic status: the prime indicator of premature death in Australia, Journal of Biosocial Science 25: 539–52.

Lazarus, R.S. 1991, Emotion and Adaptation, Oxford University Press, New York.

Le Grand, J. 1987, Inequalities in health: some international comparisons, European Economic Review 31: 182–91.

Leavitt, J.W. 1996, The Healthiest City : Milwaukee and the Politics of Health Reform, paperback edition, University of Wisconsin Press, Maddison.

Leon, D.A., Chenet, L., Shkolnikov, V.M., Zakarov, S., Shapiro, J., Rakhmanova, G., Vassin, S. & McKee, M. 1997, Huge variation in Russian mortality rates 1984–94: artefact, alcohol or what? Lancet 350: 383–8.

Leon, D.A., Lithell, H.O., Vagero, D., Koupilova, I., Mohsen, R., Berglund, L., Lithell, U.B. & McKeigue, P.M. 1998, Reduced fetal growth rate and increased risk of death from ischaemic heart disease: cohort study of 15000 Swedish men and women born 1915–29, British Medical Journal 317: 241–5.

Leon, D.A., Walt, G. & Gilson, L. 2001, International perspectives on health inequalities and policy, British Medical Journal 322: 591–4.

Lewis, J. 2000, From 'fightback' to 'biteback': The rise and fall of a national dental program, Australian Journal of Public Administration 59(1): 84–96.

Lilley, R., Feyer, A.-M., Kirk, P. & Gander, P. 2001, A survey of forest workers in New Zealand: do hours of work, rest and recovery play a role in accidents and injury? Journal of Safety Research, accepted for publication.

Lindholm, L. & Rosen, M. 2000, What is the 'golden standard' for assessing population-based interventions? Problems of dilution bias, Journal of Epidemiology and Community Health 54: 617–22.

Link, B. & Phelan, J. 1995, Social conditions as fundamental causes of disease, Journal of Health and Social Behaviour (extra issue): 80–94.

Lister, R.K. & Schrire, B.D. 1999. Save the rain forest – it saved our skin, Lancet 353: 848.

Liu, D., Diorio, J., Tannenbaum, B., Caldji, D., Francis, D., Freedman, A., Sharma, S., Pearon, D., Plotsky, J. & Meaney, M. 1997, Maternal care, hippocampal glucocorticoid receptors, and hypothalamic- pituitary-adrenal responses to stress, Science 277: 1659–62.

Lo, M.S., Ng, M.L., Azmy, B.S. & Khalid, B.A. 1992, Clinical applications of salivary cortisol measurements, Singapore Medical Journal 33: 170–3.

Lochner, K., Kawachi, I. & Kennedy, B.P. 1999, Social capital: a guide to its measurement, Health & Place 5: 259–70.

Lockwood, M., Stamper, R. & Wild, M.N. 1999, A doubling of the Sun's coronal magnetic field during the past 100 years, Nature 399: 437–9.

Loeber, R., Wei, E., Stouthamer-Loeber, M., Huizinga, D. & Thornberry, T.P. 1999, Behavioral antecedents to serious and violent offending: joint analyses from the Denver Youth Survey, Pittsburgh Youth Study and the Rochester Youth Development Study, Studies on Crime and Crime Prevention: 245–263.

Loh, J., Randers, J., MacGillivray, A., Kapos, V., Jenkins, M., Groombridge, B. & Cox, N. 1998, Living Planet Report, 1998, WWF International, New Economics Foundation, World Conservation Monitoring Centre, Gland, Switzerland.

Lomas, J. 1998, Social capital and health: implications for public health and epidemiology, Social Science & Medicine 47(9): 1181–8.

Lopez, A.D. & Ruzicka, L.T. 1983, Sex Differentials in Mortality, Department of Demography, Australian National University, Canberra.

Lopuhaa, C.E. et al. 2000, Atopy, lung function and obstructive airways disease after prenatal exposure to famine, Thorax 55(7): 555–61.

Loury, G. 1977, A dynamic theory of racial income differences, in Wallace, P.A. & Lamond, A. (Eds), Women, Minorities and Employment Discrimination, Lexington Books, Lexington, Mass.

Lucas, A., Stafford, M., Morley, R., Abbott, R., Stevenson, T., McFadian, U. & Elias-Jones, A. 1999, Efficacy and safety of long chain polyunsaturated fatty acid supplementation of infant formula milk, Lancet 354: 1948–54.

Lundberg, O. 1991, Causal explanations for class inequality in health – an empirical analysis, Social Science & Medicine 32: 385–93.

Lupien, S.J., Gaudreau, S., Tchiteya, B.M., Maheu, F., Sharma, S., Nair, N.P., Hauger, R.L., McEwen, B.S. & Meaney, M.J. 1997, Stress-induced declarative memory impairment in healthy elderly subjects: relationship to cortisol reactivity, Journal of Clinical Endocrinology and Metabolism 82: 2070–5.

Lynch, J.W. 2000, Income inequality and health: expanding the debate, Social Science & Medicine, 51: 1001–5.

Lynch, J.W., Due, P., Muntaner, C. & Davey Smith, G. 2000(a), Social capital – is it a good investment strategy for public health? Journal of Epidemiology and Community Health 54: 404–8.

Lynch, J.W., Davey Smith, G., Kaplan, G.A. & House, J.S. 2000(b), Income inequality and mortality: importance to health of individual income, psychosocial environment, or material conditions, British Medical Journal 320: 1200–4.

Lynch, J.W., Due, P., Muntaner, C. & Smith, G. 2000(c), Social capital economic capital and power: further issues for public health agenda, Journal of Epidemiology and Community Health 54: 409–10.

Lynch, J.W. & Kaplan, G.A. 1997, Understanding how inequality in the distribution of income affects health, Journal of Health Psychology 2(3): 297–314.

Lynch, J.W., Kaplan, G.A. & Salonen, J.K. 1997, Why do the poor behave poorly? Variation in adult health behaviours and psychosocial characteristics by stages of the socioeconomic lifecourse, Social Science & Medicine 44: 809–19.

Lynch, J.W., Kaplan, G.A., Cohen, R.D., Tuomilehto, J. & Salonen, J.T. 1996, Do cardiovascular risk factors explain the relation between socioeconomic status, risk of all-cause mortality, cardiovascular mortality, and acute myocardial infarction? American Journal of Epidemiology 144: 934–42.

Lynch, J.W., Kaplan, G.A., Pamuk, E.R, Cohen, R.D., Heck, K.E., Balfour, J.L. & Yen, I.H. 1998, Income inequality and mortality in metropolitan areas of the United States, American Journal of Public Health 88(7): 1074–80.

Lyon, J.L., Gardner, K. & Gress, R.E. 1994, Cancer incidence among Mormons and non-Mormons in Utah (United States) 1971–85, Cancer Causes and Control 5 (2): 149–56.

MacIntyre, S. & Ellaway, A. 2000, Ecological approaches: rediscovering the role of the physical and social environment, in Berkman, L.F. & Kawachi, I. (Eds), pp. 332–48.

MacIntyre, S., MacIver, S. & Sooman, A. 1993, Area, class and health: should we be focusing on places or people? Journal of Social Policy 22(2): 213–34.

Mackenbach, J.P. 1998, Commentary, in Arves-Pares (Ed.), 1998, Promoting Research on Inequality in Health. Proceedings from an International Expert Meeting, Stockholm, 24–25 September 1997, Swedish Council for Social Research, Stockholm.

Mackenbach, J.P. & Droomers, M. 1999, Interventions and Policies to Reduce Socioeconomic Inequalities in Health: Proceedings of the Third Workshop of the European Network on Interventions and Policies to Reduce Socioeconomic Inequalities in Health, Department of Public Health, Erasmus University, Rotterdam.

Mackenbach, J.P. 1996, The contribution of medical care to mortality decline: McKeown revisited, Journal of Clinical Epidemiology 49: 1207–13.

Mackenbach, J.P., Cavelaars, E.J.M., Kunst, A.E. & Groenhof, F. 2000, Socioeconomic inequalities in cardiovascular disease mortality, European Heart Journal 21: 1141–51.

Mackenbach, J.P., van den Bos, J., Joung, I.M.A., van de Meen, H. & Stronks, K. 1994, The determinants of excellent health: different from the determinants of health, International Journal of Epidemiology 23: 1273–81.

Mackenbach, J.P., Kunst, A.E., Cavelaars, A.E., Groenhof, F., Geurts, J. & the EU Working Group on Socioeconomic Inequalities in Health, 1997, Lancet 349: 1655–59.

Mackerras, D. 1998, Evaluation of the Strong Women, Strong Babies, Strong Culture Program, Menzies Occasional Papers 2/98, Menzies School of Health Research, Darwin.

MacMahon, S., Peto, R., Cutler, J., Collins, R., Sorlie, P., Neaton, J., Abbott, R., Godwin, J., Dyer, A. & Stamler, J. 1990, Blood pressure, stroke, and coronary heart disease. Part 1, Prolonged differences in blood pressure: prospective observational studies corrected for the regression dilution bias, Lancet 335(8692): 765–74.

MacMillan, D. & Chavis, D. 1986, Sense of community: a definition and theory, Journal of Community Psychology 14: 6–23.

Magnani, E. 2000, The Environmental Kuznets Curve, environmental protection policy and income distribution, Ecological Economics 32: 431–43.

Magnusson, D. & Bergman, L.R. 1990, A pattern approach to the study of pathways from childhood to adulthood, in Robins, L. & Rutter, M. (Eds), 1990, Straight and Devious Pathways from Childhood to Adulthood, Cambridge University Press, New York, pp. 101–15.

Manuck, S.B., Kaplan, J.R., Adams, M.R. & Clarkson, T.B. 1998, Studies of psychosocial influences on coronary artery atherogenesis in cynomolgus monkeys, Health Psychology 7: 113–24.

Mårin, P. & Björntorp, P. 1993, Endocrine-metabolic pattern and adipose tissue distribution, Hormone Research 39 (Suppl. 3): 81–5.

Marjoribanks, K. 1991, Family and social capital and young adults educational attainment and occupational aspirations, Psychological Reports 69: 237–8.

Marmot, M.G. & Wilkinson, R.G. (Eds) 1999, Social Determinants of Health, Oxford University Press, Oxford.

Marmot, M.G. 1998, Improvement in social environment to improve health, Lancet 351: 57–60.

Marmot, M.G. 1999, Epidemiology of socio-economic status and health: are determinants within countries the same as between countries? in Adler, N. E., Marmot, M., McEwen, B. S. & Stewart, J. (Eds), pp. 16–29.

Marmot, M.G. 2000, Social determinants of health: from observation to policy, Medical Journal of Australia 172: 379–82.

Marmot, M.G., Bosma H., Hemingway, H., Brunner, E. & Stansfeld, S. 1997(a), Contribution of job control and other risk factors to social variations in coronary heart disease incidence, Lancet 350(9073): 235–359.

Marmot, M.G., Bosma, H., Hemingway, H., Brunner, E., Stansfield, S. 1997(b), Comment, Lancet 350(9088): 1404–5.

Marmot, M.G., Siegrist, J., Theorell, T. & Feeney, A. 1999, Health and the psychosocial environment at work, in Marmot, M. & Wilkinson, R.G. (Eds), pp. 105–31.

Marmot, M.G. & McDowall, M.E. 1986, Mortality decline and widening social inequalities, Lancet ii: 274–6.

Marmot, M.G. & Mustard, J.F. 1994, Coronary heart disease from a population perspective, in Evans, R.G., Barer, M.L. & Marmor, T.R. (Eds), pp. 189–214.

Marmot, M.G. 1986, Social inequalities in mortality: the social environment, in Wilkinson, R.G. (Ed.), Class and Health: Research and Longitudinal Data, Tavistock, London, pp. 21–33.

Marmot, M.G., Fuhrer, R., Ettner, S.L., Marks, N.F., Bumpass, L.L. & Ryff, C.D. 1998, Contribution of psychosocial factors to socioeconomic difference in health, Milbank Quarterly 76: 403–48.

Marmot, M.G., Rose, G., Shipley, M., Hamilton, P.J. 1978, Employment grade and coronary heart disease in British civil servants, Journal of Epidemiology and Community Health 32(4): 244–9.

Marmot, M.G., Shipley, M.J. & Rose, G. 1984, Inequalities in death: specific explanations of a general pattern? Lancet 1: 1003–6.

Marmot, M.G., Smith, G.D., Stansfeld, S., Patel, C., North, F., Head, J., White, I., Brunner, E. & Feeney, A. 1991, Health inequalities among British civil servants: the Whitehall II Study, Lancet 337: 1387–93.

Marshall, J. & Watt, P. 1999, Child Behaviour Problems: A Literature Review of the Size and Nature of the Problem and Prevention Interventions in Childhood, The Interagency Committee on Children's Futures, Perth.

Martelin, T. 1994, Mortality by indicators of socioeconomic status among the Finnish elderly, Social Science & Medicine 38: 1257–78.

Martikainen, P.T. & Marmot, M.G. 1999, Socioeconomic differences in weight gain and determinants and consequences of coronary risk factors, American Journal of Clinical Nutrition 69: 719–26.

Martikainen, P. & Valkonen, T. 1999, Policies to reduce income inequalities are unlikely to eradicate inequalities in mortality, British Medical Journal 319: 319.

Martin, B., 1999, Sub-National Income Differentials, 1986–1996, Population Studies Centre, University of Waikato, Hamilton.

Martin, C.M., R.G. Attewell, M. Nisa, J. McCallum, J. & Raymond, C.J. 1997, Characteristics of longer consultations in Australian general practice, Medical Journal of Australia 167: 76–9.

Martin, H.-P. & Schumann, H. 1997, The Global Trap. Globalisation and the assault on prosperity and democracy, Zed Books, London.

Martuzzi, M., Grundy, C. & Elliott, P. 1998, Perinatal mortality in an English health region: geographical distribution and association with socio-economic factors, Paediatric and Perinatal Epidemiology 12: 263–76.

Masood, E. 2000, Global 'eco-survey' plan gets a rough ride, Nature 397: 97.

Massey, D.S. 1996, The age of extremes: concentrated affluence and poverty in the twenty-first century, Demography 33: 395–412.

Mathers, C. 1994, Health Differentials Among Adult Australians Aged 25–64 Years, Australian Institute of Health and Welfare, Health Monitoring Series No. 1, Australian Government Publishing Service, Canberra.

Mayo-Smith, W., Hayes, C.W., Biller, B.M.K., Kibanski, A., Rosenthal, H. & Rosenthal, D.I. 1989, Body fat distribution measured by CT: correlations in healthy subjects, patients with anorexia nervosa, and patients with Cushing's Syndrome, Radiology 170: 515–18.

McAvay, G.J., Seeman, T.E. & Rodin, J. 1996, A longitudinal study of change in domain-specific self-efficacy among older adults, Journals of Gerontology, Psychological and Social Sciences 51B: P243–53.

McCain, M.N., Mustard, J.F. 1999, Early Years Study: Final Report, Publications Ontario, Toronto.

McCarty, M.F. 2000, The insulin-sensitizing activity of moderate alcohol consumption may promote leaness in women, Medical Hypotheses 54: 794–7.

McClelland, A. & Scotton, R. 1998, Poverty and health, in Fincher, R. & Nieuwenhuysen, J. (Eds), Australian Poverty: Then and Now, Melbourne University Press, Melbourne, pp. 185–202.

McCoy, A.R. & Reynolds, A.J. 1999, Grade retention and school performance: an extended investigation, Journal of School Psychology 37: 273–98.

McDonough, P., Duncan, G.J., Williams, D., House, J. 1997, Income dynamics and adult mortality in the United States, 1972 through 1989, American Journal of Public Health 87: 1476–83.

McEvoy, L. & Land, G. 1981, Lifestyle and death patterns of the Missouri RLDS Church, American Journal of Public Health 71 (12): 1350–7.

McEwen, B. 1998, Protective and damaging effects of stress mediators, New England Journal of Medicine 338: 171–9.

McEwen, B.S. & Stellar, E. 1993, Stress and the individual: mechanisms leading to disease, Archives of Internal Medicine 153: 2093–101.

McEwen, B.S. 1997, Hormones as regulators of brain development: life-long effects related to health and disease, Acta Paediatrica 422 (Suppl.): 41–4.

McGlynn, G., Newman, P.W.G. & Kenworthy, J.R. 1991, Towards Better Cities, Commission for the Future, Melbourne.

McKee, M. & Jacobson, B. 2000, Public health in Europe, Lancet, 356: 665–70.

McKnight, J.L. 1985, Health and empowerment, Canadian Journal of Public Health 76: 37–8.

McMichael, A. 1989, Coronary heart disease: interplay between changing concepts of aetiology, risk distribution, and social strategies for prevention, Community Health Studies XIII(1): 5–13.

McMichael, A.J., Haines, A., Slooff, R. & Kovats, S. (Eds) 1996, Climate Change and Human Health, World Health Organization, Geneva.

McMichael, A.J. 1993, Planetary Overload: Global Environmental Change and the Health of the Human Species, Cambridge University Press, Cambridge.

McMichael, A.J. 1999, Prisoners of the proximate: loosening the constraints on epidemiology in an age of change, American Journal of Epidemiology 149: 887–97.

McMichael, A.J. 2001, Human Frontiers, Environments and Disease: Past patterns, uncertain futures, Cambridge University Press, Cambridge.

McMichael, A.J., Smith, K.R. & Corvalan, C.F. 2000, The sustainability transition: a new challenge [editorial], Bulletin of the World Health Organization 78: 1067.

Meaney, M., Aitken, D., Berkel, C., Bhatnagar, S. & Sapolsky, R. 1998, Effect of neonatal handling on age-related impairments associated with the hippocampus, Science 239: 766–8.

Mechanic, D. 2000, Rediscovering The social determinants of health: book review essay, Health Affairs May/June: 269–76.

Megalogenis, G. 2000, Death of a dream, The Australian, June 17.

Mehmet, O. 1995, Westernizing the Third World: the Eurocentricity of Economic Development Theories, Routledge, London.

Melamed, S., Ugarten, U., Shirom, A., Kahana, L., Lerman, Y. & Froom, P. 1999, Chronic burnout, somatic arousal and elevated salivary cortisol levels, Journal of Psychosomatic Research 46: 591–8.

Melchior, A., Telle, K. & Wiig, H. 2000, Globalisation and Inequality: World Income Distribution and Living Standards, 1960–1998, Royal Norwegian Ministry of Foreign Affairs, Norwegian Institute of International Affairs (NUPI) <odin.dep.no/ud> (last visited 27.2.01).

Mellor, J. & Milyo, J. 1999, Income inequality and health status in the United States: evidence from the current population survey, in Wagstaff, A. & van Doorslaer, E. (Eds) 2000, Income inequality and health: what does the literature tell us? Annual Review of Public Health 21: 543–67.

Menchek, P. 1993, Economic status as a determinant of mortality among older black and white men: does poverty kill? Population Studies 47: 427–36.

Metropolitan Life Insurance Company 1980, Statistical Bulletin 61(2): 2.

Meyer, R.J. & Haggerty, R.J. 1962, Streptococcal infection in families: factors altering individual susceptibility, Pediatrics 29: 539–49.

Miki, K., Kawamorita, K., Araga, Y., Musha, T. & Sudo, A. 1998, Urinary and salivary stress hormone levels while performing arithmetic calculation in a noisy environment, Industrial Health 36: 66–9.

Milburn, A. 2001, Breaking the link between poverty and ill health. Long-Term Medical Conditions Alliance Conference, Royal College of Physicians, 28 February, <www.doh.gov.uk/healthinequalities/speech. htm> downloaded 7/03/01).

Miller, G.E., Kemeny, M.E., Taylor, S.E., Cole, S.W. & Bisscher, B.R. 1997, Social relationships and immune processes in HIV seropositive gay and bisexual men, Annals of Behavioral Medicine 19: 139–51.

Miller, T.Q., Smith, T.W., Turner, C.W., Guijarro, M.L. & Hallet, A.J. 1996, A meta-analytic review of research on hostility and physical health, Psychological Bulletin 119: 322–48.

Mitrovica, J.X., Tamisiea, M.E., Davis, J.L., Milne, G.A. 2001, Recent mass balance of polar ice sheets inferred from patterns of global sea-level change, Nature 409: 1026–9.

Moberg, C.L. & Cohn, Z.A. 1991, René Jules Dubos, Scientific American 264(5): 32–8.

Moffitt, T. 1993, Adolescence-limited and life course-persistent antisocial behavior: a developmental taxonomy, Psychological Review 100(4): 674–701.

Monk, M. 1987, Epidemiology of Suicide, Epidemiologic Reviews 9: 51–69.

Moore, C. (Ed.) 1909, Plan of Chicago, City of Chicago, June.

Morehead, A., Steele, M., Alexander, M., Stephen, K. & Duffin, L. 1997, Changes at work: the 1995 Australian Workplace Industrial Relations Survey, Longman, Melbourne.

Morris, M., Bernhardt, A.D. & Handcock, M.S. 1994, Economic inequality: new methods for new trends, American Sociological Review 59: 205–9.

Muecke, M. 1994, Worries and worriers in Thailand, Health Care Womens International 15: 503–19.

Munasinghe, M. & Shearer, W. (Eds) 1995, Defining and measuring sustainability: The biogeophysical foundations. The World Bank, Washington.

Muntaner, C. & Lynch, J. 1999, Income inequality, social cohesion, and class relations: a critique of Wilkinson's neo-Durkheimian research program, International Journal of Health Services 29(1): 59–81.

Muntaner, C. 1999, Invited commentary: social mechanisms, race and social epidemiology, American Journal of Epidemiology 150: 121–6.

Muntaner, C., Lynch, J. & Oates, G.L. 1999, The social class determinants of income inequality and social cohesion, International Journal of Health Services 29(4): 699–732.

Murphy, J.M., Oliver, D.C., Monson, R.R., Sobol, A.M., Federman, E.B. & Leighton, A.H. 1991, Depression and anxiety in relation to social status, Archives of General Psychiatry 48: 223–9.

Murray, C.J. & Lopez, A.D. 1997(a), Mortality by cause for eight regions of the world: Global Burden of Disease Study, Lancet 349(9061): 1269–76.

Murray, C.J. & Lopez, A.D. 1997(b), Regional patterns of disability-free life expectancy and disability-adjusted life expectancy: Global Burden of Disease Study, Lancet 349(9062): 1347–52.

Murray, C.J.L. & Chen, L.C. 1993, In search of a contemporary theory for understanding mortality change, Social Science & Medicine 36: 143–55.

Murray, C.J.L. & Lopez, A.D. (Eds) 1996, The Global Burden of Disease – Summary, The Harvard School of Public Health on behalf of the World Health Organization and the World Bank, distributed by Harvard University Press.

Mustard, J.F. 1996, Health and social capital, in Blane, D., Brunner, E. & Wilkinson, R. (Eds), pp. 303–13.

Myers, D. & Diener, E. 1995, Who is happy? Psychological Science 6(1): 10–19.

Myers, D.G. 2000, The funds, friends and faith of happy people, American Psychologist 55(1): 56–67.

Myers, N. 1997, The world's forests and their ecosystem services, in Daily, G.C., Reichert, J.S. & Myers, J.P. (Eds), Nature's Services: Societal Dependence on Natural Ecosystems, Island Press, Washington, pp. 215–35.

Nader, R., Greider, W. et al. 1993, The Case Against 'Free Trade': GATT, NAFTA and the Globalisation of Corporate Power, Earth Island Press and North Atlantic Books, San Francisco and Berkeley.

Nagin, D. & Tremblay, R.E. 1999, Trajectories of boys' physical aggression, opposition and hyperactivity on the path to physically violent and non-violent juvenile delinquency, Child Development 70: 1181–96.

Nahapiet, J. & Ghoshal, S. 1998, Social capital, intellectual capital and the organisational advantage, Academy of Management Review 23(2): 242–66.

Najman, J.M. 1989, Health Care in Developing Countries, in Freeman, H.E. & Levine, S. (Eds), Handbook of Medical Sociology, Prentice-Hall, Englewood Cliffs, NJ, pp. 332–46.

Najman, J.M., Aird, R., Bor, W., O'Callaghan, M., Shuttlewood, G. & Williams, G. 2000, A Better Start For Life. Report submitted to Queensland Health, Department of Sociology, Anthropology and Archaeology, The University of Queensland, St. Lucia.

Najman, J.M., Aird, R., Bor, W., O'Callaghan, M., Williams, G., Shuttlewood, G.J. & Andersen, M.J. (Submitted 2002), Foetal and early childhood pathways to inequalities in adult health and well-being.

National Aboriginal Health Strategy Working Party Report (NAHS) 1989, The National Aboriginal Health Strategy, Commonwealth Government Publishers, Canberra.

National Advisory Committee on Health and Disability (National Health Committee) 1998, The Social, Cultural, and Economic Determinants of Health in New Zealand: Action to Improve Health, National Advisory Committee on Health and Disability, Wellington, New Zealand.

National Crime Prevention 1999, Pathways to Prevention: Developmental And Early Intervention Approaches To Crime In Australia, National Crime Prevention, Attorney-General's Department, Canberra.

National Food Survey Committee 1990, Household food consumption and expenditure 1989, Stationery Office, London.

National Health and Medical Research Council 2000, How to Use the Evidence: Assessment and Application of Scientific Evidence, Handbook series on preparing clinical practice guidelines, Biotext, Canberra.

National Health Information Management Group for the Australian Health Ministers' Advisory Council 1998, National Summary of the 1998 Jurisdictional Reports against the Aboriginal and Torres Strait Islander Health Performance Indicators. Australian Institute of Health and Welfare, Canberra.

National Health Strategy 1992, Enough to Make You Sick: How Income and Environment Affect Health. Research Paper No. 1, Treble Press, Melbourne.

National Occupational Health and Safety Commission 1998, Work-Related Traumatic Fatalities in Australia, 1989 to 1992, Ausinfo, Canberra.

NATSEM 2000(a), A Divide Between the Cities and the Bush? Income Distribution Report, Issue 12, May 2000. National Centre for Social and Economic Modelling, University of Canberra, Canberra.

NATSEM 2000(b), <www.theaustralian.com.au/extras/where/data/newspoll.pdf> (at 18 January 2001).

Navarro, V. 1998, Comment: whose globalization? American Journal of Public Health 88: 42–3.

Ness, A.R. & Powles, J.W. 1997, Fruit and vegetables and cardiovascular disease: a review, International Journal of Epidemiology 26: 1–13.

Netterstrom, B. & Sjol, A. 1991, Glycated haemoglobin (HbA$_{1c}$) as an indicator of job strain, Stress Medicine 7: 113–18.

Netterstrom, B., Danborg, L. & Olesen, H. 1988, Glycated hemoglobin as a measure of physiological stress, Behavioural Medicine 14: 13–16.

Neuman, W.L. 1994, Social Research Methods: Qualitative and Quantitative Approaches (2nd edition), Allyn and Bacon, Boston.

New Zealand Ministry of Health 1995, Population Based Funding 1996/97, Personal Health, DSS, Public Health. Technical Guides, Ministry of Health, Wellington.

New Zealand Ministry of Health 1998, Purchasing for Your Health, 1996/97, Performance Management Unit, Wellington.

New Zealand Ministry of Health 1999, Taking the Pulse, The 1996/97 New Zealand Health Survey, Ministry of Health, Wellington.

New Zealand Ministry of Health 2000(a), Our Health, Our Future. Haoura Pakari, Koiora Roa, Ministry of Health, Wellington.

New Zealand Ministry of Health 2000(b), The New Zealand Health Strategy, Discussion Document, Ministry of Health, Wellington.

Newman, P.W.G. & Hogan, T.L.F. 1981, A review of urban density models: towards a resolution of the conflict between populace and planner, Human Ecology, 9(3): 269–304.

Newman, P.W.G. & Kenworthy, J.R. 1989, Cities and Automobile Dependence: An International Sourcebook, Gower, Aldershot.

Newman, P.W.G. & Kenworthy, J.R. 1999, Sustainability and Cities: Overcoming Automobile Dependence, Island Press, Washington DC.

Newman, P.W.G. 1991(a), The Noxious Industry Transition, Fremantle Papers, ISTP, Murdoch University, Perth.

Newman, P.W.G. 1991(b), Social organisation for sustainability – towards a more sustainable settlement pattern, in Cock, Peter (Ed.), Social Structures for Sustainability, Centre for Resource and Environmental Studies, ANU, Canberra.

Newman, P.W.G. 2000(a) The Global City and the Parochial City, Minister for Planning's Discussion Paper Series on Future Perth, Ministry for Planning, Perth.

Newman, P.W.G. 2000(b) Democratising Transport, submitted to Transport Engineering in Australia.

Newman, P.W.G. et al. 1996, Human settlements, in Lowe, I. et al. (Eds), State of the Environment Australia, CSIRO Publications, Melbourne.

Newton, C.J., Samuel, D.L. & James, V.H.T. 1986, Aromatase activity and concentrations of cortisol, progesterone and testosterone in breast and abdominal adipose tissue, Journal of Steroid Biochemistry and Molecular Biology 24: 1033–9.

Newton, K. 1999, Social and political trust, in Norris, P. (Ed.), Critical Citizens: Global Support for Democratic Government, Oxford University Press, Oxford.

Nieman, L.K., Chrousos, G.P., Kellner, C., Spitz, I.M., Nisula, B.C., Cutler, G.B., Merriam, G.R., Bardin, C.W. & Loriaux, D.L. 1985, Successful treatment of Cushing's syndrome with the glucocorticoid antagonist RU 486, Journal of Clinical Endocrinology and Metabolism 61: 536–40.

Nocella, L. 1996, Strengthening Families Program: An Initiative of the Port Adelaide Central Mission – External Evaluation Report, June 1995–July 1996, University of South Australia, Adelaide.

North, F., Syme, S.L., Feeney, A., Head, J., Shipley, M.J. & Marmot, M.G. 1993, Explaining socioeconomic differences in sickness absence: the Whitehall II Study, British Medical Journal 306: 361–6.

Notzon, F.C., Komarov, Y.M., Ermakov, S.P., Senpos, C.T., Marks, J.S. & Senpos, E.V. 1998, Causes of declining life expectancy in Russia, Journal of the American Medical Association 279: 793–800.

NSW Health Department 2000, Healthy People 2005, New Directions for Public Health in New South Wales, NSW Health Department, Sydney.

O'Brien, C.M. Fox, C.J., Planque, B. & Casey, J. 2000, Fisheries: climate variability and North Sea cod, Nature 404: 142.

O'Connor, R.E., Jenkins, J.R. & Slocum, T.A. 1995, Transfer among phonological tasks in kindergarten: essential instructional content, Journal of Educational Psychology 87: 202–17.

O'Dea, D. 2000, The Changes in New Zealand's Income Distribution, Treasury Working Paper 00/13, New Zealand Treasury, Wellington.

O'Dea, K. & Walker, K.Z. 1995, Diet in the aetiology of diabetes, in Flatt, P.R. & Ioannides, C. (Eds), Drugs, Diet and Disease: Mechanistic Approaches to Diabetes (vol. 2), Prentice-Hall, Herts, pp. 121–52.

O'Dea, K. 1983, Lifestyle change and diabetes in Australian Aborigines, Aboriginal Health Project Information Bulletin 4: 17–21.

O'Dea, K. 1984, Marked improvement in carbohydrate and lipid metabolism in diabetic Australian Aborigines after temporary reversion to traditional lifestyle, Diabetes 33: 596–603.

Odber, J., Cawood, E.H. & Bancroft, J. 1998, Salivary cortisol in women with and without perimenstrual mood changes, Journal of Psychosomatic Research 45: 557–68.

OECD 1995, Income distribution in OECD countries, OECD, Paris.

OECD 1998, OECD environment ministers shared goals for action. Press Release SG/COM/NEWS(98)39, OECD, Paris.

Office of Population Censuses and Surveys 1978, Occupational Mortality: The Registrar General's Decennial Supplement for England and Wales (Series DS No. 1), Stationery Office, London.

Office of Population, Censuses and Statistics 1988, 1995, OPCS Monitor, Series DH3 Sudden Infant Deaths, OPCS, London.

Office of the Status of Women 1999, Women in Australia 1999, Office of the Status of Women, Canberra.

Okada, S., Hamada, H., Ishii, K., Ichiki, K., Tanokuchi, S. & Ota, Z. 1995, Factors related to stress in patients with non-insulin-dependent diabetes mellitus, Journal of International Medical Research 23: 449–57.

Oldenburg, B., McGuffog, I. & Turrell, G. 2000, Socioeconomic determinant of health in Australia: policy responses and intervention options, Medical Journal of Australia 172: 489–92.

Olds, D.L., Eckenrode, J., Henderson, C.R. Jr. et al. 1997, Long-term effects of home visitation on maternal life course, child abuse and neglect: fifteen year follow-up of a randomised controlled trial, Journal of the American Medical Association 278: 637–43.

Olds, D.L., Henderson, C.R. Jr., Kitzman, H.J., Eckenrode, J.J., Cole, R.E. & Tatelbaum, R.C. 1999, Prenatal and infancy home visitation by nurses: recent findings, The Future of Children 9: 44–64.

Olds, D.L., Henderson, C. Jr., Cole, R., Eckenrode, J., Kitzman, H., Luckey, D., Pettitt, L., Sidora, K., Morris, P. & Powers, J. 1998(a), Long term effects of nurse home visitation on children's criminal and antisocial behaviour: 15-year follow up of a randomized controlled trial, Journal of the American Medical Association 280: 1238–44.

Olds, D.L., O'Brien, R.A., Racine, D., Glazner, J. & Kitzman, H. 1998(b), Increasing the policy and program relevance of results from randomized trials of home visitation, Journal of Community Psychology 26: 85–100.

Oregon Progress Board 1999, Achieving The Oregon Shines Vision: The 1999 Benchmark Performance Report Highlights. Report to the Legislative Assembly, Oregon Progress Board, Salem, Oregon.

Ovretveit, J. 1998, Evaluating Health Interventions, Open University Press, Redwood Books, Trowbridge.

Pappas, G., Queen, S., Hadden, W. & Fisher, G. 1993, The increasing disparity in mortality between socioeconomic groups in the United States, New England Journal of Medicine 329: 103–9.

Parry, M.L., Rosenzweig, C., Iglesias, A., Fischer, G. & Livermore, M. 1999, Climate change and world food security: a new assessment, Global Environmental Change 9: s52–s67.

Pattenden, S., Dolk, H. & Vrijheid, M. 1999, Inequalities in birth weight: parental social class, area deprivation and 'lone mother' status, Journal of Epidemiology and Community Health 53: 355–8.

Pavaluri, M.N., Luk, S.-N. & McGee, R. 1996, Help-seeking for behavior problems by parents of preschool children: a community study, Journal of the American Academy of Child and Adolescent Psychiatry 35: 215–23.

Pearson, L.B. 1969, Commission on International Development, Praeger, New York,

Perry, B. 1995, Between a rock and a hard place: equivalence scales and inter-household welfare comparisons, Social Policy Journal of New Zealand 5: 42–162.

Perry, B.D., 1996, Incubated in terror: neurodevelopmental factors in the 'cycle of violence', in Ofosksy, J.D. (Ed.), Children Youth and Violence: Searching for Solutions, Guilford Press, New York.

Peto, R., Lopez, A.D., Boreham, J., Thun, M. & Heath, C., Jr. 1992, Mortality from tobacco in developed countries: indirect estimation from national vital statistics, Lancet 339: 1268–78.

Peto, R., Lopez, A.D., Boreham, J., Thun, M. J. & Heath, C., Jr. 1994, Mortality from Smoking in Developed Countries, 1950–2000: Indirect Estimates from National Vital Statistics, Oxford University Press, Oxford.

Pettigrew, M. & Macintyre, S. 2001, What Do We Know About the Effectiveness, and Cost-Effectiveness of Measures to Reduce Inequalities in Health? Paper presented to the Issues Panel on Equity in Health, Kings Fund, London, 29 January 2001, <www.ukheu.org.uk/ipehnotes>

Phillips, D.I.W., Barker, D.J.P., Fall, C.H.D., Seckl, J.R., Whorwood, C.B., Wood, P.J. & Walker, B.R. 1998, Elevated plasma cortisol concentrations: a link between low birth weight and the insulin resistance syndrome? Journal of Clinical Endocrinology and Metabolism 83: 757–60.

Pierce, J.P. & Gilpin, E.A. 2001, News media coverage of smoking and health is associated with changes in population rates of smoking cessation but not initiation, Tobacco Control 10(2): 145–53.

Pincus, T. & Callahan, L.F. 1995, What explains the association between socioeconomic status and health: primary access to medical care or mind-body variables? The Journal of Mind-Body Health 11(1): 4–35.

Pockley, P. 1999, Global warming 'could kill most coral reefs by 2100', Nature 400: 98.

Pollard, J.A., Hawkins, J.D. & Arthur, M.W. 1999, Risk and protection: are both necessary to understand diverse behavioral outcomes in adolescence? Social Work Research 23: 145–58.

Pollock, D. 1999, Denial and Delay: The Political History of Smoking and Health, 1951–1964, Action on Smoking and Health, London.

Popay, J. 2000, Social capital: the role of the narrative and historical research, Journal of Epidemiology and Community Health 54: 401–3.

Popay, J., Williams, G., Thomas, C. & Gatrell A. 1998, Theorising inequalities in health: the place of lay knowledge, in Bartley, M., Blane, D. & Davey Smith, G. (Eds).

Porter, L.S., Stone, A.A. & Schwartz, J.E. 1999, Anger expression and ambulatory blood pressure: a comparison of state and trait measures, Psychosomatic Medicine 61: 454–63.

Postel, S.L., Daily, G.C. & Ehrlich, P.R. 1996, Human appropriation of renewable fresh water, Science 271: 785–8.

Poulter, N.R., Chang, C.L., MacGregor, A.J., Snieder, H. & Spector, T.D. 1999, Association between birth weight and adult blood pressure in twins: historical cohort study, British Medical Journal 319: 1330–3.

Power, C., Matthews, S., Manor, O. 1996, Inequalities in self-rated health in the 1958 birth cohort: lifetime social circumstances or social mobility? British Medical Journal 313: 449–53.

Power, C., Rodgers, B. & Hope, S. 1999, Heavy alcohol consumption and marital status: disentangling the relationship in a national study of young adults, Addiction 94(10): 1477–87.

Powles, J. & Gifford, S. 1990, How healthy are Australia's immigrants? in Reid, J. & Trompf, P. (Eds), The Health of Immigrant Australia: A Social Perspective, Harcourt, Sydney, pp. 77–107.

Powles, J.W. & Gifford, S. 1993, Health of nations: lessons from Victoria, Australia, British Medical Journal 306: 125–7.

Powles, J.W. & Sanz, M.A. 1999. 'Arcadian bias' in discussions of the Mediterranean advantage. XV International Scientific Meeting of the International Epidemiological Association, Epidemiology for Sustainable Health. Florence, Italy, 31 August–4 September 1999, vol. II, Poster Sessions, p. 37.

Prentice, A.M. & Jebb, S.A. 1995(a), Obesity in Britain: gluttony or sloth? British Medical Journal 311: 437–9.

Prentice, A.M. & Jebb, S.A. 1995(b), Obesity in Britain: gluttony or sloth? [comment] British Medical Journal 311: 1568–9.

Preston, S.H. 1985, Resources, knowledge, and child mortality: a comparison of the US in the late nineteenth century and developing countries today, in Proceeedings of the International Population Conference, International Union for the Scientific Study of Population, Florence, pp. 373–86.

Price, T.D. & Feinman, G.M. (Eds) 1995, Foundations of Social Inequality, Plenum Publishing Corporation, New York.

Purvis, A. & Hector, A. 2000, Getting the measure of biodiversity, Nature 405: 2212–19.

Pusey, M. 1991, Economic Rationalism in Canberra: A Nation Building State Changes its Mind, Cambridge University Press, Cambridge.

Puska, P. 2000, Editorial: Do we learn our lessons from the population based interventions? Journal of Epidemiology and Community Health 54: 562–3.

Puska, P., Vartiainen, E., Tuomilehto, J., Salomaa, V. & Nissinen, A. 1998, Changes in premature deaths in Finland: successful long-term prevention of cardiovascular diseases, Bulletin of the World Health Organization 76(4): 419–25.

Putnam, R. 1993, Making Democracy Work: Civic Traditions in Modern Italy, Princeton University Press, Princeton, New Jersey.

Putnam, R. 1996, The strange disappearance of civic services, Policy, Autumn: 3–15.

Quinlan, M. 1999, The impact of labour market restructuring on occupational health and safety in industrialised societies, Economic and Industrial Democracy, 20(3): 42–60.

Quinlan, M., Mayhew, C. and Bohle P. 2001, The global expansion of precarious employment, work disorganisation and occupational health: a review of recent research, International Journal of Health Services 31(2): 33–414.

Raghuram, S. (Ed.) 2000, Health and Equity – Effecting Change, Technical report series 1.8, HIVOS, Bangalore.

Rainbow, R. & Tan, H. 1993, Meeting the Demand for Mobility, Selected Papers, Shell International, London.

Ravelli, A.C.J, van der Meulen, J.H.P., Osmond, C., Barker, D. J.P. & Bleker, O.P. 1999, Obesity at the age of 50 Y in men and women exposed to famine prenatally, American Journal of Clinical Nutrition 70(5): 811–16.

Reaven, G.M. 1998, Role of insulin resistance in human disease, Diabetes 37: 1595–1607.

Rebuffé-Scrive, M., Krotkiewski, M., Elfverson, J. & Björntorp, P. 1988, Muscle and adipose tissue morphology and metabolism in Cushing's syndrome, Journal of Clinical Endocrinology and Metabolism 67: 1122–28.

Rebuffé-Scrive, M., Lundholm, K. & Björntorp, P. 1985, Glucocorticoid hormone binding to human adipose tissue, European Journal of Clinical Investigation 15: 267–71.

Reich, R.B. 1992, The Work of Nations, Vintage Books, New York.

Reid, Elizabeth. 1997, Power, participation and partnerships for health promotion, in Labonte, R. (Ed.), Power Participation and Partnerships for Health Promotion, VicHealth, Melbourne, pp. 1–11.

Reilly, P.A. 1998, Balancing flexibility: meeting the interests of employer and employee, European Journal of Work and Organisational Psychology 7: 7–22.

Reul, J.M.H.M., Stec, I., Wiegers, G.J., Labeur, M.S., Linthorst, A.C.E., Arzt, E. & Holsboer, F. 1994, Prenatal immune challenge alters the hypothalamic-pituitary-adrenocortical axis in adult rats, Journal of Clinical Investigation 93: 2600–7.

Richardson, J., Macarounas, K., Milthorpe, F., Ryan, J. & Smith, N. 1991, An evaluation of the effect of increasing doctor numbers in their geographic distribution, NHMRC National Centre for Health Program Evaluation, Technical Report No. 2, Melbourne.

Richardson, S. 1998, Progress in the workplace, in Eckersley, R. (Ed.), pp. 210–21.

Rich-Edwards, J.W., Stampfer, M.J., Manson, J.E., Rosner, B., Hankinson, S.E., Colditz, G.A., Willett, W.C. & Hennekens, C.H. 1997, Birth weight and risk of cardiovascular disease in a cohort of women followed up since 1976, British Medical Journal 315: 396–400.

Ridley, M. 1996, The Origins of Virtue, Viking (Softback Preview edition, 1997).

Ringback-Weitoft, G., Haglund, B. & Rosen, M. 2000, Mortality among lone mothers in Sweden: a population study, Lancet 355(9211): 1215–19.

Ringen, K., Englund, A., Welch, L., Weeks, J.L. & Seegal, J.L. 1995, Why construction is different, Occupational Medicine: State of the Art Reviews 10: 255–9.

Rissel, C. 1994, Empowerment: the holy grail of health promotion, Health Promotion 9: 39–47.

Roberts, G. & Sherratt, T.N. 1998, Development of cooperative relationships through increasing investment, Nature 394: 175–9.

Robins, L. & Rutter, M. (Eds) 1990, Straight and Devious Pathways from Childhood to Adulthood, Cambridge University Press, New York.

Rockefeller Foundation 2000, The Equity Gauge: An Approach to Monitoring Equity in Health and Health Care in Developing Countries, Report of a meeting held in South Africa, August 17–20, 2000, <www.rockfound.org/display.asp?co>

Rodgers, B. 1994, Pathways between parental divorce and adult depression, Journal of Child Psychology and Psychiatry and Allied Disciplines 35: 1289–1308.

Rodgers, G.B. 1979, Income and inequality as determinants of mortality: an international cross-section analysis, Population Studies 33: 343–51.

Rose, G. & Marmot, M.G. 1981, Social class and coronary heart disease, British Heart Journal 45(1): 13–19.

Rose, R. 2000, Getting things done in an anti-modern society: social capital networks in Russia, in Dasgupta, P. & Serageldin, I. (Eds), Social Capital: A Multifaceted Perspective, World Bank, Washington DC, pp. 147–11.

Rosmond, R. & Björntorp, P. 1998(a), Blood pressure in relation to obesity, insulin and the hypothalamic-pituitary-adrenal axis in Swedish men, Journal of Hypertension 1612 (Pt 1): 1721–6.

Rosmond, R. & Björntorp, P. 1998(b), Endocrine and metabolic aberrations in men with abdominal obesity in relation to anxio-depressive infirmity, Metabolism 47: 1187–93.

Rosmond, R. & Björntorp, P. 2000, The hypothalamic-pituitary-adrenal axis activity as a predictor of cardiovascular disease, type 2 diabetes and stroke, Journal of Internal Medicine 247: 188–97.

Rosmond, R., Lapidus, L. & Björntorp, P. 1996, The influence of occupational and social factors on obesity and body fat distribution in middle-aged men, International Journal of Obesity 20: 599–607.

Ross, C.E. & Van Willigen, M. 1997, Education and the subjective quality of life, Journal of Health and Social Behavior 38 (September): 275–97.

Ross, N.A., Wolfson, M.C., Dunn, J.R., Berthelot, J.M., Kaplan, G.A. & Lynch, J.W. 2000, Relation between income inequality and mortality in Canada and in the United States: cross-sectional assessment using census data and vital statistics, British Medical Journal 320: 898–902.

Rossi, P.H. & Freeman, H.E. 1993, Evaluation: A Systematic Approach, Sage Publications, California.

Rousseau, D.M. & Libuser, C. 1997, Contingent workers in high-risk environments, California Management Review 39: 103–23.

Rowley, K., Daniel, M., Skinner, K., White, G. & O'Dea, K. 2000, Effectiveness of a community-directed 'health lifestyle' program in a remote Australian Aboriginal community, Australian and New Zealand Journal of Public Health 24: 136–44.

Royal Australian College of Opthalmologists 1980, National Trachoma and Eye Health Program of the Royal Australian College of Opthamologists, Sydney.

Royal College of Physicians 1962, Smoking and Health, Pitman Medical, London.

Royal Commission on Social Policy, New Zealand 1988, The April Report, vols I–IV, Wellington.

Rubio, M. 1997, Perverse social capital: Some evidence from Columbia, Journal of Economic Issues 31: 805–16.

Russell, G. & Bowman, L. 2000, Work and Family: Current Thinking, Research and Practice, Department of Family and Community Services, Canberra.

Rutter, M. & Smith, D.J. (Eds) 1995(a), Psychosocial Disorders in Young People: Time Trends and Their Causes, John Wiley & Sons, Chichester.

Rutter, M. & Smith, D.J. 1995(b), Towards causal explanations of time trends in psychosocial disorders of youth, in Rutter, M. & Smith, D.J. (Eds), pp. 782–808.

Rutter, M. 1979, Protective factors in children's responses to stress and disadvantage, in Kent, M.W. & Rolfe, J.E. (Eds), Primary Prevention of Psychopathology: Vol 3. Social Competence in Children, University Press of New England, Hanover, NH, pp. 49–74.

Rutter, M. 1990, Psychosocial resilience and protective mechanisms, in Rolf, J., Masten, A.S., Cichetti, D., Nuchterlein, K.N. & Weintraub, S. (Eds), Risk and Protective Factors in the Development of Psychopathology, Cambridge University Press, New York, pp. 181–214.

Rutter, M. 1998, Developmental catch-up and deficit following adoption and severe early global deprivation:

English and Romanian Adoptees (ERA) Study Team, Journal of Child Psychology and Psychiatry and Allied Disciplines 39: 465–76.

Rutter, M. 2000(a), Attachment disorder behaviour following early severe deprivation – extension and longitudinal follow-up, English and Romanian Adoptees (ERA) Study Team, Journal of the American Academy of Child and Adolescent Psychiatry 39: 703–12.

Rutter, M. 2000(b), Resilience reconsidered: conceptual considerations, empirical findings, and policy implications, in Shonkoff, J.P. & Meisels, S.J. (Eds), Handbook of Early Childhood Intervention (2nd edition), Cambridge University Press, Cambridge, pp. 651–82.

Rychetnik, L. & Frommer, M. 2000, A proposed schema for evaluating evidence on public health interventions, a discussion paper prepared for The National Public Health Partnership, NPHP, Melbourne.

Ryle, J. & Russel, W. 1949, The natural history of coronary disease: a clinical and epidemiological study, British Heart Journal 11: 370–89.

Sabha, J.S. 2000, What Globalisation Does to People's Health: Understanding what globalisation is all about and how it affects the health of the poor, South Vision, Chennai, India.

Saggers, S. & Gray, D. 1991, Aboriginal Health and Dociety: The traditional and contemporary Aboriginal struggle for better health, Allen and Unwin, North Sydney.

Saggers, S. & Gray, D. 1998, Dealing with Alcohol: Indigenous usage in Australia, New Zealand and Canada, Cambridge University Press, Cambridge.

Sainsbury, P. 1955, Suicide in London, Maudsley Monograph No. 1, Chapman Hall, London.

Salisbury, H.E. 1992, The New Emperors, Harper Collins, London.

Salmon, L. 1993, The non-profit sector and democracy: prerequisite, impediment or irrelevance, paper presented at Symposium, Democracy and the Non-profit Sector sponsored by The Aspen Institute Non-profit Research Fund, Washington, DC.

Salvaris, M., Hogan, D., Ryan, R. & Burke, T. 2000, Tasmania Together: Benchmarking community progress, Final Report, March 2000, Institute of Social Research, Swinburne University of Technology, Melbourne, and Centre for Civics and Education, University of Tasmania, Hobart.

Sampson, R.J. & Laub, J.H. 1994, Urban poverty and the family context of delinquency: a new look at structure and process in a classic study, Child Development 65: 523–40.

Sampson, R.J. 1997, Neighbourhoods and violent crime: a multilevel study of collective efficacy, Science 227: 918–24.

Samuels, S.C., Furlan, P.M., Boyce, A. & Katz, I.R. 1997, Salivary cortisol and daily events in nursing home residents, American Journal of Geriatric Psychiatry 5: 172–6.

Sapolsky, R.M. & Mott, G.E. 1987, Social subordination in wild baboons is associated with suppressed high-density lipoprotein-cholesterol concentrations: the possible role of chronic social stress, Endocrinology 121: 1605–10.

Sapolsky, R.M. 1989, Hypercortisolism among socially subordinate wild baboons originates at the CNS level, Archives of General Psychiatry 46: 1047–51.

Sapolsky, R.M. 1998, Why Zebras Don't Get Ulcers: A guide to stress, stress-related disease and coping (2nd edition), W.H. Freeman, New York.

Sapolsky, R.M., Uno, H., Rebert, C.S., & Finch, C.E. 1990, Hippocampal damage associate with prolonged glucocorticoid exposure in primates, Journal of Neuroscience 10: 2897–902.

Sarason, S. 1974, The Psychological Sense of Community: Prospects for Community Psychology, Josey-Bass, San Francisco, CA.

Saul, J.R. 1997, The Unconscious Civilization, Free Press, New York.

Saunders, P. 1996, Poverty, Income Distribution and Health: An Australian Study, Report No. 128, Reports and Proceedings, Social Policy Research Centre, University of New South Wales, Sydney.

Saunders, P. 1997, Do inequalities in income cause inequalities in health? in Crampton, P.& Howden-Chapman, P. (Eds), Socioeconomic Inequalities and Health, Proceedings of the Socioeconomic Inequalities and Health Conference, Wellington, 9–10 December 1996, Institute of Policy Studies, Wellington, pp. 9–36.

Saunders, P. 1998, Poverty and health: exploring the links between financial stress and emotional stress in Australia, Australian and New Zealand Journal of Public Health 22(1): 11–16.

Saunders, S. & Munro, D. 2000, The construction and validation of a consumer orientation questionnaire (SCOI) designed to measure Fromm's (1995) 'marketing character' in Australia, Social Behaviour and Personality 28 (3): 219–40.

Schiermeier, Q. 2001, Assessment ups the ante on climate change, Nature 409: 445.

Schlefer, J. 1998, Today's most mischievous misquotation, Atlantic Monthly 281(3): 16–19.

Schoen, C., Davis, K., DesRoches, C., Donelan, K. & Blendon, R.J. 2000, Health insurance markets and income inequality: findings from an international health policy survey, Health Policy 51: 67–85.

Schoenbach, V.J., Kaplan, B.H. et al. 1985, Social ties and mortality in Evans County Georgia, American Journal of Epidemiology 123(4): 577–91.

Schofield, D. 1997, The Distribution and Determinants of Private Health Insurance in Australia, 1990, Discussion Paper No. 17, Canberra: National Centre for Social and Economic Modelling, University of Canberra.

Schofield, D. 1999, Ancillary and specialist health services: the relationship between income, user rates and equity of access, Australian Journal of Social Issues 34(1): 79–96.

Schore, A.N. 1994, Affect Regulation and the Origin of Self: The Neurobiology of Emotional Development, Erlbaum, Hillsdale, New Jersey.

Schuck, P. 1998, Glycated hemoglobin as a physiological measure of stress and its relations to some psychological stress indicators, Behavioural Medicine 24: 89–94.

Schulkin, J., McEwen, B. & Gold, P.W. 1994, Allostasis, amygdala, and anticipatory angst, Neuroscience and Biobehavioral Reviews 18: 385–96.

Schwabb, R.G. & Anderson, I. 1998, Indigenous Participation in Health Sciences Education: Recent Trends in the Higher Rducation Dector, Centre for Aboriginal Economic Policy Research, The Australian National University, Canberra.

Schwartz, B. 2000, Self-determination: the tyranny of freedom, American Psychologist 55 (1): 79–88.

Schweinhart, L.J. & Weikart, D.P. 1997, Lasting Differences: The High/Scope Perry Preschool Curriculum Comparison Through Age 23, High Scope Press, Ypsilanti, Michigan.

Schweinhart, L.J., Barnes, H.V., Weikhart, D.P., Barnett, W.S. & Epstein, A.S. 1993, Significant benefits: the High/Scope Perry Preschool Study through age 27, Monographs of the High/Scope Educational Research Foundation Number 10, High/Scope Educational Research Foundation, Ypsilanti, Michigan.

Scott, K.G., Mason, C.A. & Chapman, D.A. 1999, The use of epidemiological methodology as a means of influencing public policy, Child Development 70: 1263–72.

Scott, M.-A. 1997, Equity in the distribution of health care in Australia, in Harris, A.H. (Ed.), Economics and Health 1996, Proceedings of the 18th Annual Conference of Health Economists, School of Health Services Management, University of New South Wales, Sydney, pp. 319–58.

Scotton, R.B. & Macdonald, C.R. 1993, The Making of Medibank, School of Health Services Management, University of NSW, Sydney.

Scott-Samuel, A. & Sihto, M. 2000, Editorial: Health inequality 2000, Critical Public Health 10(2): 105–6.

Seagert, S. & Whinkel, G. 1998, Social capital and the revitalization of New York's distressed inner city housing, Housing Policy Debate 9: 17–60.

Seeman, T.E. & McEwen, B.S. 1996, Impact of social environment characteristics on neuroendocrine regulation, Psychosomatic Medicine 58: 459–71.

Seeman, T.E. 1996, Social ties and health: the benefits of social integration, Annals of Epidemiology 6: 442–51.

Seeman, T.E., Berkman, L.F., Gulanski, B.I., Robbins, R.J., Greenspan, S.L., Charpentier, P.A. & Rowe, J.W. 1995, Self-esteem and neuroendocrine response to challenge: MacArthur studies of successful aging, Journal of Psychosomatic Research 39: 69–84.

Seeman, T.E., Bruce, M.L. & McAvay, G.J. 1996, Social network characteristics and onset of ADL disability: MacArthur studies of successful aging, Journals of Gerontology. Series B, Psychological Sciences and Social Sciences 51B:S191–S200.

Seeman, T.E., Singer, B.H., Rowe, J.W., Horwitz, R.I. & McEwen, B.S. 1997, Price of adaptation-allostatic load and its health consequences: MacArthur studies of successful aging, Archives of Internal Medicine 157: 2259–68.

Seligman, M. 1990, Why is there so much depression today? The waxing of the individual and the waning of the commons, in Ingram, R.E. (Ed.), Contemporary Psychological Approaches to Depression – Theory, research and treatment, Plenum Press, New York.

Selye, H. 1956, The Stress of Life, McGraw-Hill, New York.

Sen, A. 1999, Development As Freedom, Oxford University Press, Oxford.

Serageldin, I. 1996, Sustainability and the Wealth of Nations: First Steps in an Ongoing Journey, Environmentally sustainable development studies and monographs series no.5, The World Bank, Washington DC.

Shanahan, D. 2000, Make money and be proud: Reith, The Weekend Australian, June 17–18.

Shaw, M., Dorling, D., Gordon, D., Davey Smith, G. (Eds) 1999, The Widening Gap: Health Inequalities and Policy in Britain, The Policy Press, Bristol.

Shetty, P.S., Henry, C.J., Black, A.E. & Prentice, A.M. 1996, Energy requirements of adults: an update on basal metabolic rates (BMRs) and physical activity levels (PALs), European Journal of Clinical Nutrition 50: Suppl. 1, S11–S23.

Shindell, D.T., Rind, D. & Lonergan, P. 1998, Increased polar stratospheric ozone losses and delayed eventual recovery owing to increasing greenhouse-gas concentrations, Nature 392: 589–92.

Shinkai, S., Watanabe, S., Kurokawa, Y. & Torii, J. 1993, Salivary cortisol for monitoring circadian rhythm variation in adrenal activity during shiftwork, International Archives of Occupational and Environmental Health 64: 499–502.

Shonkoff, J. & Phillips, D. (Eds) 2000. From Neurons To Neighbourhoods: The Science Of Early Development, Committee on Integrating the Science of Early Childhood Development, Board on Children, Youth, and Families, National Academy Press, Washington DC.

Shonkoff, J.P., Phillips, D.A. & Keilty, B. (Eds) 2000, Early Childhood Intervention: Views from the Field, Report of a Workshop, Committee on Integrating the Science of Early Childhood Development, Board on Children, Youth, and Families, National Research Council, Institute of Medicine, National Academy Press, Washington.

Shouls, S., Congdon, P. & Curtis, S. 1996, Modelling inequality in reported long term illness in the UK: combining individual and area characteristics, Journal of Epidemiology and Community Health 50: 366–76.

Shutt, H. 1998, The Trouble with Capitalism: An Enquiry into the Causes of Global Economic Failure, Zed Books, London and New York.

Sigfusson, N., Sigvaldason, H., Steingrimsdottir, L., Gudmundsdottir, I.I., Stefansdottir, I., Thorsteinsson, T. & Sigurdsson, G. 1991, Decline in ischaemic heart disease in Iceland and change in risk factor levels, British Medical Journal 302(6789): 1371–5.

Sihto, M. & Keskimaki, I. 2000, Does a policy matter? Assessing the Finnish health policy in relation to its equity goals, Critical Public Health 10(2): 273–86.

Silburn, S.R., Zubrick, S.R., Garton, A., Gurrin, L., Burton, P., Dalby, R., Carlton, J. Shepherd, C. & Lawrence, D. 1996, Western Australian Child Health Survey: Family and Community Health, Australian Bureau of Statistics and the TVW Telethon Institute for Child Health Research, Perth, WA.

Simon, D., Senan, C., Garnier, P., Saint-Paul, M. & Papoz, L. 1989, Epidemiologic features of glycated hemoglobin A1c -distribution in a healthy population: The Telecom study, Diabetologia 32: 864–9.

Simon, J.L. & Kahn, H. 1984, The Resourceful Earth, Blackwell, Oxford, UK.

Singer, M. 1989, Passage to a Human World: The Dynamics of Creating Global Wealth, Transaction Publishers, New Brunswick, USA.

Singh, R.B., Sharma, J.P., Rastogi, V., Niaz, M.A., Ghosh, S., Beegom, R. & Janus, E.D. 1997, Social class and coronary disease in rural population of north India: The Indian Social Class and Heart Survey, European Heart Journal 18(4): 588–95.

Smaglik, P. 2000, Climate change expert stirs new controversy, Nature 407: 7.

Smeed, R.J. 1972, The usefulness of formulae in traffic engineering and road safety, Accident Analysis and Prevention 4: 303–12.

Smeeding, T.M. & Gottschalk, P. 1999, Cross national income inequality: how great is it and what can we learn from it? International Journal of Health Services 29(4): 733–41.

Smith, A. 1776 (1979), An Inquiry into the Nature and Causes of the Wealth of Nations, Clarendon Press, Oxford.

Smith, D., Taylor, R., Coates, M. 1996, Socio-economic differentials in cancer incidence and mortality in NSW, Australian and New Zealand Journal of Public Health 20(2): 129–37.

Smith, D.J. & Rutter, M. 1995, Time trends in psychosocial disorders of youth, in Rutter, M. & Smith, D.J. (Eds), pp. 763–81.

Smith, P.J., Moffatt, M.E.K., Gelskey, S.C., Hudson, S. & Kaita, K. 1997, Are community health interventions evaluated appropriately? A review of six journals, Journal of Clinical Epidemiology, 50(2): 137–46.

Smith, T. 1997, Factors relating to misanthropy in contemporary American society, Social Science Research 26: 170–96.

Smyth, J., Ockenfels, M.C., Porter, L., Kirschbaum, C., Hellhammer, D.H. & Stone, A.A. 1998, Stressors and mood measured on a momentary basis are associated with salivary cortisol secretion, Psychoneuroendocrinology 23: 353–70.

Snow, C.E., Burns, M.S. & Griffin, P. 1999, Preventing Reading Difficulties in Young Children, National Academy Press, Washington, DC.

Soobader, M-J & LeClere, F.B. 1999, Aggregation and the measurement of income inequality: effects on morbidity, Social Science & Medicine 48: 733–44.

South Western Sydney Area Health Service, 2000, Health Outcomes Resource Unit Data, Sydney.

Spitz, R. 1965, The First Year of Life, International Universities Press, New York.

Spurgeon, A., Harrington, J.M. & Cooper, C.L. 1997, Health and safety problems associated with long working hours: a review of the current position, Occupational and Environmental Medicine 54: 367–75.

Sroufe, L.A. 1995, Emotional Development: The Organisation of Emotional Life in the Early Years, Cambridge University Press, London.

Sroufe, L.A. 1997, Psychopathology as an outcome of development, Development and Psychopathology 9: 251–68.

Stallone, D.D., Brunner, E.J., Bingham, S.A. & Marmot, M.G. 1997, Dietary assessment in Whitehall II: the influence of reporting bias on apparent socioeconomic variation in nutrient intakes, European Journal of Clinical Nutrition 51: 815–25.

Stamp, K., Duckett, S. & Fisher, D. 1998, Hospital use for potentially preventable conditions in Aboriginal and Torres Strait Islander and other Australian populations, Australian and New Zealand Journal of Public Health 22: 673–8.

Stanistreet, D., Scott-Samuel, A., Bellis, M.A. 1999, Income inequality and mortality in England, Journal of Public Health Medicine 21(2): 205–7.

Stansfeld, S.A., Head, J. & Marmot, M.G. 1998, Explaining social class differences in depression and well-being, Social Psychiatry and Psychiatric Epidemiology 33: 1–9.

Stansfeld, S.A., North, F.M., White, I. & Marmot, M.G. 1995, Work characteristics and psychiatric disorder in civil servants in London, Journal of Epidemiology and Community Health 49: 48–53.

Statistics New Zealand 1990, The Fiscal Impact on Income Distribution 1987/88, Statistics New Zealand, Wellington.

Statistics New Zealand 1998, The New Zealand Official Yearbook 1998, Statistics New Zealand, Wellington.

Statistics New Zealand 1999, New Zealand Now.Incomes, Statistics New Zealand, Wellington.

Statistics New Zealand 2000(a), Labour Market Statistics 1999, Statistics New Zealand, Wellington.

Statistics New Zealand 2000(b), New Zealand Yearbook 2000, Statistics New Zealand, Wellington.

Steckel, R.H. 1995, Stature and the standard of living, Journal of the Economic Literature 33: 1903–40.

Stefanski, V. 1998, Social stress in loser rats: opposite immunological effects in submissive and subdominant males, Physiology and Behavior 63: 605–13.

Steiner, C. 1997, Achieving Emotional Literacy, Bloomsbury Publishing, London.

Steketee, M. & Haslem, B. 2000, Wealth divide to widen, The Australian, June 19.

Stephens, B. & Waldegrave, C. 1996, Measuring poverty in New Zealand, in Crampton, P. & Howden-Chapman, P. (Eds), Social Inequalities and Health, Proceedings of the Socioeconomic Inequalities and Health Conference, 9–10 December 1996, Wellington, pp. 105–20.

Sterling, P. & Eyer, I. 1988, Allostasis: A new paradigm to explain arousal pathology, in Fisher, S. & Reason, J. (Eds), Handbook of Life Stress, Cognition and Health, John Wiley & Son, London, pp. 629–49.

Stewart-Weeks, M. 2000, Trick or treat? Social capital, leadership and the new public policy, in Winter, I. (Ed.), Australian Institute for Family Studies, Melbourne.

Stolle, D. & Rochon, T. 1998, Are all associations alike? Members diversity, associational type and the creation of social capital, American Behavioural Scientist 42: 41–65.

Street, A. & Duckett, S. 1996, Are waiting lists inevitable? Health Policy 36: 1–15.

Strickland, P., Morris, R., Wearden, A. & Deakin, B. 1998, A comparison of salivary cortisol in chronic fatigue syndrome, community depression and healthy controls, Journal of Affective Research 471: 191–4.

Strickland, S. & Shetty, P. (Eds) 1998, Human Biology and Social Inequality, Society for the Study of Human Biology, Symposium 39, Cambridge University Press, Cambridge.

Stronks, K., Dike van de Mheen, H., Looman, C.W.N. & Mackenbach, J.P. 1997, Cultural, material, and psychosocial correlates of the socioeconomic gradient in smoking behavior among adults, Preventative Medicine 265 (Pt 1): 754–66.

Stronks, K., van de Mheen, H.D., Looman, C.W.N. & Mackenbach, J.P. 1996, Behavioural and structural factors in the explanation of socioeconomic inequalities in health: an empirical analysis, Sociology of Health and Illness 18(5): 653–74.

Sugden, R. 1993, Welfare, resources and capabilities: a review of Inequality Reexamined by Amartya Sen, Journal of Economic Literature 31: 1947–62.

Summers, R. & Heston, A. 1991, The Penn World Table (Mark 5): An expanded set of international comparisons, 1950–1988, Quarterly Journal of Economics 106: 327–68.

Susser, M. 1995, The tribulations of trials – intervention in communities, Editorial, American Journal of Health Promotion 85(2): 156–60.

Susser, M. 1998, Does risk factor epidemiology put epidemiology at risk? Peering into the future, Journal of Epidemiology and Community Health 52: 612–13.

Sverke, M., Gallagher, D.G. & Hellgren, J. 2000, Alternative work arrangement: job stress, well-being and work attitudes among employees with different employment contracts, in Isaksson, K., Hogstedt, C., Eriksson, C. & Theorell, T. (Eds), pp. 145–67.

Swales, J. 2000, Inequalities: A challenge to science and politics, New Zealand Medical Journal, 11: 324–5.

Swidler, A. 1986, Culture in action: symbols and strategies, American Sociological Review 51: 273–86.

Sylva, K. & Colman, P. 1998, Preschool intervention to prevent behaviour problems and school failure, in Buchanan, A. & Hudson, B.L. (Eds), Parenting, Schooling and Children's Behaviour, Ashgate, Sydney, pp. 178–91.

Syme, S.L, 1996(a), Rethinking disease: Where do we go from here? Annals of Epidemiology 6: 464–8.

Syme, S.L. & Berkman, L.F. 1976, Social class, susceptibility and sickness, American Journal of Epidemiology, 104(1): 1–8.

Syme, S.L. 1996(b), To prevent disease: the need for a new approach, in Blane, D., Brunner, E. & Wilkinson, R. (Eds), pp. 21–31.

Syme, S.L. 1998, Social and economic disparities in health: thoughts about intervention, The Milbank Quarterly 76(3): 493–505.

Szreter, S. 1988, The importance of social intervention in Britain's mortality decline c.1850–1914: a reinterpretation of the role of public health, Journal of the Society for the Social History of Medicine 1: 1–37.

Szreter, S. 1997, Economic growth, disruption, deprivation, disease and death: on the importance of the politics of public health, Population and Development Review 23: 693–728.

Szreter, S. 1999, Rapid economic growth and 'the four Ds' of disruption, deprivation, disease and death: public health lessons from nineteenth century Britain for twenty-first century China? Tropical Medicine and International Health 4: 146–52.

Szwarcwald, C.L., Bastos, F.I., Viacava, F. & de Andrade, C.L.T. 1999, Income inequality and homicide rates in Rio de Janeiro, Brazil, American Journal of Public Health 89: 845–50.

Tanne, J.H. 1998, Biodiversity loss threatens new treatments, British Medical Journal 316: 1261.

Tarlov, A.R., 1999, Public policy grameworks for improving population health, in Adler, N.E., Marmot, M., McEwen, B.S. & Stewart, J. (Eds).

Taylor, C. & Jolly, R. 1988. The straw men of primary health care, Social Science & Medicine 26: 971–7.

Taylor, R., Chey, T., Bauman, A. & Webster, I. 1999, Socio-economic, migrant and geographic differentials in coronary artery disease in NSW, Australian and New Zealand Journal of Public Health 23(1): 20–6.

Taylor, R., Morrell, S., Slaytor, E. & Ford, P. 1998, Suicide in urban New South Wales, Australia 1985–1994: socio-economic and migrant interactions, Social Science & Medicine 47(11): 1677–86.

Taylor, R., Quine, S., Lyle, D. & Bilton, A. 1992, Socioeconomic correlates of mortality and hospital morbidity differentials by local government area in Sydney 1985–88, Australian Journal of Public Health 16(3): 305–14.

Taylor, S.E. & Repetti, R.L. 1997, Health Psychology: what is an unhealthy environment and how does it get under the skin? Annual Review of Psychology 48: 411–47.

Taylor, S.E. & Seeman, T.E. 1999, Psychosocial resources and the SES–health relationship, in Adler, N.E., Marmot, M., McEwen, B.S. & Stewart, J. (Eds), pp. 210–25.

Taylor, V. 1999, Informing Strategic Directions for Food and Nutrition in Aboriginal and Torres Strait Islander Populations, Discussion Paper, Office for Aboriginal and Torres Strait Islander Health, Commonwealth Department of Health and Aged Care, Canberra.

Temkin, K. & Rohe, W. 1998, Social capital and neighbourhood stability: an empirical investigation, Housing Policy Debate 9: 61–88.

Theorell, T., Haggmark, C. & Kallner, A. 1988, Elevation of glycosylated hemoglobin in a severe crisis situation – cancer in a close relative, Behavioural Medicine 14: 125–8.

Thiel, C., Minh Thai, D. & Heinemann, L. 1994, Vitaminaufnahme vor und nach der Wende in Ostdeutschland, Vitaminspur 9: 32–4.

Tidey, J.W. & Miczek, K.A. 1996, Social defeat stress selectively alters mesocorticolimbic dopamine release: an in vivo microdialysis study, Brain Research 7211: 140–9.

Tominaga, S. & Kuroishi, T. 1997, An ecological study on diet/nutrition and cancer in Japan, International Journal of Cancer Suppl.: 102–6.

Tomison, A. 2000, Evaluating Child Abuse Prevention Programs, Issues in Child Abuse prevention, National Clearinghouse Issues Paper No. 12, National Child Protection Clearinghouse, Melbourne.

Tomison, A.M. & Wise, S. 1999, Community-based Approaches in Preventing Child Maltreatment, National Child Protection Clearinghouse Issues Paper 11, pp. 1–19.

Tones, K. 1992, Health promotion, self-empowerment and the concept of control, in Colquhoun, D., (Ed.), Health Education: Politics and Practice, Deakin University, Geelong, Victoria.

Toohey, B. 1994, Tumbling Dice: The Story of Modern Economic Policy, William Heinemann Australia, Melbourne.

Totaro, P. & Brown, M. 2000, Greed: It's an epidemic, Sydney Morning Herald, April 22.

Toumborou, J.W. 1999, Implementing Communities that Care in Australia: A community mobilisation approach to crime prevention, Trends and Issues in Crime and Criminal Justice No. 122, Australian Institute of Criminology, Canberra.

Townsend, P. & Davidson, N. (Eds) 1982, Inequalities in Health: The Black Report, Penguin, London.

Townsend, P. 1993, The International Analysis of Poverty, HarvEster Wheatsheaf, Hemel Hempstead, UK.

Tremblay R, 1999, When children's social development fails, in Keating, D. & Hertzman, C. (Eds), pp. 55–71.

Tremblay, R., Kurtz, L., Masse, L.C., Vitaro, F., & Phil, R.O. 1995, A bimodal preventive intervention for disruptive kindergarten boys: its impact through mid-adolescence, Journal of Consulting and Clinical Psychology 63: 560–8.

Tremblay, R., Pihl, R., Vitaro, F. & Dobkin, P. 1994, Predicting early onset of male antisocial behaviour from preschool behaviour, Archives of General Psychiatry 51: 732–9.

Troy, P. 1996, The Perils of Urban Consolidation, The Federation Press, Sydney.

Tunstall-Pedoe, H., Vanuzzo, D., Hobbs, M., Mahonen, M., Cepaitis, Z., Kuulasmaa, K. & Keil, U. 2000, Estimation of contribution of changes in coronary care to improving survival, event rates, and coronary heart disease mortality across the WHO MONICA Project populations, Lancet 355: 688–700.

Turrell, G. & Mathers, C. 2000, Socioeconomic status and health in Australia, Medical Journal of Australia 172: 434–8.

Turrell, G. & Mathers, C. 2001, Socioeconomic inequalities in all-cause and specific-cause mortality in Australia: 1985–1987 and 1995–1997, International Journal of Epidemiology 30: 231–9.

Turrell, G. 2000, Income non-response: implications for health inequalities research, Journal of Epidemiology and Community Health 54: 207–14.

Turrell, G., Oldenburg, B., McGuffog, I. & Dent, R. 1999, Socio-economic Determinants of Health: Towards a National Research Program and a Policy and Intervention Agenda, Queensland University of Technology, School of Public Health, Ausinfo, Canberra.

Twenge, J.M. 2000, The age of anxiety? Birth cohort change in anxiety and neuroticism, 1952–1993, Journal of Personality and Social Psychology 79(6): 1007–21.

UK Office for National Statistics 1998, Health Inequalities, Decennial Supplement.

UNICEF 2000, A league table of Child Poverty in Rich Nations, Innocenti Report Card Issue Number 1, United Nations Children's Fund, Innocenti Research Centre, Florence.

Union of Concerned Scientists 1992, World Scientists' Warning to Humanity, Union of Concerned Scientists, Cambridge, Mass. <www.ucsusa.org/about/warning.html> (last visited 14.01.01).

United Nations 1995, The Copenhagen Declaration and Programme of Action: World Summit for Social Development, 6–12 March 1995, United Nations Department of Publications, New York.

United Nations Development Program (UNDP) 1999, Human Development Report 1999, Oxford University Press, New York.

United Nations Environment Programme 1998, Environmental Effects of Ozone Depletion 1998 Assessment, Elsevier, Lausanne.

United Nations Population Division 1998, World Population Prospects: The 1998 Revision, The Demographic Impact of HIV/AIDS, Department of Economic and Social Affairs, United Nations, New York.

United Nations Research Institute for Social Development. 1995, States of Disarray: The Social Effects of Globalisation, UNRISD, London.

Uno, H., Tarara, R., Else, J.G., Suleman, M.A, & Sapolsky, R.M. 1989, Hippocampal damage associated with prolonged and fatal stress in primates, Journal of Neuroscience 9: 1705–11.

US Department of Health and Human Services, Office of Disease Prevention and Health Promotion. 2000, Healthy People 2010: Understanding and Improving Health (2nd edition), US Government Printing Office, Pittsburg, PA.

US Surgeon General 1964, Smoking and Health: Report of the Advisory Committee to the Surgeon General of the Public Health Service, US Department of Health, Education and Welfare, Washington.

Vague, J., Boyer, J., Jubelin, J., Nicolino, C. & Pinto, C. 1969, Adipomuscular ratio in human subjects, in Vague, J. & Denton, R.M. (Eds), Physiopathology of Adipose Tissue, Excerpta Medica, Amsterdam, pp. 360–86.

van Beeck, E.F., Borsboom, G.J.J. & Mackenbach, J.P. 2000, Economic development and traffic accident mortality in the industrialised world, International Journal of Epidemiology 29: 503–9.

Van den Boom, D.C. 1994, The influence of temperament and mothering on attachment and exploration: an experimental manipulation of sensitive responsiveness among lower-class mothers with irritable infants, Child Development 65: 1449–69.

van der Meer, J.B.W. & Mackenbach, J.P. 1998, Course of health status among chronically ill persons: differentials according to level of education, Journal of Clinical Epidemiology 51: 171–9.

van Eck, M., Berkhof, H., Nicolson, N. & Sulon, J. 1996, The effects of perceived stress, traits, mood states, and stressful daily events on salivary cortisol, Psychosomatic Medicine 58: 447–58.

Van Ijzendoorn, M.H., Goldberg, S., Kroonenberg, P.M. & Frenkel, O.J. 1992, The relative effects of maternal and child problems on the quality of attachment: a metaanalysis of attachment in clinical samples, Child Development 59: 147–56.

Van Loon, A., Brug, J., Goldbohm, R., van den Brandt, P. & Brug, J. 1995, Differences in cancer incidence and mortality among socio-economic groups, Scandinavian Journal of Social Medicine 23(2): 110–20.

van Rossum, C.T.M., Shipley, M.J., van de Mheen, H., Grobbee, D.E. & Marmot, M.G. 2000, Employment grade differences in cause specific mortality: A 25 year follow up of civil servants from the first Whitehall study, Journal of Epidemiology and Community Health 54: 178–84.

Vanier Institute of the Family, 1998, From the Kitchen Table to the Board Room Table, Vanier Institute, Ottawa.

Vartiainen, E., Puska, P., Pekkanen, J., Tuomilehto, J. & Jousilahti, P. 1994, Changes in risk factors explain changes in mortality from ischaemic heart disease in Finland, British Medical Journal 309(6946): 23–7.

Veenhoven, R. 1999, Quality of life in individualistic society, Social Indicators Research 48: 157–86.

Veenhoven, R. 2000, Well-being in the welfare state: level not higher, distribution not more equitable, Journal of Comparative Policy Analaysis 2: 91–125.

Veizer, J., Godderis, Y., François, L.M. 2000, Evidence for decoupling of atmospheric CO_2 and global climate during the Phanerozoic eon, Nature 408: 698–701.

VicRoads (multiple years). Road Traffic Accidents Involving Serious Casualties, VicRoads, Melbourne.

Vinson, T. & Homel, R. 1975, Crime and disadvantage: the coincidence of medical and social problems in an Australian city, The British Journal of Criminology 15: 21–31.

Vinson, T. 1999, Unequal in Life: The Distribution of Social Disadvantage in Victoria and New South Wales, Jesuit Social Services, Melbourne.

Virgin, C.E.J. & Sapolsky, R.M. 1997, Styles of male social behavior and their endocrine correlates among low-ranking baboons, American Journal of Primatology 42: 25–39.

Vitousek, P.M., Ehrlich, P.R., Ehrlich, A.H. & Mateson, P.A. 1986, Human appropriation of the products of photosynthesis, Bioscience 34: 368–73.

Vitousek, P.M., Mooney, H.A., Lubchenko, J. & Melillo, J.M. 1997, Human domination of the Earth's ecosystems, Science 277: 494–9.

Waaler, H.T. 1984, Height, weight and mortality: the Norwegian experience, Acta Medica Scandinavica Supplement: 679.

Wagstaff, A. & van Doorslaer, E. 2000. Income inequality and health: what does the literature tell us? Annual Review of Public Health 21: 543–567.

Wagstaff, A., E. van Doorslaer, E, van der Burg, E.H., Calonge, S., Christiansen, T., Citoni, G., Gerdtham, U.G, Gerfin, M., Gross, L., Hakinne, U., John, P., Johnson, P., Klavus, J., Lachaud, C., Lauritsen, J., Leu, R., Nolan, B., Peran, E., Pereira, J., Propper, C., Puffer, F., Rochaix, L., Rodriguez, M., Schellhorn, M., Sundberg, G. & Winkelhake, O. (1999). Equity in the finance of health care: Some further international comparisons, Health Economics 19: 263–90.

Waitzman, N.J. & Smith, K.R. 1998, Separate but lethal: the effects of economic segregation on mortality in metropolitan areas, The Milbank Quarterly 76(3): 341–73.

Waldmann, R.J. 1992, Income distribution and infant mortality, Quarterly Journal of Economics 107: 1283–302.

Waldon, S., Young, L., Harris, E. 1998, Household Survey Report, Centre for Health Equity Training Research & Evaluation, Sydney.

Wallerstein, N. 1992, Powerlessness, empowerment and health: implications for health promotion programs, American Journal of Health Promotion 6: 197–205.

Walsh, P. & Brosnan, P. 1999, Re-designing industrial relations: the Employment Contracts Act and its consequences, in Walsh, P. & Brosnan, P. (Eds), Re–designing the Welfare State in New Zealand: Problems, Policies and Prospects, Oxford University Press, Auckland, pp. 117–35.

Walt, G. 1998, Health Policy: An introduction to process and power, Witwatersrand University Press, Johannesburg.

Wareham, N.J., Wong, M.Y. & Day, N.E. 2000, Glucose intolerance and physical inactivity: the relative importance of low habitual energy expenditure and cardiorespiratory fitness, American Journal of Epidemiology 152: 132–9.

Wasserman, G.A. & Miller, L.S. 1998, The prevention of serious and violent juvenile offending, in Loeber, R & Farrington, D.P. (Eds), Serious and Violent Juvenile Offenders, Sage, London, pp. 197–247.

Waters, A.-M. & Bennett, S. 1995, Risk Factors for Cardiovascular Disease: A Summary of Australian Data, Cardiovascular Disease Series No.1, Australian Institute of Health and Welfare (AIHW) and the University of Newcastle, Australia, AIHW, Canberra.

Watson, C. 2000, Social Anxiety and Health, Public Health Association Conference, Inequality as a Health Hazard, Perth.

Wearing, A. & Headey, B. 1998, Who enjoys life and why: measuring subjective well-being, in Eckersley, R. (Ed.), pp. 169–82.

Wedekind, C. & Milinski, M. 2000, Cooperation through image scoring in humans, Science 288: 850–2.

Weikart, D. & Schweinhart, L. 1992, High/Scope preschool program outcomes, in McCord, J. & Tremblay, R. (Eds), Preventing Antisocial Behaviour: Interventions From Birth Through Adolescence, Guilford, New York, pp. 67–86.

Welsh, B.C. & Farrington, D.P. 1999, Delinquency prevention using family-based interventions, Children and Society 13(4): 287–303.

Wennemo, I. 1993, Infant mortality, public policy and inequality – a comparison of 18 industrialised countries, 1950–85, Sociology of Health and Illness 15(4): 429–46.

Went, R. 2000, Globalisation: Neoliberal Challenge, Radical Responses, Pluto Press with International Institute for Research and Education, London.

Werner, D. & Sanders, D. 1997, Questioning the Solution: The Politics of Primary Health Care and Child Survival, HealthWrights, Palo Alto, CA.

Werner, E.E. 1987, Vulnerability and resiliency in children at risk for delinquency: a longitudinal study from birth to adulthood, in Burchard, J.D. & Burchard, S.N. (Eds), Primary Prevention of Psychopathology: Vol 10. Prevention of Delinquent Behavior. Sage, Newbury Park, CA, pp. 16–43.

Western, J.S. 1983, Social Inequality in Australian Society, Macmillan, Melbourne.

Whalley, L.J. & Deary, I.J. 2001, Longitudinal cohort study of childhood IQ and survival up to age 76, British Medical Journal 322(7290): 819.

White, M. 1997, Comment, Lancet 350(9073): 231–2.

White, S. 1996, Russia Goes Dry: Alcohol, State and Society, Cambridge University Press, Cambridge.

Whitehead, M. 1990, The Concepts and Principles of Equity and Health, World Health Organization, Copenhagen.

Whitehead, M. 1995, Tackling inequalities: a review of policy initiatives, in Benzeval, M., Judge, K. & Whitehead, M. (Eds), Tackling Inequalities in Health: An Agenda for Action, King's Fund Publishing, London, pp. 22–52.

Whitehurst, G.J., Arnold, D.S., Epstein, J.N., Angell, A.L., Smith, M. & Fischel, J.E. 1994, A picture book reading intervention in day care and home for children from low-income families, Developmental Psychology 30: 679–89.

WHO (World Health Organization) – see under World Health Organization (WHO).

Wiggers, J.H. & Sanson-Fisher, R. 1997, Duration of general practice consultations: Association with patient occupational and educational status, Social Science & Medicine 44(7): 925–34.

Wikström, P. & Loeber, R. 1999, Do disadvantaged neighborhoods cause well-adjusted children to become adolescent delinquents? A study of male juvenile serious offending, individual risk and protective factors, and neighborhood context, Unpublished paper, Institute of Criminology, University of Cambridge.

Wilkinson, R.G. & Marmot, M. 1998, The Solid Facts, WHO, WHO Regional Office for Europe.

Wilkinson, R.G. 1986, Income and mortality, in Wilkinson, R.G. (Ed.), Class and Health: Research and Longitudinal Data, Tavistock, London.

Wilkinson, R.G. 1989, Class mortality differentials, income distribution and trends in poverty 1921–1981, Journal of Social Policy 18: 307–35.

Wilkinson, R.G. 1990, Income distribution and mortality: a 'natural' experiment, Sociology of Health and Illness 12(4): 391–412.

Wilkinson, R.G. 1992(a), Income distribution and life expectancy, British Medical Journal 304: 165–68.

Wilkinson, R.G. 1992(b), National Mortality Rates: The impact of inequality? American Journal of Public Health 82(8): 1082–4.

Wilkinson, R.G. 1994(a), The epidemiological transition: from material scarcity to social disadvantage? Daedalus 123(4): 61–77.

Wilkinson, R.G. 1994(b), Health, redistribution and growth, in Glyn, A. & Miliband, D. (Eds), Paying for Inequality: The Economic Cost of Social Injustice, Rivers Oram Press, London.

Wilkinson, R.G. 1995, Commentary: A reply to Ken Judge: mistaken criticisms ignore overwhelming evidence, British Medical Journal 311: 1285–7.

Wilkinson, R.G. 1996(a), Unhealthy Societies: The Afflictions of Inequality, Routledge, London.

Wilkinson, R.G. 1996(b), How can secular improvements in life expectancy be explained? In Blane, D., Brunner, E. & Wilkinson, R. (Eds), pp. 109–24.

Wilkinson, R.G. 1997(a), Comment: Income, inequality, and social cohesion, American Journal of Public Health 87(9): 1504–6.

Wilkinson, R.G. 1997, Commentary: Income inequality summarises the health burden of individual relative deprivation, British Medical Journal 314: 1727–8.

Wilkinson, R.G. 1997(b), Health inequalities: relative or absolute material standards? British Medical Journal 314: 591–5.

Wilkinson, R.G. 1998(a), Equity, social cohesion and health, in Strickland, S. & Shetty, P. (Eds), pp. 58–75.

Wilkinson, R.G. 1998(b), Letter to the Editor, Social Science & Medicine 47(3): 411–12.

Wilkinson, R.G. 1999(a), Putting the picture together: prosperity, redistribution, health, and welfare, in Marmot, M. & Wilkinson, R.G. (Eds), pp. 256–74.

Wilkinson, R.G. 1999(b), Income inequality, social cohesion, and health: clarifying the theory – a reply to Muntaner and Lynch, International Journal of Health Services 29(3): 525–43.

Wilkinson, R.G. 1999(c), The culture of inequality, in Kawachi, I., Kennedy, B.P., & Wilkinson, R.G., (Eds), Income Inequality and Health: The Society and Population Health Reader vol.1, The New Press, New York.

Wilkinson, R.G. 2000, Inequality and the social environment: a reply to Lynch et al., Journal of Epidemiology and Community Health 54: 411–13.

Wilkinson, R.G., Kawachi, I. & Kennedy, B.P. 1998, Mortality, the social environment, crime and violence, Sociology of Health and Illness 20(5): 578–97.

Willcox, S. 1991, A Healthy Risk? Use of Private Insurance, Background Paper No. 4, National Health Strategy.

Williams, D. 1997, Race and health: basic questions, emerging directions, Annals of Epidemiology 7: 322–33.

Williams, D., Lavizzo-Mourey, R. & Warren, R. 1994, The concept of race and health status in America, Public Health Reports 109(1): 26–43.

Williams, N. 1998, Overfishing disrupts entire ecosystems, Science 279: 809.

Wilson, M. & Daly, M. 1997, Life expectancy, economic inequality, homicide, and reproductive timing in Chicago neighbourhoods, British Medical Journal 314: 1271–4.

Winkelby, M.A. 1994, The future of community-based cardiovascular disease intervention studies, American Journal of Public Health 84(9): 1369–72.

Winkleby, M.A., Barr Taylor, C., Jatulis, D. & Fortmann, S.P. 1996, The long-term effects of a cardiovascular disease prevention trial: the Stanford five-city project, American Journal of Public Health 86(12): 1773–9.

Wisner, B. 1988, GOBI Versus PHC? Some dangers of selective primary health care, Social Science & Medicine 26: 963–9.

Wolcott, I. & Glezer, H. 1995, Work and Family Life: Achieving Integration, Australian Institute of Family Studies, Melbourne.

Wolfson, M., Kaplan, G., Lynch, J., Ross, N. & Backlund, E. 1999, Relationship between income inequality and mortality: empirical demonstration, British Medical Journal 319: 953–5.

Wooden, M., Holton, R., Hugo, G. & Sloan, J. 1994, Australian Immigration: A Survey of the Issues, Australian Government Publishing Service, Canberra.

Woodward, A. & Kawachi, I. 1998, Why should we reduce health inequalities? Background Paper 2 for National Health Committee, National Advisory Committee on Health and Disability, Wellington.

World Bank 1993, Investing in Health: World Development Report 1993, Oxford University Press for the World Bank, Oxford.

World Bank 1997(a), The State in a Changing World: World Development Report 1997, Oxford University Press for the World Bank, Oxford.

World Bank 1997(b), Expanding the Measure of Wealth: Indicators of Environmentally Sustainable Development, The World Bank, Washington DC.

World Bank 1999(a), Entering the 21st Century: World Development Report 1999/2000, Oxford University Press, for the World Bank, Oxford.

World Bank 1999(b), 1999 World Development Indicators, World Bank, Washington DC.

World Bank 2000(a), Attacking Poverty: World Development Report 2000/2001, The World Bank, Washington.

World Bank 2000(b), Voices of the Poor, World Bank, Geneva.

World Health Organization (WHO) 1986(a), The role of intersectorial collaboration in national strategies for Health For All, Health Promotion 1(2): 239–51.

World Health Organization (WHO) 1986(b), The Ottawa Charter for Health Promotion, Health Promotion International 1(4): i–v.

World Health Organization (WHO) 1998, Taskforce on Equity: Strategies to Promote Equity in Health and Health Care, Discussion paper, World Health Organization.

World Health Organization (WHO) 1999, World Health Report 1999: Making a Difference, World Health Organization, Geneva.

World Health Organization (WHO) 2000, Bulletin of the World Health Organization, Special Theme – Inequalities in Health, Vol. 78(1).

Wright, B.R.E., Caspi, A., Moffitt, T.E. & Silva, P.A. 1999, Low self control, social bonds and crime: social causation, social selection, or both? Criminology 37(3): 479–514.

Wrigley, E.A., Davies, R.S., Oeppen, J.E. & Schofield, R.S. 1997, English Population History from Family Reconstitution 1580–1837, Cambridge University Press, Cambridge.

Wulsin, L.R., Vaillant, G.E. & Wells, V.E. 1999, A systematic review of the mortality of depression, Psychosomatic Medicine 61: 6–17.

Xu, L.C. & Zou, H. 2000, Explaining the changes of income distribution in China, China Economic Review 11: 149–70.

Yen, I.H. & Kaplan, G.A. 1999, Neighborhood social environment and risk of death: multilevel evidence from the Alameda County Study, American Journal of Epidemiology 149(10): 898–907.

Yen, I.H. & Syme, S.L. 1999, The social environment and health: a discussion of the epidemiologic literature, Annual Review of Public Health 20: 287–308.

Yoshikawa, H. 1994, Prevention as cumulative protection: effects of early family support and education on chronic delinquency and its risks, Psychological Bulletin 115: 28–54.

Young, J.B. & Morrison, S.F. 1998, Effects of fetal and neonatal environment on sympathetic nervous system development, Diabetes Care, 21 (Suppl. 2): B156–60.

Young, M. & Willmott, P. 1962, Family and Kinship in East London, Penguin Books, Harmondsworth.

Youniss, J., McLellan & Yates, M. 1997, What we know about engendering civic identity, American Behavioural Scientist 40: 620–31.

Yudkin, J.S., Forrest, R.D., Jackson, C.A., Ryle, A.J., Davie, S. & Gould, B.J. 1990, Unexplained variability of glycated haemoglobin in nondiabetic subjects not related to glycaemia, Diabetologia 33: 208–15.

Zatonski, W.A., McMichael, A.J. & Powles, J.W. 1998, Ecological study of reasons for sharp decline in mortality from ischaemic heart disease in Poland since 1991, British Medical Journal 316 (7137): 1047–51.

Zika, S. & Chamberlain, K. 1992, On the relation between meaning in life and psychological well-being, British Journal of Psychology 83: 133–45.

Zimmerman, M.A. 1990, Taking aim on empowerment research: on the distinction between individual and psychological conceptions, American Journal of Community Psychology 18: 169–77.

Zubrick, S., Silburn, S., Vimpani, G. & Williams, A. 1999, Emergent demand for measurement indicators of social and family functioning, in Report of a National Workshop on Indicators of Social and Family Functioning, 12–12 April 1999, Commonwealth Department of Family and Community Services, Canberra, pp. 11–38.

Index

Page references followed by *fig* indicate figures; those
followed by *tab* indicate tables

Aboriginal health, 118–20
   diabetes, 214
   expenditure on, 155
   extent of disadvantage, 118tab, 247
   governmental policy and interventions, 248,
      250–4
   housing quality and, 252
   primary health care, 251–2
   and traditional lifestyle, 241
Aboriginality, 250, 254, 256
access to health care, 149–56
Adelaide Health Development and Social Capital
   Study, 197–202
alcohol consumption, 20–1, 233
allostasis, 237, 239
appropriable organisations, 93–4
area characteristics, 94–9
areas, *see* localities
attachment, 210–11
Australia/New Zealand health comparisons,
   114–28
automobile dependence, 163, 164–8figs, 167–72

Barker, D.J., 79
belonging, 65
Berkman, L.F., 91, 93
biodiversity decline, 40
biological embedding, 209
birth weight, 225–6, 226tab
   as cause of later disease, 225, 229–30, 230,
      238–9
   correlations with SES, 226–9, 227tab, 228tab,
      229tab
Björntorp, P., 239–41
body size, 4–5, 5fig, 6fig
Bourdieu, P., 191
brain development, 209–10, 211

breast cancer, 108
bulk billing, 150, 151fig

Canada, 88, 97, 261
capital stock, 8–9, 43
capitalism, 34, 36–7
cardiovascular disease, 10–11, 16, 20fig
   foetal origins, 225, 226tab
causal pathways, 75, 76fig, 80–2, 81fig
causation, 54, 292
CHD, *see* coronary heart disease
child-friendly neighbourhoods, 271–2
child mortality, 8–9, 23, 25, 26tab
child poverty, 207–8
childhood
   attachment experiences, 210–11
   developmental pathways, 209, 216–17, 275
   early brain development, 209–10, 211–12
   effect of parenting, 210–11
   influence on later health, 107, 207–14
   intervention programs, 213–14, 219–23
   maltreatment in, 210, 271
   protective processes, 217–18, 219tab, 272–3
   risk exposure, 217–18, 219tab, 220–1
   transitions, 216, 222
childhood services, 213–14
cities
   health impact, 159–63, 173, 176
   segregated land use, 162–3
   see also automobile dependence
civic participation, 193, 197–202, 199tab, 201fig
climate change, 40–1, 45
Coleman, J, 190
communities, 271–4
   see also disadvantaged communities; localities
Communities That Care, 273
community, sense of, 173, 176, 195
community action, 193, 274
community development, 274
'constitutional' susceptibility theory, 106–9